Updates in Clinical Dermatology

Series Editors:

John Berth-Jones
Chee Leok Goh
Howard I. Maibach

More information about this series at http://www.springer.com/series/13203

Prasad Kumarasinghe
Editor

Pigmentary Skin Disorders

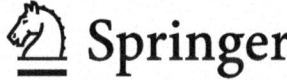 Springer

Editor
Prasad Kumarasinghe, MBBS, MD, FCCP, FAMS, FACD
Clinical Professor
Department of Dermatology
Fiona Stanley Hospital and University of Western Australia
Perth, WA, Australia

ISSN 2523-8884   ISSN 2523-8892   (electronic)
Updates in Clinical Dermatology
ISBN 978-3-030-09956-5   ISBN 978-3-319-70419-7   (eBook)
https://doi.org/10.1007/978-3-319-70419-7

Dedicated to my late parents

Preface

Pigmentary disorders have received increasing attention in the last two decades. The psychological effects of hyperpigmentation or hypopigmentation can be enormous in a given patient. The impact is not only due to the extent of the disease but also due to the individual patient's expectations and the sociocultural implications. Improving the quality of life of each individual should be a treatment goal. While arrest of the disease and reversal of the dyspigmentation are the main treatment goals, when they are not possible, camouflage also plays an important role. The psychological impact of pigmentary disorders such as vitiligo, melasma and macular pigmentation of uncertain aetiology can be severe in dark-skinned patients.

The study of melanocyte has attracted a lot of attention in the recent past. Progress in the management of advanced melanoma has been tremendous in the last few years. Dermoscopy and reflectance confocal microscopy are useful tools in diagnosis of early malignant melanomas where available. Because of greater awareness by communities with fairer skin, melanomas are diagnosed relatively early. In dark-skinned communities, due to lower prevalence and lack of awareness, melanomas are often diagnosed late, leading to poorer outcomes. It is also heartening to note that there are a lot of promising, ongoing research projects now on diseases such as vitiligo giving patients more hope for effective treatment.

This book attempts to address many important topics of skin disorders with dyspigmentation. We do not intend for this to be a textbook that covers the A–Z of all pigmentary disorders. It covers the most important hyperpigmentary and hypopigmentary disorders, discusses skin colour measuring devices and techniques such as reflectance confocal microscopy and proposes a practical, comprehensive clinical classification for pigmentary disorders. This book highlights the recent advances in the field of pigmentary disorders. We believe it will be a valuable aid to young doctors, clinical researchers, dermatology trainees and dermatologists.

The authors of the chapters are from 12 countries in many diverse regions of the world, making this truly an international effort. The contributions by the world leaders in disorders of pigmentation are outstanding. I am grateful to all the authors of the chapters and Springer staff for doing an excellent job in making this book project a success. I am also thankful to Prof Chee Leok Goh of Singapore for encouraging me to take on this task.

I hope that this book will serve as a useful reference and a valuable complement to the publications in the field of pigmentary disorders.

Perth, WA, Australia   Prasad Kumarasinghe

Contents

Contributors

Sharnika Abeyakirthi, MBBS, MD (Derm), MMedSci (Edin UK) Department of Dermatology, Panadura Base Hospital, Panadura, Sri Lanka

Ana Sofía Ayala-Cortés, MD Dermatology Department, Hospital Universitario Dr. José Eleuterio González de la Universidad Autónoma de Nuevo León, Monterrey, NL, México

Shivani Bansal, MD, DNB Kaya Skin Clinic, Preet Vihar, India

Ankit M. Bharti, MD Department of Dermatology, Seth GS Medical College & KEM Hospital, Mumbai, Maharashtra, India

Riti Bhatia, MD Department of Dermatology and Venereology, All India Institute of Medical Sciences, New Delhi, Delhi, India

Nesrine Brahimi, MD Melanoma Diagnostic Centre, Royal Prince Alfred Hospital, Sydney, NSW, Australia

Benjamin Carew, BPhty., MBBS, FRACGP, FACD Department of Medicine (Dermatology), Mater Hospital South Brisbane, Brisbane, QLD, Australia

Thiam Seng Colin Theng, MBBS, MMed, MRCP(UK), FAMS(Derm) The Skin Specialists & Medical Clinic, Mount Alvernia Medical D, Singapore, Singapore

Johannes F. Dayrit, MD Department of Dermatology, Research Institute for Tropical Medicine, Metro Manila, Philippines

Department of Internal Medicine, De La Salle Health Sciences Institute, Cavite, Philippines

Priyadarshani Galappatthy, MBBS, MD, FCCP, FRCP(Lond) Department of Pharmacology, Faculty of Medicine, University of Colombo, Colombo, Sri Lanka

Pascale Guitera, MD, PhD Department of Dermatology, Melanoma Diagnostic Centre, Royal Prince Alfred Hospital and Melanoma Institute Australia, University of Sydney, Sydney, NSW, Australia

Iltefat H. Hamzavi, MD Department of Dermatology, Henry Ford Hospital, Detroit, MI, USA

Masahiro Hayashi, MD, PhD Department of Dermatology, Yamagata University Faculty of Medicine, Yamagata, Japan

Hee Young Kang, MD, PhD Department of Dermatology, Ajou University School of Medicine, Suwon, Korea

Uday S. Khopkar, MD, DNB Department of Dermatology, Seth GS Medical College & KEM Hospital, Mumbai, Maharashtra, India

Prasad Kumarasinghe, MBBS, MD, FCCP, FAMS, FACD Department of Dermatology, Fiona Stanley Hospital and University of Western Australia, Perth, WA, Australia

Melissa Levoska, BS Department of Dermatology, Henry Ford Hospital, Detroit, MI, USA

Tasneem F. Mohammad, MD Department of Dermatology, Henry Ford Hospital, Detroit, MI, USA

James Muir, MBBS, FACD, FACRRM Department of Dermatology, Mater Hospital South Brisbane, Brisbane, QLD, Australia

Sanjeev V. Mulekar, MD National Center for Vitiligo & Psoriasis, Riyadh, Saudi Arabia

Deepani Munidasa, MBBS, MD (Derm) Department of Dermatology, Anuradhapura Teaching Hospital, Anuradhapura, Sri Lanka

Nisansala Mahenthi Nagodavithana, MBBS, MD-Dermatology Department of Dermatology, Sir Charles Gairdner Hospital, Nedlands, WA, Australia

Kyoung-Chan Park, MD, PhD Department of Dermatology, Seoul National University Bundang Hospital, Seongnam, Korea

Davinder Parsad, MD Department of Dermatology, Venereology and Leprology, Postgraduate Institute of Medical Education and Research, Chandigarh, India

M. Ramam, MD Department of Dermatology and Venereology, All India Institute of Medical Sciences, New Delhi, Delhi, India

Deepani Rathnayake, MBBS, MD, FACD Sinclair Dermatology, East Melbourne, Victoria, Australia

Muhammed Razmi T, MD, DNB Department of Dermatology, Venereology and Leprology, Postgraduate Institute of Medical Education and Research, Chandigarh, India

Germaine Nathalie Relyveld, MD, PhD Antoni van Leeuwenhoek – Netherlands Cancer Institute, Amsterdam, The Netherlands

Mauritskliniek Amsterdam, Amsterdam, The Netherlands

Bernadette Ricciardo, MBBS (Hons), DCH, FACD Department of Dermatology, Fiona Stanley Hospital, Murdoch, WA, Australia

Michelle Rodrigues, MBBS (Hons), FACD Department of Dermatology, St. Vincent's Hospital, Fitzroy, VIC, Australia

Rashmi Sarkar, MD Department of Dermatology, Maulana Azad Medical College, New Delhi, India

Gerrit Schlippe, MD, PhD Dermatest GmBH, Münster, Germany

Tamio Suzuki, MD, PhD Department of Dermatology, Yamagata University Faculty of Medicine, Yamagata, Japan

Eugene Sern-Ting Tan, MBBS, Dip Derm, DPD, FAMS(Derm) Department of Dermatology, National Skin Centre, Singapore, Singapore

A Clinical Classification of Pigmentary Disorders

Bernadette Ricciardo and Prasad Kumarasinghe

Introduction

Background

Human skin colour is determined by pigment located in the epidermis and the dermis. The most critical of these pigments is melanin, produced by the epidermal melanocytes. Haemoglobin plays a role, especially in lightly pigmented skin where slight variations in perfusion are clearly visible as erythema. Other pigments such as bilirubin and beta-carotene also play a minor role in physiological and pathological pigmentation [1]. Occasionally certain metals (e.g. iron, silver, gold), drugs and deposits of drug-melanin complexes can cause altered skin pigmentation. Areas of skin indentation can sometimes appear 'hyperpigmented' as an optical illusion, and skin overlying venous structures can appear bluish in colour due to the Tyndall effect.

Melanocytes are located in the basal layer of the epidermis, and their main function is melanin synthesis (melanogenesis). This takes place in special-

B. Ricciardo (✉)
Department of Dermatology, Fiona Stanley Hospital, Murdoch, WA, Australia
e-mail: bernadette.haak@gmail.com

P. Kumarasinghe
Department of Dermatology, Fiona Stanley Hospital and University of Western Australia, Perth, WA, Australia

ized organelles called melanosomes, with tyrosinase being the key enzyme in the melanin biosynthetic pathway. Mature melanosomes are transferred to the surrounding keratinocytes. There is on average one melanocyte for each 36 keratinocytes, this is referred to as the multicellular epidermal melanin unit [2]. The ratio of melanocytes to basal cells is 1:4 to 1:9 depending on the region of the body but irrespective of ethnic origin. It is the number and size of mature melanosomes, and not the number of melanocytes, that results in the variations in skin colour seen among different ethnicities [3, 4].

There are two main types of melanin that influence the colour of the human skin: eumelanins that are brown-black and phaeomelanins that are yellow-orange. These melanins are found in different proportions in different populations. In most of the Caucasians, the Indians and the Africans, the predominant pigment is eumelanin. In the Mongoloids and the red-headed Caucasians, the predominant pigment is phaeomelanin [5].

The main influence on melanin synthesis is genetics [6]. The inherent genetic coding expressed by the melanocyte is the most important determinant in a given person's general pigmentation. Other factors that can stimulate or inhibit skin pigmentation include exposure to UV light, hormonal influences (i.e. MSH, ACTH) and biochemical substances (e.g. melatonin, β-lipoprotein).

In different pigmentary disorders, melanin synthesis, transfer, deposition or degradation may be defective.

© Springer International Publishing AG, part of Springer Nature 2018
P. Kumarasinghe (ed.), *Pigmentary Skin Disorders*, Updates in Clinical Dermatology,
https://doi.org/10.1007/978-3-319-70419-7_1

Definitions

The pigmentary disorders include those where there is a lightening in skin colour, a darkening in skin colour, a mixed pattern of lightening and darkening in skin colour, or the development of an unusual skin colour. The vast majority of pigmentary disorders are due to quantitative or qualitative defects in the synthesis, transfer, deposition and degradation of melanin. Abnormal skin colour can also result from disturbances in both endogenous and exogenous pigments. On broad terms, changes of skin colour can be called dyschromias. However, in this chapter, we use the terms hypopigmentation, hyperpigmentation and mixed type of pigmentation (hyper- and hypopigmentation) as the main categories of pigmentary disorders.

Hypopigmentation refers to any form of reduced pigmentation, whereas hypomelanosis refers specifically to a decrease in melanin content. Hypomelanosis may be due to decreased melanin production or defective melanosome function despite a normal number of epidermal melanocytes (melanopaenic hypomelanosis), or it may be due to a decreased number of epidermal melanocytes (melanocytopenic hypomelanosis). *Depigmentation* or leukoderma describes total loss of pigmentation resulting in a whitish appearance of the lesional skin. It is almost always due to a deficiency in melanin [7].

Hyperpigmentation on the other hand refers to any form of increased pigmentation, with hypermelanosis or melanoderma specifically referring to an increase in melanin content. Epidermal melanin excess produces a brownish skin colour and may be due to increased melanin production by a quantitatively normal melanocyte density in the epidermis (melanotic hypermelanosis), or it may be due to an increased number of epidermal melanocytes (melanocytic hypermelanosis). Dermal melanin excess produces a blue-grey skin colour and may be due to production of melanin by ectopic dermal melanocytes (dermal melanocytosis) or due to an abnormal transfer of melanin from epidermal cells to the dermis (pigmentary incontinence) [8].

Abnormal skin colour may also result from disturbances in non-melanin pigments [8]. Examples of this include:

- Variations in the haemoglobin content within the skin (e.g. anaemia) or localized vascular disorders (e.g. Bier spots and naevus anaemicus) causing the skin to appear pale (hypopigmented).
- Haemosiderin deposition resulting in a red-brown discolouration, a common sequel of chronic venous insufficiency.
- Xanthoderma resulting in a yellow-orange skin discolouration and most commonly due to jaundice and carotenoderma.
- Heavy metals (e.g. iron, silver, gold) and traumatic, aesthetic or medical tattoos.
- Increased epidermal thickness leading to diffuse, patchy or reticulated light to dark brown hyperpigmentation.
- Chronic avoidance of washing inducing hyperpigmented, and often keratotic, papules and plaques (e.g. retention hyperkeratosis).
- Abnormal colouration of the sweat (i.e. chromhidrosis or pseudo-chromhidrosis).

Approaching the Patient

History

When taking a history from a patient presenting with a pigmentary disorder, it is important to determine the age of onset of the skin changes. For changes that are present from birth or develop in the first 1 to 2 years of life, the skin disorder is likely to be congenital and represent a genodermatosis, whereas pigmentation changes that develop after this time are more typically acquired, and the aetiology is more varied [1].

For pigmentary disorders presenting at any age, it is important to elicit the following information:

- Was the pigmentation preceded by injury, inflammation or pruritus?
- What was the evolution/development of the pigmentation?

Table 1.1 Acquired hyperpigmented dermatoses with prominent involvement of sun-exposed skin

Acquired brachial cutaneous dyschromatosis
Ashy dermatosis
Carcinoid syndrome
Chronic liver disease
Chronic renal insufficiency
Drug-induced hyperpigmentation – photoallergic and phototoxic drug reactions, heavy metals (including silver and gold), drugs (including amiodarone, chlorpromazine and related phenothiazines, hydroxychloroquine, minocycline, phenytoin)
Ephelides
Endocrine disorders – acromegaly, Addison's disease
Erythromelanosis follicularis faciei et colli
Erythrose peribuccale of Brocq
Haemochromatosis
Lichen planus pigmentosus
Linea fusca
Melasma
Nutritional deficiencies – vitamin B12, vitamin B3, vitamin C, folic acid
Ochronosis – alkaptonuria, exogenous ochronosis
Phytophotodermatitis
Poikiloderma of Civatte
Porphyrias – hereditary coproporphyria, porphyria cutanea tarda, porphyria variegata
Post-inflammatory hyperpigmentation – especially acne, atopic dermatitis, cutaneous lupus, dermatomyositis, infections (including chikungunya), physical or chemical injuries
Riehl's melanosis

- Is the pigmentation persistent and stable, or is it transient and intermittent?
- Is the pigmentation related to sun exposure? (Table 1.1.)
- Is the pigmentation symptomatic?
- Is there pathology involving other organs?
  - For pigmentation that develops within the first 1 to 2 years of life (i.e. congenital disorders), specifically consider musculoskeletal, cardiac, ocular, neurodevelopmental and endocrine anomalies.
  - For pigmentation that develops after the first 1 to 2 years of life (i.e. acquired disorders), specifically consider neoplastic (including melanoma), endocrine, nutritional, metabolic and autoimmune disorders.
- Is there a family history of similar pigmentation?
- Is there a history of parental consanguinity?

Table 1.2 Physiological pigmentation in skin of colour

Familial periorbital hyperpigmentation
Hyperpigmentation of the tongue
Inherited patterned lentiginosis in black people
Longitudinal melanonychia (multiple)
Pigmentary demarcation lines
Pigmentation of the gingiva
Pigmented plantar and palmar macules
Transient pigmentary lines of the newborn

- Are there any offending drugs?
- Is there a relevant occupational history (e.g. contact with phenolic substances)?
- Is there a relevant travel history (e.g. to areas endemic for treponematoses, leishmaniasis, leprosy or onchocerciasis)?
- Is there a relevant sexual health history (e.g. risk factors for syphilis or HIV/AIDS)?

Examination

Examination should begin with an assessment of the patient's normal constitutive skin colour. Some lesions are more common in certain skin types (races), e.g. ashy dermatosis and progressive macular hypomelanosis in dark-skinned races. In addition, certain skin changes are considered physiological in skin of colour (Table 1.2.).

Clinical examination can then determine whether the skin changes are hypopigmented/depigmented, hyperpigmented or mixed pigmentation (hypopigmented and hyperpigmented). The specific features of the pigmentary change must then be assessed:

- Is it generalized and diffuse (i.e. contiguous)?
  - If so, is there pigmentary dilution (hypochromia), concentration (hyperchromia) or both?
- Is it circumscribed (i.e. non-contiguous)?
  - If so,
    - Is it solitary or multiple?
      - If multiple, are they widespread or localized to a certain area of the body? For example, some hyperpigmented dermatoses have predominant flexural pigmentation (Table 1.3).

Table 1.3 Hyperpigmented dermatoses with predominant flexural pigmentation

Acanthosis nigricans
Atopic dermatitis – 'dirty neck'
Confluent and reticulated papillomatosis
Dowling-Degos disease
Dyskeratosis congenita
Flexural pigmentation with multiple lentigines
Galli-Galli disease
Granular parakeratosis
Harber's syndrome
Infections – especially erythrasma
Neurofibromatosis – Crowe's sign
Post-inflammatory hyperpigmentation – especially contact dermatitis

- What is the morphology, e.g. punctate/guttate, patchy, linear, whorled, segmental, reticulate or flagellate?
- Is it macular (i.e. flat) or associated with textural change of the skin?
- For hyperpigmented disorders, what colour is the pigmentation?
- In the setting of circumscribed hyperpigmented lesions, it is important to assess for Darier's sign, which is positive in urticaria pigmentosa and solitary mastocytoma.

It is then important to examine the patient beyond the skin to assess whether:

- The hair colour is altered (Table 1.4.).
- The nail colour is altered (Table 1.5.).
- The oral mucosa (Table 1.6.) and/or other mucosal sites are affected [9].
- The eyes are affected.
- Dysmorphic features are present.
- Other organs are involved.

If the individual lesions or the pattern of pigmentation change are atypical, the search for other features in history and a detailed systemic examination becomes very important to arrive at the correct diagnosis.

Bedside investigations can be useful and include:
- *Alcohol swabbing* [8]
  - While exogenous pigmentation, sweat discolouration and dirt pigmentation (terra

firma-forme dermatosis) can be resistant to a regular wash with soap and water, they can be removed by alcohol swabbing. In dirt pigmentation, it is typically necessary to exert substantial shearing force when alcohol swabbing.
- *Diascopy* [7, 8, 10]
  - Diascopy can be used to identify vascular disorders. Using diascopy, non-melanotic lesions such as naevus anaemicus, Bier's spots and Woronoff's ring can be made to blend into the surrounding blanched skin. In addition, these lesions do not display the reflex vasodilatory response upon application of pressure and heat.
- *Wood's lamp examination* [3, 8, 11]
  - Wood's lamp examination can be a useful adjunct when diagnosing disorders of pigmentation. Naevus anaemicus is not accentuated by Wood's lamp, in contrast to hypomelanotic causes of hypopigmentation where the lesions are enhanced. On Wood's lamp examination, vitiligo lesions typically show chalky-white accentuation. Hypermelanosis due to epidermal pigmentation is enhanced by Wood's lamp examination, whereas it remains unchanged when it is due to dermal pigmentation. In erythrasma, corynebacteria cause a pigmented rash in skin folds that fluoresces a coral-pink colour with Wood's lamp examination. The slightly scaly hypo- or hyperpigmented rash seen over the torso in pityriasis versicolour typically emits a yellow-green glow when active. Patients with progressive macular hypomelanosis show small specs of red fluorescence in a follicular pattern inside the hypopigmented lesional skin when examined under Wood's lamp.
- *Skin scrapings and potassium hydroxide examination*
  - Under a microscope 'spaghetti- and meatball-like' structures (representing mycelia and oval yeasts, respectively) may be seen in pityriasis versicolour. In tinea nigra light to dark brown septal hyphae are typically observed.

Table 1.4 Disorders with altered hair colour

Hypopigmented/depigmented		Hyperpigmented	Other colours
Circumscribed	Diffuse		

Inherited
  Isolated occipital
  white lock
  Isolated white
  forelock
  Piebaldism
  Tuberous sclerosis
  Waardenburg
  syndrome
  White forelock with
  multiple
  malformations
  White forelock with
  osteopathia striata
Naevoid
  Angora hair naevus
  Associated with
  naevus comedonicus
  Scalp heterochromia
  secondary to
  mosaicism
Inflammatory or
autoimmune
  Alezzandrini
  syndrome
  Alopecia areata
  Halo naevus
  Post-inflammatory
  (i.e. discoid lupus)
  Post-traumatic
  Vitiligo
  Vogt-Koyanagi-
  Harada syndrome
	Inherited
	  Book syndrome
	  Down syndrome
	  Fanconi syndrome
	  Hallermann-Streiff
	  syndrome
	  Prolidase deficiency
	  Treacher-Collins
	  syndrome
	Drugs
	  Antimalarials
	  Tyrosine kinase
	  inhibitors
	Nutritional/endocrine
	  Chronic protein loss or
	  deficiency ('flag sign')
	  Copper deficiency
	  Hyperthyroidism
	  Vitamin B12 deficiency
		Metabolic
		  Porphyria cutanea tarda
		Drugs
		  Dithranol (topical)
		  Methotrexate
		  Prostaglandin
		  analogues, e.g.
		  latanoprost (topical)
			Silvery hair syndromes
			  Chediak-Higashi
			  syndrome
			  Elejalde syndrome
			  Griscelli syndrome
			  Oculocerebral
			  hypopigmentation
			  syndrome, Cross type
			Premature greying
			Inherited
			  Ataxia telangiectasia
			  "Bird-headed" dwarfism
			  Fisch syndrome
			  Hereditary premature
			  canities
			  Oasthouse disease
			  Piebaldism
			  Progeria
			  Prolidase deficiency
			  Rothmund-Thomson
			  syndrome
			  Waardenburg syndrome
			  Werner syndrome
			Inflammatory or
			autoimmune
			  Sudden whitening of hair
			  (alopecia areata)
			  Myotonic dystrophy
			  Vitiligo
			Green
			Exogenous copper
			deposition

Investigations

Investigations are dependent on the diagnosis suspected.

In congenital pigmentary disorders, karyotyping and molecular genetic analysis of the skin and blood may be considered, especially when the child has associated developmental delay or structural abnormalities.

Laboratory investigations may include nutritional, autoimmune, infectious, endocrine, renal, hepatic and haematologic screens.

Quantitative spectrophotometric skin colour measurements are not required for clinical diagnosis, but it is useful for monitoring and comparing improvement of various forms of treatments (refer to Chap. 3: Measurements of Skin Color).

Skin biopsy for histopathology can be a useful investigation in some, but not all disorders of pigmentation. In hypopigmented disorders, histology is most important in acquired conditions where inflammation, infection (e.g. tuberculoid leprosy), sarcoidosis, clear cell papulosis, dyschromic amyloidosis or mycosis fungoides are suspected. In hyperpigmented disorders, melanophages in the dermis suggest post-inflammatory hyperpigmentation or a lichenoid reaction pattern (which can be due to numerous causes), melanocytes in the dermis suggest conditions such as Mongolian blue spot or Hori's naevus, and deeper naevoid cells suggest a lesion such as a blue naevus. In cases where an inflammatory cause is suspected, biopsies should be taken from an advancing edge of the lesion as well as an older lesion. In disorders with

Table 1.5 Disorders with altered nail colour

Hypopigmented/depigmented	Hyperpigmented	Other colours

True leukonychia
  Completely white (leukonychia totalis)
    Acquired: cirrhosis, cytotoxic drugs, infection (typhoid, leprosy, trichinosis), onychophagia
    Hereditary: associated with cheilitis, dental changes, keratosis pilaris, knuckle pads, hypoparathyroidism, koilonychia, LEOPARD syndrome, palmoplantar keratoderma, peeling skin, pilar cysts, pili torti, sebaceous cysts, sensorineural deafness, renal calculi
  Incompletely white (leukonychia partialis, striata, punctata)
    Acquired: chronic arsenic poisoning (Mee's lines), trauma
    Hereditary: Darier-White disease
Apparent leukonychia
  Hepatic failure, cirrhosis, diabetes mellitus, CHF, hyperthyroidism, malnutrition (Terry's nails)
  Hypoalbuminaemia (Muehrcke's nails)
  Onycholysis
  Renal failure (half and half nails)
Pseudoleukonychia
  Fungal nail infection – dermatophyte and yeast
  Trauma
	Longitudinal melanonychia
	  Physiologic causes: racial, pregnancy
	  Local or regional causes: trauma, onychotillomania, onychophagia, carpel tunnel syndrome, subungual foreign body, radiation, fungi, bacteria, neoplasm
	  Dermatologic causes: onychomycosis, chronic paronychia, psoriasis, lichen planus, lichen striatus, amyloidosis, chronic radiation, systemic lupus erythematosus, localized scleroderma, Bowen's disease, onychomatricoma, myxoid pseudocyst, basal cell carcinoma, subungual fibrous histiocytoma, periungual verruca, subungual linear keratosis
	  Systemic causes: Addison's disease, Cushing's syndrome, Nelson's syndrome, hyperthyroidism, acromegaly, alkaptonuria, nutritional disorders, haemosiderosis, porphyria, hyperbilirubinaemia, graft versus host disease, AIDS
	  Syndromes: Laugier-Hunziker, Peutz-Jeghers, Touraine
	  Melanocytic hyperplasia: lentigo, naevus, melanoma
	Transverse melanonychia
	  Drugs (especially chemotherapeutics)
	  Phototherapy
	  Radiation
	Diffuse melanonychia
	  Drugs (especially chemotherapeutics)
		Splinter haemorrhage
		  Antiphospholipid syndrome
		  Peptic ulcer disease
		  Malignancies
		  Oral contraceptive use
		  Psoriasis
		  Pregnancy
		  Rheumatoid arthritis
		  Systemic lupus erythematosus
		  Subacute bacterial endocarditis
		  Trauma
		Greenish-black nails
		  Pseudomonas aeruginosa
		Yellow nail
		  Chronic use of nail enamel
		  Yellow nail syndrome
		Exogenous pigmentation
		  Food colourings
		  Industrial chemicals
		  Nail lacquers
		  Topical medications (e.g. potassium permanganate)
		Abnormal lunula Colour
		  Blue/azure – Wilson disease, silver poisoning, bacterial paronychia, quinacrine, zidovudine
		  Blue, pale – diabetes mellitus
		  Brown black – excessive fluoride ingestion
		  Red – heart failure, chronic obstructive pulmonary disease, collagen vascular disease, haematologic malignancy
		  Yellow – tetracycline

Table 1.6 Disorders with altered mucosal colour

Hypopigmented/depigmented	Hyperpigmented
Aphthous ulceration	Congenital melanotic macules of the tongue
Chronic mucocutaneous candidiasis	Dowling-Degos disease
Contact stomatitis – e.g. cinnamon	Drugs – especially chemotherapeutics
Dyskeratosis congenita	Endocrinopathies – e.g. Addisons disease
Darier-White disease	Exogenous material – e.g. tattoos
Howel-Evans syndrome	Familial lentiginoses – e.g. Peutz-Jeghers, Carney
Morsicatio buccarum (chronic cheek chewing)	complex
Neoplasic – oral leucoplakia, SCC, verrucous carcinoma	Haemochromatosis
Nicotine stomatitis	Hairy tongue
Oral submucous fibrosis	Heavy metal poisoning – e.g. argyria
Pachyonychia congenita (leucokeratosis)	Hyperpigmentation of the tongue/gingiva (racial)
Post-inflammatory hypopigmentation	Laugier-Hunziker syndrome
Systemic sclerosis	Lentigines
Vitiligo	Mucosal melanotic macules
White sponge nevus	Neoplastic – melanocytic naevus, melanoma
	Post-inflammatory hyperpigmentation: lichen planus, fixed drug eruption
	Smoker's melanosis
	Vascular anomalies – e.g. haemangioma, purpura

Table 1.7 Pigmentary disorders where histopathology is helpful in the diagnosis

Hypopigmented dermatoses	Hyperpigmented dermatoses
Amyloidosis dyschromia cutis	Acanthosis nigricans
Chronic arsenic poisoning	Blue naevus
Clear cell papulosis	Chronic arsenic poisoning
Connective tissue naevi	Colloid milium
Darier-White disease-associated hypopigmented macules	Congenital melanocytic naevus
	Dermatomyositis
Epidermal naevus	Dermatosis papulosa nigra
Epidermodysplasia verruciformis-associated pityriasis versicolor-like lesions	Dowling-Degos disease
	Flexural pigmentation with multiple lentigines
Grover disease-associated hypopigmented macules	Galli-Galli disease
	Granular parakeratosis
Halo naevi	Hori's naevus
Leprosy – tuberculoid, borderline tuberculoid	Lentigo maligna
Lichen sclerosus et atrophicus	Lichen planus pigmentosus
Lichen striatus	Lichenoid drug eruption
Microcystic lymphatic malformation	Maculopapular cutaneous mastocytosis
Molluscum contagiosum	Melanoacanthoma/seborrhoeic keratosis
Morphea	Ochronosis – exogenous
Mucinoses	Pigmented purpuric dermatosis (capillaritis)
Mycosis fungoides	Pityriasis versicolour
Pityriasis versicolour	Porphyria cutanea tarda
Plane warts	Primary cutaneous amyloidosis – macular / lichenoid
Post-kala-azar dermal leishmaniasis	Siderosis (e.g. due to extravasated iron)
Sarcoidosis	Talon noir
Vitiligo	Tattoos – accidental (e.g. carbon)
White fibrous papulosis	Tinea nigra

patchy pigmentation change, a biopsy from a comparable area of normal skin is helpful to evaluate subtle changes in pigmentation. Special stains are useful in establishing the diagnosis in some cases, e.g. clear cell papulosis. Table 1.7 provides a list of pigmentary disorders where histopathology becomes helpful in the diagnosis.

Classification of Pigmentary Disorders

There are several ways that pigmentary disorders can be classified, including pathological, aetiological and clinical.

A comprehensive pathological classification based on structural and ultrastructural details is not yet possible due to non-availability of comparable histopathological, immunohistochemical and electron microscopic data of many conditions. Basic light microscopic histopathological features alone are not diagnostic of many pigmentary disorders.

A classification based on aetiology is also difficult as often times the aetiology is unknown. When the genetic cause of a pigmentary disorder is known, the disease may be categorized on a genetic basis. In the Online Mendelian Inheritance of Man (OMIM), each disease is given a six-digit code. [12]

Where exact aetiology is unknown, and the pathology is non-specific, a clinical classification based on clinical features is useful to the clinician. [13]

The classification presented in this discussion is based on clinical features. There are several classifications in journal articles and textbooks; however, many articles are not comprehensive, focusing only on the common conditions. [1, 6, 13–15]

Here, an attempt has been made to include most known disorders that are hypopigmented/depigmented, hyperpigmented and mixed pigmentation (hypopigmented and hyperpigmented). Not only pigmentation due to melanin, but also other agents causing a 'hyperpigmented appearance' (hyperchromia), are included for a clear understanding of the numerous anomalies that afflict human skin and result in discolouration of the skin (dyschromia).

When classified by clinical features, some diseases may be listed more than once as the clinical appearance can vary in different skin types and depending on the stage of evolution/resolution of the skin disorder.

There are certain skin disorders that have been only minimally included in this classification. This includes the ichthyotic disorders, as although the scale is often dyschromic in the ichthyotic disorders the primary clinical feature is scale. Likewise, we have elected to exclude a number of skin neoplasms that display (secondary) pigmentary change. However, for completeness, these disorders have been tabulated (Table 1.8). [16]

As the main thrust of this classification is clinical, we first divide the pigmentary disorders in to whether the lesions are (Fig. 1.1):

- *Hypopigmented/depigmented*
- *Hyperpigmented*
- *Mixed pigmentation (hypopigmented and hyperpigmented)*

Each primary division is then broken down into whether the lesions have their:

- *Onset in early childhood*
  - This includes disorders that are either present at birth or develop in the first 1 to 2 years of life. The vast majority of these disorders have a genetic aetiology.
- *Onset in later childhood through to adulthood*
  - This includes disorders that typically present after the first 1 to 2 years of life. Most of these are acquired in origin; however some are genetically determined disorders manifesting many years after birth.

Within these categories, we group the pigmentary disorders on the nature of distribution and whether the skin changes are (Figs 1.2 and 1.3):

- *Generalized and diffuse (contiguous)*
  - This refers to pigmentary disorders that affect the entire skin surface confluently.
  - It includes disorders of pigmentary dilution (e.g. oculocutaneous albinism) and pig-

Table 1.8 Neoplasms with pigmentary changes or discolouration

Hypopigmented neoplastic conditions	Hyperpigmented neoplastic conditions
Arsenical keratoses and associated neoplasms with rain drop depigmentation Halo naevi Melanoma with regression and associated leucoderma Microcystic lymphatic malformation Mycosis fungoides – hypopigmented Porokeratosis Stucco keratosis White fibrous papulosis White sponge naevus of oral mucosa Sebaceoma Xanthomas	Acrochordons Actinic keratosis – pigmented variant Angiokeratoma Basal cell carcinoma – pigmented variant Bowenoid papulosis Chloroma/cutaneous myeloid sarcoma Dermatofibroma Dermatosis papulosa nigra Glomus tumour Haemangioma – deep Kaposi's sarcoma Lymphomatoid papulosis Malignant melanoma, lentigo maligna, melanosis secondary to advanced melanoma Mastocytoma Melanoacanthoma Melanocytic naevus Merkel cell carcinoma (can appear purplish or reddish in colour) Mycosis fungoides – pigmented variant Neurofibroma Paget's disease – pigmented variant Pilomatricoma (bluish in colour) Squamous cell carcinoma – pigmented variant Seborrhoeic keratosis Syringomas (in dark-skinned persons) Tumours with rapid growth and internal haemorrhage

Modified from Kumarasinghe and Hewitt [17]

mentary concentration (e.g. melanosis diffusa congenita).

  - These disorders tend to be macular, without significant infiltration or epidermal change.
  - Within this group there may be accentuation of pigmentation in certain areas, e.g. more prominent pigmentation in the skin creases in Addison's disease.
  - This category is variably grouped according to *aetiology* or *associated extracutaneous signs/organ involvement*.
- *Circumscribed (non-contiguous)*
  - This refers to pigmentary disorders that do not affect the entire skin surface.

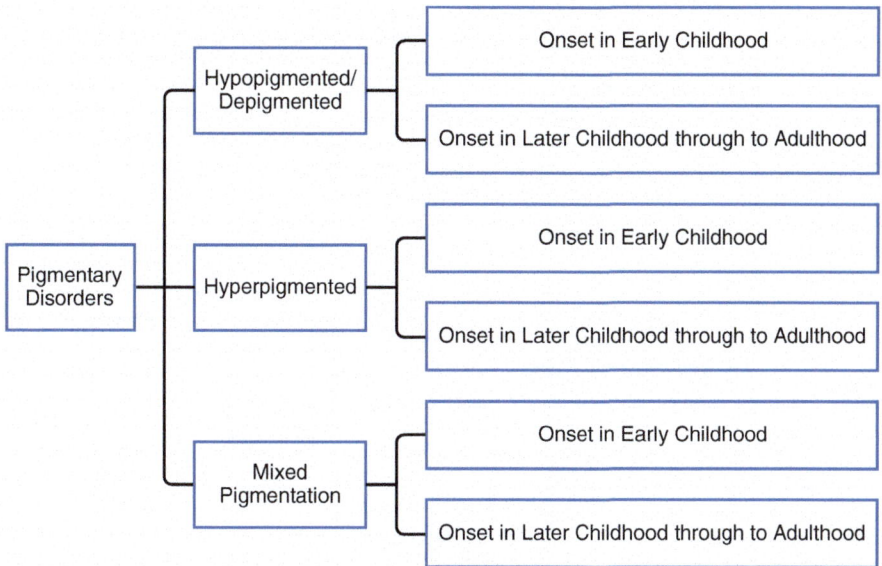

Fig. 1.1 Onset in Later Childhood though to Adulthood Clinical classification of pigmentary disorders

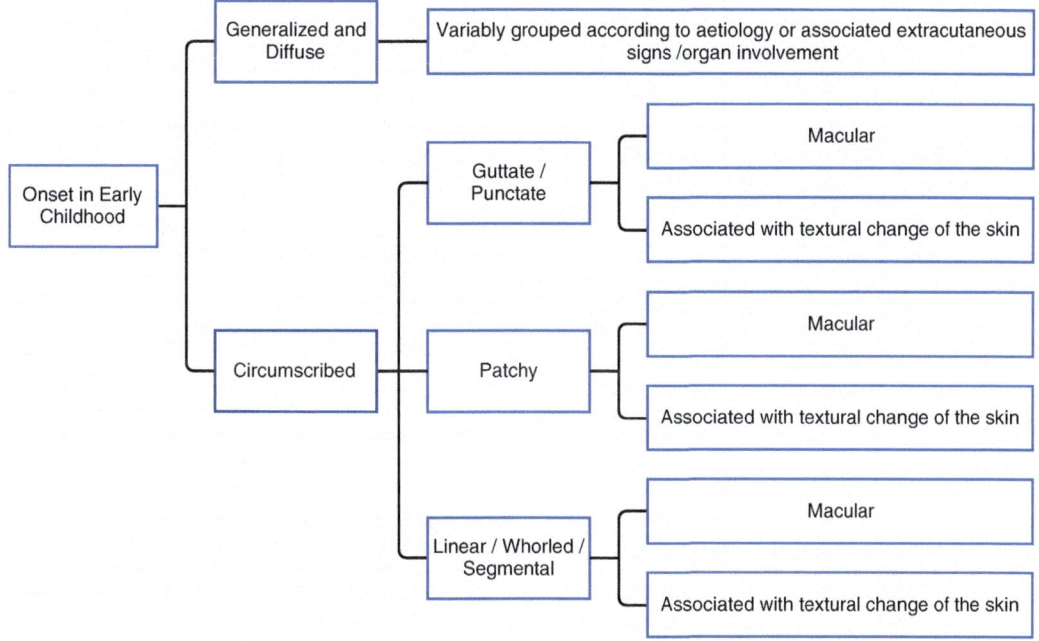

Fig. 1.2 Clinical classification of pigmentary disorders continued from Fig. 1.1

– The individual lesions are well demarcated.
– These circumscribed lesions can be widespread or localized to certain areas.
– Different morphological patterns of pigmentation are seen in circumscribed pigmentary disorders including:

- *Guttate/punctate*: < 1cm in diameter.
- *Patchy*: ≥1cm in diameter.
- *Linear/whorled/segmental*: including blaschkoid, zosteriform and flagellate pigmentation.

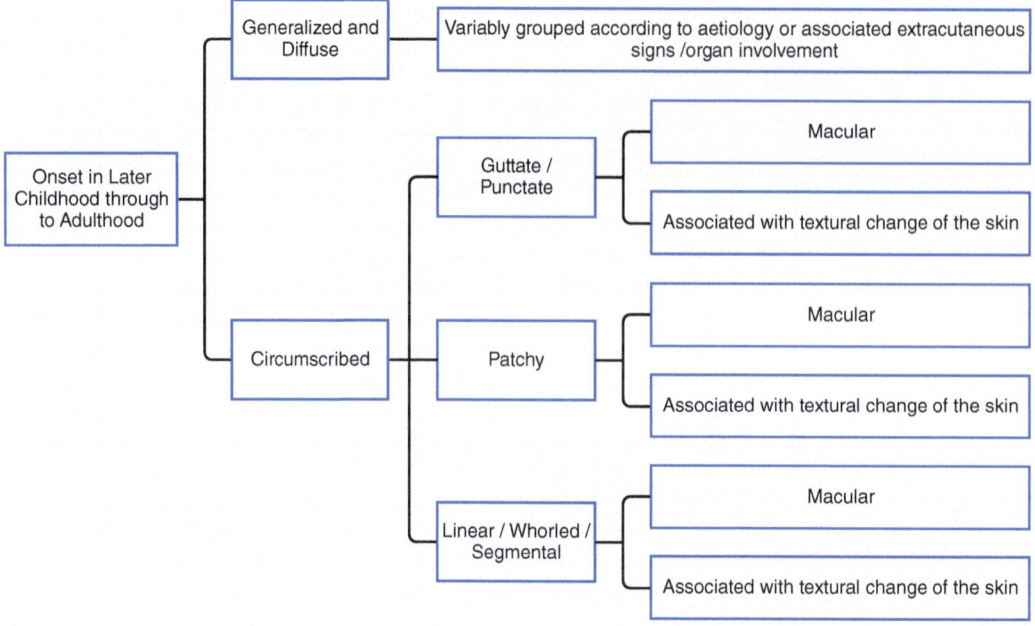

Fig. 1.3 Clinical classification of pigmentary disorders continued from Fig. 1.1

– These patterns of pigmentation can then be further categorized based on whether they are:
  • *Macular*: flat with no associated textural change of the skin.
  • *Associated with textural change of the skin*: including papular change/infiltration, epidermal atrophy, skin induration and scale.

Finally, in the hyperpigmented and mixed pigmentation groups, we variably group the circumscribed lesions into subcategories based on further clinical features including:

• *Reticulate* – this includes skin disorders showing hyperpigmented and/or hypopigmented macules leading to a blotchy appearance, as well as skin disorders characterized by a lacy or net-like pattern of hyperpigmentation. [16, 18]
• *Flagellate* – figurate dermatoses characterized by a parallel linear or curvilinear arrangement simulating the marks of whiplashes.
• *Grey-blue hypermelanosis* (*dermal hypermelanosis, ceruloderma*) – skin disorders characterized by collections of dermal melanocytes and clinically appearing as grey-blue lesions.

• *Red-brown hypermelanosis* (*haemosiderosis*) – skin disorders characterized by haemosiderin or iron deposition in the dermis resulting in a red-brown discolouration of the skin.
• *Poikiloderma* – skin disorders characterized by hypopigmentation, hyperpigmentation, telangiectasia and skin atrophy.

Key	
☉	Dermatoses that are more common/conspicuous in skin of colour
*	Non-melanin pigmentation

Hypopigmented/Depigmented

Onset in Early Childhood [3, 7, 12, 15, 19, 20]

Generalized and Diffuse Hypopigmentary Disorders (Pigment Dilution/Hypochromia)

Affecting Eyes, Skin and Hair
  In isolation
• Oculocutaneous albinism, types IA, IB, II-VII [OMIM # 203100, 606952, 203200, 203290, 606574, 615312, 113750, 615179]

- Histidinaemia (*syn. histidine ammonia-lyase deficiency*) [OMIM #235800]

Associated with bleeding diathesis
- Hermansky-Pudlak syndrome, types 1–10 [OMIM # 203300, 608233, 606118, 606682, 607521, 607522, 614076, 614077, 614171, 617050]

Associated with deafness
- ABCD syndrome (*syn. albinism, black lock, cell migration disorder of the neurocytes of the gut and deafness*) [OMIM #600501]
- Tietze syndrome (*syn. albinism-deafness of Tietze*) [OMIM #103500]

Associated with immunological disease
- Chediak-Higashi syndrome [OMIM #214500]

Associated with neurological disease and/or intellectual disability
- Angelman syndrome [OMIM #105830]
- Homocystinuria (*syn. methylenetetrahydrofolate reductase deficiency*) [OMIM #236200]
- Infantile nephropathic cystinosis [OMIM #219800]
- Oculocerebral hypopigmentation syndrome of Preus [OMIM #257790]
- Oculocerebral syndrome with hypopigmentation (*syn. Cross syndrome, Kramer syndrome*) [OMIM #257800]
- Phenylketonuria (*syn. phenylalanine hydroxylase deficiency*) [OMIM #261600]
- Prader-Willi syndrome [OMIM #176270]

Affecting the Skin and Hair
In isolation
- Griscelli syndrome, type 3 [OMIM #609227]

Associated with cardiorespiratory disease
- Selenium deficiency (e.g. due to total parenteral nutrition)

Associated with defects in other ectodermal structures
- Ectodermal dysplasias (including Hypohidrotic ectodermal dysplasia and Ectrodactyly ectodermal dysplasia)

Associated with immunological disease
- Griscelli syndrome, type 2 [OMIM #607624]

Associated with neurological disease and/or intellectual disability
- Copper deficiency (e.g. in premature or severely malnourished infants)
- Elejalde disease (*syn. neuroectodermal melanolysosomal disease*) [OMIM #256710]
- Griscelli syndrome, type 1 [OMIM #214450]
- Menkes disease (*syn. kinky hair disease, steely hair disease*) [OMIM #309400]

Affecting the Skin
Endocrinopathies
- Hypogonadism
- Hypothyroidism *
- Hypopituitarism
- Pernicious anaemia (B12 deficiency)

Variations in the haemoglobin content and vascular disorders
- Anaemia *
- Cutaneous oedema *
- Vasoconstriction *

Metabolic
- Infantile sialic acid storage disease [OMIM #269920]

Nutritional
- Protein-energy malnutrition – marasmus and kwashiorkor ⊙

Circumscribed Hypopigmentary Disorders

Depigmented
Guttate/punctate
- Vitiligo ponctue

Patchy
- *In isolation*
  - Piebald trait (*syn. piebaldism*) [OMIM #172800]
  - Vitiligo
- *Associated with deafness*
  - Albinism-deafness syndrome (*syn. Ziprkowski-Margolis Syndrome; Woolf syndrome*) [OMIM #300700]

– Ermine phenotype (*syn. Pigmentary Disorder with Hearing Loss*) (includes Black locks with albinism and deafness syndrome, BADS) [OMIM #227010]
– Waardenburg syndrome, types 1, 2a–2e, 3 and 4a–4c [OMIM #193500, 193510, 600193, 606662, 608890, 148820, 277580, 613265, 613266]
• *Associated with neurological disease and/or intellectual disability*
– Piebald trait with neurologic defects [OMIM #172850]

Linear/whorled/segmental
• Vitiligo: segmental, blaschkoid and koebnerized

Hypopigmented
Guttate/punctate
• *Macular*
– Cole disease (*syn. guttate hypopigmentation and punctate palmoplantar keratoderma*) [OMIM #615522]
– Post-inflammatory hypopigmentation° – especially herpes virus infection (HSV, VZV) and guttate psoriasis
– Tuberous sclerosis, types 1 and 2: confetti-like hypomelanotic macules [OMIM #191100, 613254]
• *Associated with textural change of the skin*
– Clear cell papulosis of the skin *
– Cutaneous papular mucinosis of infancy *
– Infection – especially molluscum contagiosum*, plane warts* and pityriasis versicolour
– Microcystic lymphatic malformation (*syn. lymphangioma circumscriptum*)
– Mucopolysaccharidosis, type 2: ivory-white reticulate pebbling (*syn. Hunter syndrome*) [OMIM #309900] *

Patchy
• *Macular*
– Naevus depigmentosus (*syn. achromic naevus, hypopigmented naevus*):
  • Isolated naevus depigmentosus
  • Systematized naevus depigmentosus

• Naevus depigmentosus-associated syndromes:
– Ataxia telangiectasia [OMIM #208900]
– Capillary malformations arteriovenous malformations (CM-AVMs): hypoemic halos [OMIM #608354]
– Fanconi anaemia [OMIM #227650]
– Neurofibromatosis, type 1: oval spots [OMIM #162200]
– Phakomatosis pigmentovascularis, type I
– Proteus syndrome [OMIM #176920]
– Trisomy 13 – phylloid hypomelanosis
– Tuberous sclerosis, types 1 and 2: ash-leaf and polygonal macules [OMIM #191100, 613254]
– Naevus anaemicus *
  • Isolated naevus anaemicus
  • Naevus anaemicus-associated syndromes * –
– Neurofibromatosis, type 1 [OMIM #162200]
– Phakomatosis pigmentovascularis, types II, III and IV
– Post-inflammatory hypopigmentation° – especially eczema (including molluscum contagiosum-associated perilesional eczema), neonatal lupus erythematosus, pityriasis alba and psoriasis
• *Associated with textural change of the skin*
– Apert syndrome: hypopigmentation and hyperkeratosis of plantar surfaces [OMIM #101200]
– Infection – especially pityriasis versicolour and leprosy

Linear/whorled/segmental

• *Macular*
– Hypomelanosis of Ito [OMIM #300337]
– Linear and figurated hypopigmented naevus (*syn. linear and whorled naevoid hypomelanosis*)
– Menkes disease – female carrier (*syn. kinky hair disease, steely hair disease*) [OMIM #309400]

- Naevus depigmentosus (*syn. achromic naevus, hypopigmented naevus*) – linear, blaschkoid or segmental
- Pigmentary demarcation lines
- Post-inflammatory hypopigmentation[⊙] – especially herpes zoster infection, lichen striatus
- *Associated with textural change of the skin*
  - Conradi-Hunermann-Happle syndrome: atrophoderma vermiculatum following Blaschko's lines (*syn. X-linked dominant chondrodysplasia punctata*) [OMIM #302960] [*]
  - Epidermal naevus/comedonal naevus [*]
  - Focal dermal hypoplasia (*syn. Goltz syndrome*) [OMIM #305600]
  - Microphthalmia with linear skin defect syndrome (*syn. MIDAS syndrome – microphthalmia, dermal aplasia, sclerocornea*) [OMIM #309801] [*]
  - Lichen striatus (in darker skin types) [*⊙]
  - Infection – especially plane warts (koebnerized)[*]

Onset in Later Childhood Through to Adulthood [3, 7, 10–16, 19–22]

Generalized and Diffuse Hypopigmentary Disorders (Pigment Dilution/Hypochromia)

Depigmented
- Drug-induced depigmentation
  - Programmed death-1 (PD-1) inhibitors in patients with metastatic melanoma (pembrolizumab) [21]
- Vitiligo universalis

Hypopigmented
  Endocrinopathies
- Hypogonadism (e.g. in castrated human males)
- Hypothyroidism [*]
- Hypopituitarism
- Pernicious anaemia (B12 deficiency)

Variations in the haemoglobin content and vascular disorders
- Anaemia [*]
- Cutaneous oedema [*]
- Vasoconstriction [*]

Iatrogenic
- Drug-induced hypopigmentation
  - Glutathione – topical and oral [22]
  - Tyrosine kinase inhibitors (dasatinib, imatinib, gefitinib, nilotinib, pazopanib, sorafenib, sunitinib)
- Haemodialysis

Nutritional
- Copper deficiency
- Kwashiorkor
- Selenium deficiency (e.g. due to total parenteral nutrition)

Circumscribed Hypopigmentary Disorders

Depigmented
  Guttate/punctate
- Chemical leucoderma: confetti-like macules – phenol/catechol derivatives (especially monobenzyl ether of hydroquinone and hydroquinone), sulfhydryls, other (mercury, arsenic, cinnamic aldehyde, paraphenylenediamine)
- Halo naevi
- Leukoderma punctata (e.g. following PUVA, nbUVB and laser)
- Symmetrical progressive leukopathy
- Vitiligo ponctue

  Patchy
- Alezzandrini syndrome
- Chemical leukoderma – phenol/catechol derivatives (especially monobenzyl ether of hydroquinone and hydroquinone), sulfhydryls, mercury, arsenic, cinnamic aldehyde, paraphenylenediamine
- Drug-induced depigmentation

- Anti-neoplastic agents (doxorubicin, interferon-α, interferon-β, interleukin-2, survivin inhibitor)
- Programmed death-1 (PD-1) inhibitors in patients with metastatic melanoma (pembrolizumab, ipilimumab, nivolumab) [21]
- Topical/intralesional agents (azelaic acid, benzoyl peroxide, corticosteroids, 5-fluouracil, hydroquinone, imiquimod, tretinoin)
- Melanoma-associated leukoderma
- Vitiligo
- Vogt-Koyanagi-Harada disease

Linear/whorled/segmental

- Intralesional injection of corticosteroids: white line along lymphatic drainage
- Vitiligo: koebnerized, blaschkoid or segmental

Hypopigmented
Guttate/punctate
- *Macular*
  - Amyloidosis dyschromica cutis
  - Bier's spots *
  - Darier-White disease: hypopigmented macules (*syn. Darier disease, keratosis follicularis*) [OMIM #124200]
  - Epidermodysplasia verruciformis: pityriasis versicolour-like lesions *
  - Grover disease: hypopigmented macules (*syn. transient acantholytic dermatosis*)
  - Idiopathic guttate hypomelanosis
  - Multiple endocrine neoplasia, type 1 (MEN1): confetti-like macules [OMIM #131100]
  - Post-inflammatory hypopigmentation° – especially acne vulgaris and acne excoriee, cutaneous infections, lichen planus, physical or chemical injuries, pityriasis rosea, pityriasis lichenoides chronica, (guttate) psoriasis
  - Sarcoidosis: hypopigmented variant
- *Associated with textural change of the skin*
  - Clear cell papulosis of the skin *
  - Infection – especially molluscum contagiosum*, plane warts*, pityriasis versicolour and onchocerciasis

- Lichen sclerosus et atrophicus: guttate lesions
- Morphea: guttate lesions
- Mucinoses – follicular mucinosis (*alopecia mucinosa*) or papular mucinosis (*lichen myxoedematosus*) *
- Mycosis fungoides: hypopigmented variant°
- Sarcoidosis: hypopigmented variant
- White fibrous papulosis

Patchy
- *Macular*
  - Drug-induced depigmentation – topical agents including azelaic acid, benzoyl peroxide, corticosteroids (topical, intralesional), 5-fluouracil, glutathione, imiquimod and tretinoin
  - Endocrine disorders – especially Addison's disease and thyroid disease (more typically cause hyperpigmentation)
  - Infection – especially pityriasis versicolour following treatment, late-stage pinta and pintoid dyschromia of yaws
  - Multiple endocrine neoplasia, type 1 (MEN1) [OMIM #131100]
  - Pityriasis rotunda (hypopigmented in patients with darker skin)
  - Post-inflammatory hypopigmentation° – especially acne vulgaris and acne excoriee, atopic dermatitis, cutaneous lupus, dermatomyositis, drug reactions, infections, immunobullous diseases, lichen planus, lymphomatoid papulosis, mycosis fungoides, pityriasis alba, pityriasis lichenoides chronica, pityriasis rosea, physical or chemical injuries and psoriasis
  - Progressive macular hypomelanosis
  - Sarcoidosis: hypopigmented variant
  - Woronoff's ring *
- *Associated with textural change of the skin*
  - Infection – especially pityriasis versicolour, leprosy, post-kala-azar dermal leishmaniasis (PKDL), onchocerciasis, secondary syphilis and pinta
  - Lichen sclerosus et atrophicus: plaque lesions

- Morphea: plaque lesions
- Mucinoses – follicular mucinosis (*alopecia mucinosa*) or papular mucinosis (*lichen myxoedematosus*)*
- Mycosis fungoides: hypopigmented variant°
- Sarcoidosis: hypopigmented variant
- Systemic sclerosis

Linear/whorled/segmental

- *Macular*
  - Intralesional injection of corticosteroids: white line along lymphatic drainage
  - Pigmentary demarcation lines
  - Post-inflammatory hypopigmentation° – especially herpes zoster infection, lichen striatus
- *Associated with textural change of the skin*
  - Darier-White disease: linear variant (*syn. Darier disease, keratosis follicularis*) [OMIM #124200]
  - Incontinentia pigmenti – Stage 4 (*syn. Bloch-Sulzberger syndrome*) [OMIM #308300]
  - Infection – especially plane warts (koebnerized)*
  - Lichen sclerosus et atrophicus: linear variant
  - Linear unilateral basaloid follicular hamartoma
  - Morphea: linear lesions, en coup de sabre and segmental
  - Striae distensae

Hyperpigmented

Onset in Early Childhood [3, 12, 18–20, 23–28]

Generalized and Diffuse Hyperpigmentary Disorders (Pigment Concentration/Hyperchromia)

- Cardiofaciocutaneous syndrome [OMIM #115150]
- Costello syndrome (*syn. faciocutaneoskeletal syndrome*) [OMIM #218040]

- Familial progressive hyperpigmentation [OMIM #614233]
- Fanconi anaemia: melanoderma [OMIM #227650]
- Folic acid deficiency (seen in infants on exclusive goats milk)
- Gaucher disease, types 1–3 [OMIM #230800, 230900, 231000]
- Gastrointestinal stromal tumour (*syn. GIST*) [OMIM #60674] [25]
- Grey baby syndrome (following chloramphenicol exposure in neonates)
- Ichthyosis-associated (e.g. ichthyosis vulgaris, X-linked ichthyosis, autosomal recessive congenital ichthyosis, bullous ichthyosiform erythroderma)
- Universal acquired melanosis (*syn. carbon baby syndrome*)
- Vitamin B12 deficiency (due to decreased levels of B12 in maternal milk or malnutrition in infancy)

Circumscribed Hyperpigmentary Disorders

Guttate/punctate

- *Macular*
  - Bannayan-Riley-Ruvalcaba syndrome: penile lentiginosis [OMIM #153480]
  - Carney complex (*syn. NAME syndrome, LAMB syndrome*) [OMIM #160980]
  - Centrofacial lentigines (*syn. centrofacial neurodysraphic lentiginosis*)
  - Congenital melanocytic naevi – small
  - Flexural pigmentation with multiple lentigines [26]
  - Gastrointestinal stromal tumour (*syn. GIST*) [OMIM #60674] [25]
  - Isolated generalized lentigines (*syn. diffuse non-syndrome lentiginosis*)
  - Inherited patterned lentiginosis in black people °
  - Lentigo simplex
  - LEOPARD syndrome, types 1–3 (*syn. multiple lentigines syndrome*) [OMIM #151100, 611554, 613707]
  - Peutz-Jeghers syndrome (*syn. periorificial lentiginosis*) [OMIM #175200]

- Segmental lentiginosis (*syn. lentiginous naevus, partial unilateral lentiginosis, agminated lentigines, lentiginous mosaicism*)
- Transient neonatal pustular melanosis (*syn. lentigines neonatorum*) ⊙
- Xeroderma pigmentosum, groups A-G [OMIM #278700, 610651, 278720, 278730, 278740, 278760, 278780]
- *Associated with textural change of the skin*
  - Cardiofaciocutaneous syndrome: multiple pigmented naevi [OMIM #115150]
  - Congenital melanocytic naevi – small
  - Turner syndrome: multiple pigmented naevi

Patchy

- *Macular*
  - Acromelanosis progressiva
  - Bronze baby syndrome (following phototherapy)
  - Café-au-lait macules (CALM)
    - Isolated CALM
    - CALM-associated syndromes
      - Ataxia telangiectasia [OMIM #208900]
      - Bloom syndrome [OMIM #210900]
      - Familial progressive hyperpigmentation with or without hypopigmentation (*syn. FPHH; melanosis universalis hereditaria*) [OMIM #145250]
      - Fanconi anaemia [OMIM #227650]
      - Gastrointestinal stromal tumour (*syn. GIST*) [OMIM #60674] [25]
      - Legius syndrome (*syn. NF-1-like syndrome*) [OMIM #611431]
      - LEOPARD syndrome, types 1–3 (*syn. multiple lentigines syndrome*) [OMIM #151100, 611554, 613707]
      - McCune-Albright syndrome [OMIM #174800]
      - Mismatch repair cancer syndrome (*syn. constitutional mismatch repair deficiency syndrome, Turcot syndrome*) [OMIM #276300]
      - Multiple endocrine neoplasia, type 1 (MEN1) [OMIM #131100]
      - Neurofibromatosis, types I-IV and VI [OMIM #162200, 101000, 162260, 162270, 114030]
      - Neurofibromatosis, type V (*syn. segmental neurofibromatosis, mosaic-localized neurofibromatosis*)
      - Niemann-Pick disease, types A, B, C1, C2 [OMIM #257200, 607616, 257220, 607625]
      - Noonan syndrome [OMIM #163950]
      - Piebald trait (*syn. piebaldism*) [OMIM #172800]
      - Proteus syndrome [OMIM #176920]
      - Silver-Russell syndrome [OMIM #180860]
      - Tuberous sclerosis, types 1 and 2 [OMIM #191100, 613254]
      - Von Hippel-Lindau syndrome [OMIM #193300]
      - Watson syndrome (*syn. CALM with pulmonary stenosis*) [OMIM #193520]
  - Grey-blue hypermelanosis (dermal hypermelanosis, ceruloderma)
    - Mongolian spot ⊙
    - Naevus of Ito ⊙
    - Naevus of Ota ⊙ (*syn. oculodermal melanocytosis*)
    - Dermal hypermelanosis-associated syndromes –
      - GM1-gangliosidosis, type 1 [OMIM # 230500]
      - Hurler syndrome (*syn. mucopolysaccharidosis, type 1H*) [OMIM #607014]
      - Mucopolysaccharidosis, type 2 (*syn. Hunter syndrome*) [OMIM #309900]
      - Niemann-Pick disease, types A, B, C1, C2 [OMIM #257200, 607616, 257220, 607625]
      - Phakomatosis pigmentovascularis, types II, IV and V
      - Sjogren-Larsson syndrome [OMIM #270200]
      - Trisomy 20 mosaicism
  - Hyperpigmented macules on the face of young children [27]

- Maculopapular cutaneous mastocytosis (*syn. urticaria pigmentosa*) [OMIM #154800] *
- Pigmented plantar and palmar macules [⊖]
- Periungual hyperpigmentation of the newborn [⊖]
- Post-inflammatory hyperpigmentation[⊖] – especially atopic dermatitis, cutaneous lupus, infections, physical or chemical injuries.
- Reticulate –
  • Dermatopathia pigmentosa reticularis [OMIM #125595]
  • Dyskeratosis congenita, autosomal dominant 1 [OMIM#127550]
  • Dyskeratosis congenita, autosomal recessive 1 and 5 [OMIM #224230, 615190]
  • Epidermolysis bullosa simplex with mottled pigmentation [OMIM # 131960]
  • Fanconi anaemia [OMIM #227650]
  • Naegeli syndrome (*syn. Naegeli-Franceschetti-Jadassohn syndrome*) [OMIM #161000]
  • Revesz syndrome (*syn. Dyskeratosis congenita, autosomal dominant 5*) [OMIM #268130]
- Speckled lentiginous naevus: macular (*syn. naevus spilus*)
  • Isolated speckled lentiginous naevus
  • Speckled lentiginous naevus-associated syndromes
    – Phakomatosis pigmentovascularis, types III, IV and V
• *Associated with textural change of the skin*
- Congenital melanocytic naevus: medium and giant
- Maculopapular cutaneous mastocytosis (*syn. urticaria pigmentosa*) [OMIM #154800] *
- Speckled lentiginous naevus: papular (*syn. naevus spilus*)
  • Isolated speckled lentiginous naevus
  • Speckled lentiginous naevus-associated syndromes
    – Phakomatosis pigmentovascularis, types III, IV and V

Linear/whorled/segmental

• *Macular*
- Café-au-lait macules (CALM): blaschkoid
- Conradi-Hunermann-Happle syndrome (*syn. X-linked dominant chondrodysplasia punctata*) [OMIM #302960]
- Human chimerism
- Linear and figurated hyperpigmented naevus (*syn. linear and whorled naevoid hypermelanosis*)
  • Isolated linear and figurated hyperpigmented naevus
  • Linear & figurated hyperpigmented naevus-associated syndromes –
    – Cohen syndrome [OMIM #216550]
    – MELAS syndrome (mitochondrial myopathy, encephalopathy, lactic acidosis, stroke-like episodes) [OMIM #540000]
    – Pallister-Killian syndrome (*syn. Mosaic tetrasomy 12p*) [OMIM #601803]
- Pigmentary demarcation lines [⊖]
- Reticulate
  • Incontinentia pigmenti - stage 3 (*syn. Bloch-Sulzberger syndrome*) [OMIM #308300]
  • X-linked reticulate pigmentary disorder with systemic manifestations – female carriers (*syn. familial cutaneous amyloidosis, Partington disease, X-linked cutaneous amyloidosis*) [OMIM #301220]
- Socks line pigmentation [28]
- Speckled lentiginous naevus: blaschkoid (*syn. naevus spilus*)
- Transient pigmentary lines of the newborn [⊖]
• *Associated with textural change of the skin*
- Congenital melanocytic naevus: blaschkoid
- Epidermal naevus/epidermal naevus syndrome
- Focal dermal hypoplasia (*syn. Goltz syndrome*) [OMIM #305600]
- Phakomatosis pigmentokeratotica

- Reticulate –
  - Castori-Paradisi epidermal naevus syndrome
  - Hong-Lee eccrine naevus

Onset in Later Childhood Through to Adulthood [3, 6, 8, 12, 18, 19, 23, 24, 29, 30]

Generalized and Diffuse Hyperpigmentary Disorders (Pigment Concentration/Hyperchromia)

Brownish or Accentuated Dark Pigmentation

Autoimmune disorders
- Dermatomyositis
- Felty syndrome
- Primary biliary cirrhosis
- Systemic sclerosis °

Chronic liver disease
Chronic renal insufficiency
Drug-induced hyperpigmentation

- ACTH administration (high dose)
- Antiretroviral therapy (e.g. zidovudine)
- Arsenic
- Busulfan °
- Minocycline (diffuse type)
- Quinine and quinidine
- Tyrosine kinase inhibitors (dasatinib, imatinib, nilotinib)

Endocrine disorders
- Acromegaly
- Addison's disease
- Cushing's syndrome (inappropriate secretion of ACTH)
- Hyperthyroidism °
- Nelson's syndrome

Genetic disorders
- Haemochromatosis, types 1-5
- Ichthyosis-associated (e.g. ichthyosis vulgaris, X-linked ichthyosis, autosomal recessive congenital ichthyosis, bullous ichthyosiform erythroderma)

- Multiple endocrine neoplasia syndrome, type 2B (MEN 2B) [OMIM #162300]
- Porphyria cutanea tarda, types 1–3 [OMIM #176100]
- Wilson's disease (*syn. hepatolenticular degeneration*) [OMIM #277900]

Infections and infestations
- *Diphyllobothrium latum* fish tapeworm infestation (leading to B12 deficiency)
- HIV/AIDS
- Tuberculosis

Nutritional
- Folic Acid deficiency (due to pregnancy, dialysis, drugs including methotrexate, or concurrent vitamin B12 deficiency)
- Malabsorption syndromes (resulting in multiple vitamin and trace element deficiencies)
- Vitamin B3 deficiency (*syn. Pellagra*) (due to chronic alcoholism, anorexia nervosa, malabsorption syndromes, Hartnup's syndrome, tuberculosis or drugs)
- Vitamin B12 deficiency (due to fatty stool or malabsorption syndromes, including pernicious anaemia)
- Vitamin D overdose (>100 000 IU daily over prolonged period)

Malignancy
- Carcinoid syndrome (gastric and thymic carcinoid)
- Cachectic states
- Generalized malignant acanthosis nigricans
- Hodgkin's and non-Hodgkin's lymphoma
- Lymphatic leukaemia
- Lymphosarcoma
- Mycosis fungoides
- Oat cell carcinoma of the bronchus (results in ectopic ACTH syndrome)
- Phaeochromocytoma
- POEMS syndrome
- Polyposis, skin pigmentation, alopecia and fingernail changes (*syn. Cronkhite-Canada syndrome*) [OMIM #175500]
- Primary systemic amyloidosis

Sarcoid
Tanning with UV light

Grey, Slate or Bluish Pigmentation
Cyanosis *
    Drug-induced hyperpigmentation *

- Amiodarone
- Argyria (silver)
- Bismuth (bismuth)
- Chrysiasis (gold)
- Lead

    Genetic disorders
- Haemochromatosis (including the Juvenile subtype)

    Malignancy
- Metastatic melanoma and melanogenuria

Orange or Reddish Pigmentation *
    Drug-induced hyperpigmentation
- Clofazimine
- Dihydroxyacetone (primary ingredient in sunless tanning products)

    Haemosiderosis

Yellowish Pigmentation (Xanthoderma) *
    Drug-induced hyperpigmentation
- Mepacrine
- Other – picric acid, dinitrophenol, trinitrotoluene, santonin, acriflavine

    Hyperbilirubinaemia (icterus)
- Acute or chronic liver disease (e.g. hepatitis, decompensated cirrhosis, liver failure)

    Nutritional
- Carotonaemia
- Riboflavinaemia

Circumscribed Hyperpigmentary Disorders
    Guttate/punctate
- *Macular*
  - Acquired melanocytic naevi

- Acquired pigmented macules on friction areas in red hair patients [8]
- Agminated lentiginoses
- Bannayan-Riley-Ruvalcaba syndrome: penile lentiginosis [OMIM #153480]
- Carney complex (*syn. NAME syndrome, LAMB syndrome*) [OMIM #160980]
- Cowden syndrome: penile pigmentary macules (syn. *PTEN hamartoma syndrome*) [OMIM #158350]
- Ephelides (*syn. freckles*)
- Eruptive lentiginosis (paraneoplastic, post-chemotherapy, post-radiotherapy, post-sunburn)
- Genital melanosis
- Isolated generalized lentigines
- Inherited patterned lentiginosis in black people ⊙
- Laugier-Hunziker syndrome
- Lentigo simplex
- Mismatch repair cancer syndrome: axillary freckling (*syn. constitutional mismatch repair deficiency syndrome, Turcot syndrome*) [OMIM #276300]
- Neurofibromatosis, types I, III and IV: Crowe's sign [OMIM #162200, 162260, 162270]
- Peutz-Jeghers syndrome (*syn. periorificial lentiginosis*) [OMIM #175200]
- Polyposis, skin pigmentation, alopecia and fingernail changes (*syn. Cronkhite-Canada syndrome*) [OMIM #175500]
- Post-inflammatory hyperpigmentation⊙ – especially acne, infections (including chikungunya), lichen planus, physical or chemical injuries, pityriasis rosea, pityriasis lichenoides chronica and (guttate) psoriasis
- PUVA lentigines
- Reticulate –
  - Dowling-Degos disease 1 (*syn. reticular pigment anomaly of the flexures*) [OMIM #179850]
  - Dowling-Degos disease 3 [OMIM #615674]
  - Dowling-Degos disease 4 [OMIM #615696]

- Galli-Galli disease (a variant of Dowling-Degos disease)
- Harber's syndrome
- Reticulate acropigmentation of Kitamura – early [OMIM #615537]
  - Solar lentigines
  - Tattoos – accidental and decorative
- *Associated with textural change of the skin*
  - Acquired melanocytic naevi
  - Dermatosis papulosa nigra [*][o]
  - Infection – especially pityriasis versicolour
  - Morphea: guttate lesions [*]

Patchy
- *Macular*
  - Acquired bilateral telangiectatic macules [29]
  - Acquired brachial cutaneous dyschromatosis (*syn. ABCD, melasma of the arms*)
  - Acrogeria (*syn. Gottron's acrogeria*) [OMIM #201200]
  - Ashy dermatosis (*syn. erythema dyschromicum perstans*) [o]
  - Carcinoid syndrome
  - Drug-induced hyperpigmentation – chlorpromazine and related phenothiazines, chloroquine and hydroxychloroquine, cytostatic drugs (i.e. cyclophosphamide, bleomycin, fluorouracil), imipramine and other TCAs, latanoprost/bimatoprost, mercury (topical), minocycline, oestrogen (i.e. combined oral contraceptive pill), phenytoin
  - Grey-blue hypermelanosis (dermal hypermelanosis, ceruloderma)
    - Acquired bilateral naevus of Ota-like macules (ABNOM) [o]
    - Acquired dermal hypermelanocytosis
    - Hori's naevus [o]
    - Progressive dermal melanocytosis
  - Familial periorbital hyperpigmentation [o]
  - Idiopathic eruptive macular pigmentation
  - Infections – especially chikungunya, erythrasma, tinea nigra
  - Lentigo maligna: large (*syn. Hutchinson's melanotic freckle*)
  - Lichen planus pigmentosus [o]

- Linea fusca (*syn. brown forehead ring of Andersen, Wernoe and Haxthausen*)
- Macular arteritis (*syn. lymphocytic thrombophilic arteritis, macular lymphocytic arteritis*)
- Maculopapular cutaneous mastocytosis (*syn. urticaria pigmentosa*) [OMIM #154800] [*]
- Macular pigmentation of uncertain aetiology [30]
- Melasma (*syn. chloasma, mask of pregnancy*)
- Mycosis fungoides: pigmented purpuric variant
- Nutritional –
  - Folic acid deficiency (due to pregnancy, dialysis, drugs including methotrexate, or with concurrent vitamin B12 deficiency)
  - Vitamin B2 deficiency: hyperpigmentation of scrotum or vulva
  - Vitamin B3 deficiency (*syn. pellagra*): hyperpigmentation of hands, neck and feet
  - Vitamin B6 deficiency: hyperpigmentation of the scrotum or vulva
  - Vitamin B12 deficiency (due to fatty stool or malabsorption syndromes, including pernicious anaemia)
  - Vitamin C deficiency (*syn. scurvy*): melasma-like hyperpigmentation
  - Zinc deficiency: hyperpigmentation of scrotum or vulva
- Ochronosis [*] –
  - Alkaptonuria (*syn. hereditary ochronosis, homogentisic acid oxidase deficiency*) [OMIM #203500]
  - Exogenous ochronosis (commonly due to hydroquinone)
- Phototoxic reactions
  - Berloque dermatitis
  - Phytophotodermatitis
- Pigmented peribuccal pigmentation of Brocq (*syn. erythrose péribuccale pigmentaire of Brocq*) [31]
- Pigmented plantar and palmar macules [o]
- Pityriasis rotunda (hyperpigmented in patients with fair skin) [32]

- Porphyrias –
  - Hereditary coproporphryia [OMIM #121300]
  - Porphyria cutanea tarda [OMIM #176100]
  - Variegate porphyria [OMIM #176200]
- Post-inflammatory hyperpigmentation° – especially acne, atopic dermatitis, cutaneous lupus, dermatomyositis, drug reactions (i.e. phototoxic drug eruption, fixed drug eruption, lichenoid drug eruption, SJS/TEN), immunobullous diseases, lichen planus, mycosis fungoides, physical or chemical injuries
- Pregnancy-associated hyperpigmentation: nipples and anogenital skin
- Red-brown hypermelanosis (haemosiderosis) * –
  - Diabetic dermopathy – late (*syn. shin spots, pigmented pretibial patches*)
  - Haemolytic anaemias
  - Shamberg's disease and other pigmented purpuric dermatoses
  - Sickle-cell anaemia
- Reticulate –
  - Acquired atopic hyperpigmentation (*syn. atopic dirty neck*) [33]
  - Dowling-Degos disease 1 (*syn. reticular pigment anomaly of the flexures*) [OMIM #179850]
  - Dowling-Degos disease 3 [OMIM #615674]
  - Dowling-Degos disease 4 [OMIM #615696]
  - Drug-induced reticulate pigmentation – especially diltiazem
  - Dyskeratosis congenita, X-linked [OMIM #305000]
  - Dyskeratosis congenita, autosomal dominant 1 [OMIM#127550]
  - Dyskeratosis congenita, autosomal recessive 1 & 5 [OMIM #224230, 615190]
  - Erythema ab Igne
  - Galli-Galli disease (a variant of Dowling-Degos disease) [34]
  - Harber's syndrome [35]

- Hoyeraal-Hreidarsson syndrome (severe variant of dyskeratosis congenita, X-linked) [OMIM # 305000]
- Lichen planus pigmentosus: reticulate pattern
- Pigmentatio reticularis faciei et colli [36]
- Poikiloderma of Civatte
- Primary cutaneous amyloidosis: macular variant (rippled appearance)
- Reticulate acropigmentation of Kitamura – early [OMIM #615537]
- Wilson's disease (*syn. Hepatolenticular degeneration*) [OMIM #277900]
- Riehl's melanosis (*syn. pigmented cosmetic dermatitis, female facial melanosis, melanodermatitis toxica*)
- Solar lentigo: large
- Sweat discolouration *
  - Chromhidrosis (yellow, green, blue, brown or black)
  - Pseudo-chromhidrosis
- Talon noir *
- Tattoos – accidental and decorative *
- *Associated with textural change of the skin*
  - Acanthosis nigricans
  - Atrophoderma of Pierini and Pasini
  - Colloid milia: pigmented variant * (associated with exogenous ochronosis)
  - Diabetic dermopathy – late (*syn. shin spots, pigmented pretibial patches*)
  - Erythromelanosis follicularis faciei et colli [37]
  - H syndrome (*syn. hyperpigmentation and hypertrichosis, hepatosplenomegaly, heart anomalies, hearing loss, low height, hormonal disturbances, haematologic illness and hyperglycaemia syndrome*) [OMIM #602782]
  - Infection – especially chikungunya, erythrasma, pityriasis versicolour, tinea nigra, secondary syphilis and onchocerciasis (*mal morado*)
  - Maculopapular cutaneous mastocytosis (*syn. urticaria pigmentosa*) [OMIM #154800] *
  - Melanoacanthoma/seborrhoeic keratosis
  - Morphea: plaque lesions

- Muckle-Wells syndrome [OMIM #191900]
- Notalgia paraesthetica
- Reticulate –
  • Confluent and reticulated papillomatosis (*syn, Gougerot Carteaud disease*) *
  • Dirt pigmentation (*syn. dermatosis neglecta, terra firma-forme dermatosis*)*
  • Erythema ab Igne
  • Granular parakeratosis
  • Lichen planus pigmentosus – reticulate pattern
  • Pigmentatio reticularis faciei et colli [36]
  • Primary cutaneous amyloidosis: lichenoid variant (rippled appearance)
  • Prurigo pigmentosa
  • Systemic sclerosis ⊖

Linear/whorled/segmental
• *Macular*
  – Becker naevus – early (*syn. hypermelanosis naeviformis*)
  – Black dermographism
  – Flagellate pigmentation
    • Chemotherapy induced: bleomycin, peplomycin, docetaxel, bendamustine
    • Idiopathic flagellate pigmentation
    • Mechanical (true flagellation): religious punishment, torture, sexual pleasure, child/partner abuse, dermatitis artefacta
    • Rheumatological disorders: adult onset Still's disease, dermatomyositis
    • Toxin-induced: shiitake mushroom ingestion, cnidarian stings, *Paederus* and other insects
    • Other pruritic dermatoses: excoriations by pruritic conditions, phytophotodermatitis, hypereosinophilic syndrome
  – Phototoxic reactions
    • Berloque dermatitis
    • Phytophotodermatitis
  – Pigmented purpuric dermatosis: linear variant *
  – Post-inflammatory hyperpigmentation⊖ – especially physical trauma and intravenous drug use ("track marks")

- Pregnancy-associated hyperpigmentation – linea nigra
- Progressive cribriform and zosteriform hyperpigmentation (a unilateral, late-onset variant of Linear and figurated hyperpigmented naevus) [38]
- Neurofibromatosis, type V: CALM/freckling (*syn. segmental neurofibromatosis, mosaic-localized neurofibromatosis*)
- Segmental lentiginosis (*syn. lentiginous naevus, partial unilateral lentiginosis, agminated lentigines, lentiginous mosaicism*)
• *Associated with textural change of the skin*
  – Becker naevus – late (*syn. hypermelanosis naeviformis*)
  – Lichen planus / Lichen planus pigmentosus – blaschkoid or zosteriform
  – Lichenoid drug eruption – blaschkoid
  – Linear atrophoderma of Moulin
  – Morphea: linear lesions, en coup de sabre
  – Neurofibromatosis, type V: CALM/freckling and neurofibromas (*syn. segmental neurofibromatosis, mosaic-localized neurofibromatosis*)
  – Striae distensae

Mixed Pigmentation (Hypopigmented and Hyperpigmented)

Onset in Early Childhood [3, 12, 19, 20]

Generalized and Diffuse Mixed Pigmentation Disorders
• Dyschromatosis universalis hereditaria, types 1–3 (*syn. DUH*) [OMIM #127500, 612715, 615402]
• Familial progressive hyperpigmentation with or without hypopigmentation (*syn. FPHH; melanosis universalis hereditaria*) (includes Westerhof syndrome) [OMIM #145250]
• Spastic paraplegia 23 (*syn. SPG23; spastic paraplegia with pigmentary abnormalities; spastic paraparesis, vitiligo, premature greying and characteristic facies; Lison syndrome*) [OMIM #270750]

- X-linked reticulate pigmentary disorder with systemic manifestations – affected males (*syn. familial cutaneous amyloidosis, Partington disease, X-linked cutaneous amyloidosis*) [OMIM #301220]

Circumscribed Mixed Pigmentation Disorders

Guttate/punctate

- *Associated with textural change of the skin*
  - Poikiloderma -
    - Xeroderma pigmentosum, groups A-G [OMIM #278700, 610651, 278720, 278730, 278740, 278760, 278780]

Patchy

- *Macular*
  - Albinism-deafness syndrome (*syn. Ziprkowski-Margolis syndrome; Woolf syndrome*) [OMIM #300700]
  - Ermine phenotype (*syn. pigmentary disorder with hearing loss*) (includes Black locks with albinism and deafness syndrome, BADS) [OMIM #227010]
  - Fanconi anaemia [OMIM #227650]
  - Piebald trait (*syn. piebaldism*) [OMIM #172800]
  - Piebald trait with neurologic defects [OMIM #172850]
  - Post-inflammatory hyper- and hypopigmentation ⊙ – especially neonatal lupus erythematosus
  - Protein-energy malnutrition – marasmus and kwashiorkor ⊙ (likely due to phenylalanine deficiency)
  - Reticulate –
    - Dyschromatosis symmetrica hereditaria (*syn. DSH, reticulate acropigmentation of Dohi*) [OMIM #127400]
- *Associated with textural change of the skin*
  - Poikiloderma
    - Ataxia telangiectasia [OMIM #208900]
    - Bloom syndrome [OMIM #210900]
    - Hutchinson-Gilford progeria syndrome (*syn. progeria*) [OMIM #176670]
    - Kindler syndrome (*syn. Weary-Kindler syndrome, Poikiloderma with bullae*) [OMIM # 173650]

- Poikiloderma with neutropenia (*syn. poikiloderma with neutropenia, Clericuzio-type*) [OMIM #604173]
- Porphyrias
  - Congenital erythropoietic porphyria (*syn. Gunther's disease*) [OMIM #263700]
  - Hepatoerythropoietic porphyria [OMIM #176100]
- Rothmund-Thomson syndrome (*syn. hereditary congenital poikiloderma*) [OMIM #268400]
- Sclerotylosis (*syn. Huriez syndrome*) [OMIM #181600]

Linear/whorled/segmental

- *Macular*
  - Cutis tricolour – (i) as a purely cutaneous trait; (ii) as a part of a complex malformation phenotype (Ruggieri-Happle syndrome); (iii) as a distinct type with multiple, disseminated smaller skin macules (cutis tricolour parvimaculata); (iv) in association with other skin disturbances (e.g. cutis marmorata telangiectasia congenita, ataxia-telangiectasia, phacomatosis pigmentovascularis) [39]
- *Associated with textural change of the skin*
  - Focal dermal hypoplasia (*syn. Goltz syndrome*) [OMIM #305600]

Onset in Later Childhood Through to Adulthood [3, 12, 19, 23, 24]

Generalized and Diffuse Mixed Pigmentation Disorders

Autoimmune disorders

- Systemic sclerosis: salt and pepper appearance ⊙
- Vitiligo (trichrome)

Chronic renal insufficiency
Drug-induced hyperpigmentation

- Chronic arsenic poisoning

Endocrine disorders

- Addison's disease: with vitiligo

Genetic disorders

- Dyschromatosis universalis hereditaria, types 1–3 (*syn. DUH*) [OMIM #127500, 612715, 615402]
- X-linked reticulate pigmentary disorder with systemic manifestations – affected males (*syn. Familial cutaneous amyloidosis, Partington disease, X-linked cutaneous amyloidosis*) [OMIM #301220]

Primary cutaneous amyloidosis

- Amyloidosis cutis dyschromica (ACD) [40]

Circumscribed Mixed Pigmentation Disorders

Guttate/punctate

- *Macular*
  - Amyloidosis cutis dyschromica (ACD) [40]
  - Chronic arsenic poisoning
  - Reticulate –
    - Dowling-Degos disease 2 [OMIM #615327]

Patchy

- *Macular*
  - Dermatomyositis
  - Genital melanosis associated with localized depigmentation [41]
  - Infections – especially late-manifesting pinta, pintoid dyschromia of yaws
  - Post-inflammatory hyper- and hypopigmentation ⁰ – especially discoid lupus erythematosus, systemic lupus erythematosus
  - Protein-energy malnutrition – marasmus and kwashiorkor ⁰ (likely due to phenylalanine deficiency)
  - Reticulate
    - Dyskeratosis congenita, X-linked [OMIM #305000]
    - Dyskeratosis congenita, autosomal dominant 1 [OMIM #127550]
    - Dyskeratosis congenita, autosomal recessive 1 & 5 [OMIM #224230, 615190]
    - Hoyeraal-Hreidarsson syndrome (severe variant of dyskeratosis congenita, X-linked) [OMIM # 305000]

- Reticulate genital pigmentation associated with localized vitiligo [42]
- Vagabond's disease (*syn. Vagabond's leucoderma*)
- Vitiligo: trichrome variant, quadrichrome variant
- *Associated with textural change of the skin*
  - Infections – especially pityriasis versicolour, onchocerciasis (*leopard skin*), secondary syphilis (*leucoderma syphiliticum*), pinta
  - Morphea
  - Poikiloderma
    - Cockayne syndrome A [OMIM #216400]
    - Graft versus host disease (GVHD)
    - Hartnup disease [OMIM #234500]
    - Mycosis fungoides: poikilodermic variant (*syn. poikiloderma vasculare atrophicans*) [43]
    - Poikiloderma of Civatte
    - Porphyrias
      - Hereditary coproporphryia [OMIM #121300]
      - Porphyria cutanea tarda, types 1–3 [OMIM #176100]
      - Variegate porphyria [OMIM #176200]
      - Werner syndrome (*syn. adult progeria*) [OMIM #277700]

Conclusion

The colour of human skin is mainly due to melanin and haemoglobin, but it can be altered in non-physiological conditions such as jaundice, carotenoderma and drug intake. Melanin is produced by epidermal melanocytes, where it is synthesized in specialized organelles called melanosomes. Variations in individual skin colour and between people of various ethnicities are not due to the number of melanocytes but rather are due to the number, size and type of melanosomes and the dispersion of the melanin pigment.

The pigmentary disorders include those where there is a lightening in skin colour, a darkening in skin colour, a mixed pattern of lightening and darkening in skin colour or the development of an unusual skin colour. The vast majority of pigmentary disorders are due to quantitative or qualitative defects in the synthesis, transfer, deposition and degradation of melanin. Abnormal skin colour can also result from disturbances in both endogenous and exogenous pigments.

When approaching a patient with abnormal skin colour, it is important to perform a thorough history, examination and relevant bedside investigations (often including diascopy and Wood's lamp examination). Investigations are dependent on the diagnosis suspected, but in many cases investigations (including histopathology) are not diagnostic. For this reason, it is important to have a systematic approach for the pigmentary disorders.

In this chapter we have presented a comprehensive clinical classification of the pigmentary disorders.

References

1. Fistarol SK, Itin PH. Disorders of pigmentation. JDDG. 2010;8:187–202.
2. Nordlund JJ, Boissy RE. The biology of melanocytes. In: Freinkel RK, Woodley DT, editors. The biology of the skin. New York: Parthenon Publishing; 2001. p. 113–31.
3. Anstey AV. Disorders of skin colour. In: Burns T, Breathnach S, Cox N, Griffiths C, editors. Rook's textbook of dermatology. West Sussex: Wiley; 2010. p. 58.1–58.59.
4. Park HY, Pongpudpunth M, Lee J, Yaar M. Biology of melanocytes. In: Wolff K, Goldsmith LA, Katz SI, Gilchrest BA, Paller AS, Leffell DJ, editors. Fitzpatrick's dermatology in general medicine. US: The McGraw-Hill Companies; 2008. p. 591–608.
5. Bolognia JL, Orlow SJ. Melanocyte biology. In: Bolognia JL, Jorizzo JL, Schaffer JV, editors. Dermatology. US: Elsevier Limited; 2012. p. 1011–22.
6. Nieuweboer-Krobotova L. Hyperpigmentation: types, diagnostics and targeted treatment options. 2012;27(1):2–4
7. Ortonne JP, Passeron T. Vitiligo and other disorders of hypopigmentation. In: Bolognia JL, Jorizzo JL, Schaffer JV, editors. Dermatology. US: Elsevier Limited; 2012. p. 1023–48.
8. Passeron T, Ortonne JP. Atlas of pigmentary disorders (eBook). Switzerland: Springer International Publishing; 2016.
9. Allen CM, Camisa C. Oral disease. In: Bolognia JL, Jorizzo JL, Schaffer JV, editors. Dermatology. US: Elsevier Limited; 2012. p. 1149–70.
10. Halder RM, Taliaferro SJ. Vitiligo. In: Wolff K, Goldsmith LA, Katz SI, Gilchrest BA, Paller AS, Leffell DJ, editors. Fitzpatrick's dermatology in general medicine. US: The McGraw-Hill Companies; 2008. p. 616–22.
11. Mollet I, Ongenae K, Naeyaert JM. Origin, clinical presentation, and diagnosis of hypomelanotic skin disorders. Dermatol Clin. 2007;25:363–71.
12. Online Mendelian Inheritance in Man, OMIM (TM). McKusick-Nathans Institute of Genetic Medicine, Johns Hopkins University (Baltimore, MD) and National Center for Biotechnology Information, National Library of Medicine (Bethesda, MD). Retrieved from http://www.ncbi.nlm.nih.gov/omim/
13. Kumarasinghe P, Chio MTW. Pigmentary disorders. In: Goh CL, Chua SH, Ng SK, editors. The Asian skin. A reference colour atlas of dermatology. Singapore: McGraw-Hill Education; 2005. p. 48–74.
14. Tey HL. Approach to hypopigmentation disorders in adults. J Clin Exp Dermatol. 2010;35:829–34.
15. Tey HL. A practical classification of childhood hypopigmentation disorders. Acta Derm Venereol. 2010;90:6–11.
16. Lahiri K, Chatterjee M, Sarkar R. Pigmentary disorders. A comprehensive compendium. 1st ed. New Delhi: Jaypee Brothers Medical Publishers (P) Ltd; 2014.
17. Kumarasinghe P, Hewitt D. Neoplasms with pigmentary changes or discolouration. In: Lahiri K, Chatterjee M, Sarkar R, editors. Pigmentary disorders. A comprehensive compendium. 1st ed. New Delhi: Jaypee Brothers Medical Publishers (P) Ltd; 2014. p. 95–6.
18. Vachiramon V. Approach to reticulate hyperpigmentation. J Clin Exp. Dermatol. 2011;36:459–66.
19. Tadini G, Brena M, Gelmetti C, Pezzani L. Atlas of genodermatoses. 2nd ed. Florida: CRC Press; 2015.
20. Hornyak TJ. Albinism and other genetic disorders of pigmentation. In: Wolff K, Goldsmith LA, Katz SI, Gilchrest BA, Paller AS, Leffell DJ, editors. Fitzpatrick's dermatology in general medicine. US: The McGraw-Hill Companies; 2008. p. 608–16.
21. Hua C, Boussemart L, Mateus C, Routier E, Boutros C, Cazenave H, et al. Association of vitiligo with tumour response in patients with metastatic melanoma treated with Pembrolizumab. JAMA Dermatol. 2016;152(1):45–51.
22. Sonthalia S, Daulatabad D, Sarkar R. Glutathione as a skin whitening agent: facts, myths, evidence and controversies. Indian J Dermatol Venereol Leprol. 2016;82:262–72.
23. Lapeere H, Boone B, De Schepper S, Verhaeghe E, Ongenae K, Van Geel N, et al. Hypomelanosis and hypermelanosis. In: Wolff K, Goldsmith LA, Katz SI, Gilchrest BA, Paller AS, Leffell DJ, editors. Fitzpatrick's dermatology in general medicine. US: The McGraw-Hill Companies; 2008. p. 622–40.

24. Change MW. Disorders of hyperpigmentation. In: Bolognia JL, Jorizzo JL, Schaffer JV, editors. Dermatology. US: Elselvier Limited; 2012. p. 1049–74.

25. Gupta D, Chandrashekar L, Larizza L, Colombo E, Fontana L, Gervasini C, et al. Familial gastrointestinal stromal tumors, lentigines, and café-au-lait macules associated with germline *c-kit* mutation treated with imatinib. Int. J. Dermatol. 2017;56:195–201.

26. Ho JC, Chan YC, Giam YC, Ong BH, Kumarasinghe SP. Flexural pigmentation with multiple lentigines: a new primary pigmentary disorder? Br J Dermatol. 2006;154(2):382–4.

27. Hernández-Martín A, Gilliam AE, Baselga E, Vicente A, Lam J, González-Enseñat M, et al. Hyperpigmented macules on the face of young children: a series of 25 cases. J Am Acad Dermatol. 2014;70:288–90.

28. Berk DR, Tapia B, Lind A, Bayliss SJ. Sock-line hyperpigmentation: case series and literature review. Arch Dermatol. 2007;143:428–30.

29. Park JH, Lee DJ, Lee YJ, Jang YH, Kang HY, Kim YC. Acquired bilateral telangiectatic macules: a distinct clinical entity. JAMA Dermatol. 2014;150:974–7.

30. Kumarasinghe SP. Understanding macular pigmentation of uncertain aetiology. Indian J Dermatol Venereol Leprol. 2015;81:581–3.

31. Perez-Bernal A, Munoz-Perez MA, Camacho F. Management of facial hyperpigmentation. Am J Clin Dermatol. 2000;1(5):261–8.

32. Mirsky L, Watters K, Jafarian F. Chronic hyperpigmented scaly plaques. Pityriasis rotunda. Arch Dermatol. 2012;148(9):1073–8.

33. Seghers AC, Lee JS, Tan CS, Koh YP, Ho MS, Lim YL, et al. Atopic dirty neck or acquired atopic hyperpigmentation? An epidemiological and clinical study from the National Skin Centre in Singapore. Dermatology. 2014;229(3):174–82.

34. Ho J, Bhawan J. Mimickers of classic acantholytic diseases. J Dermatol. 2017;44(3):232–42.

35. McCormack CJ, Cowen P. Harber's syndrome. Australas J Dermatol. 1997;38(2):82–4.

36. Rebora A, Crovato F. Pigmentatio reticularis faciei et colli. Arch Dermatol. 1985;121(8):968.

37. Rather S, Yaseen A, Mukhija M. Erythromelanosis follicularis faciei et colli – a cross-sectional, descriptive study. Indian J Dermatol. 2016;61(3):308–13.

38. Kim JY, GN O, Seo SH, Ahn HH, Kye YC, Choi JE. Progressive cribriform and zosteriform hyperpigmentation. Cutis. 2015;96(1):E4–6.

39. Ruggieri M, Polizzi A, Schepis C, Morano M, Strano S, et al. Cutis tricolor: a literature review and report of five new cases. Quant Imaging Med Surg. 2016;6(5):525–34.

40. Mahon C, Oliver F, Purvis D, Agnew K. Amyloidosis cutis dyschromica in two siblings and review of the epidemiology, clinical features and management in 48 cases. Australas J Dermatol. 2016;57(4):307–11.

41. Harmelin Y, Cardot-Leccia N, Ortonne JP, Bahadoran P, Lacour JP, et al. Localized depigmentation on genital melanosis. Br J Dermatol. 2013;168(3):663–4.

42. Romero-Mate A, Minano-Medrano R, Najera-Botello L, Castano-Pascual A, Martiinez-Moran C, et al. Reticulate genital pigmentation associated with localized vitiligo. Arch Dermatol. 2010;146(5):574–5.

43. Bloom B, Marchbein S, Fischer M, Kamino H, Patel R, et al. Poikilodermatous mycosis fungoides. Dermatol Online J. 2012;18(12):4.

Dermatopathology Clues in Pigmentary Disorders

2

Riti Bhatia and M. Ramam

Pigmentary disorders are a group of diseases characterized by a reduction, increase or alteration of pigment in the skin. Several diseases show a pigmentary change in addition to other findings, particularly in dark skin, but this chapter will focus on those diseases in which pigmentary change is the primary, if not exclusive feature.

There is a kaleidoscopic range of pigmentary disorders, some common, some uncommon. These conditions usually present with macules and are diagnosed significantly more easily on clinical examination than on biopsy primarily because many of the diagnostic clinical findings do not have histopathological counterparts. In these almost two-dimensional macular lesions, there is very little more for the dermatopathologist to see *in* the skin beyond what is *on* the skin. Typically, hypopigmented lesions show a reduction of melanin in basal epidermal cells. In some conditions, there may be an accompanying reduction in the number of melanocytes. Hyperpigmented lesions show an increase in basal layer melanin with some melanophages in the upper dermis. The ash leaf macule of tuberous sclerosis, nevus depigmentosus, hypomelanosis of Ito, progressive macular hypomelanosis, macular post-kala-azar dermal

leishmaniasis and melasma, freckles, café-au-lait macules, raindrop pigmentation of arsenicism and dyschromatoses are some of the clinical conditions that show these relatively non-diagnostic histopathological changes.

Additionally, these changes can be difficult to appreciate in biopsies from pigmented skin as there is a wide variation in the degree of normal epidermal melanization, so much so that it may be difficult to say if a particular biopsy was obtained from a hypopigmented or hyperpigmented macule.

The clinical findings in pigmentary disorders are described throughout the rest of this book. Our focus in this chapter is on histopathological clues that can help make a diagnosis. These clues fall into three groups: those related to melanocytes and melanin, those related to the identification of non-melanin pigments and those not related to the pigmentary system but distinctive enough to allow a diagnosis.

I Clues Related to Melanocytes and Melanin

While melanocytes are the cells that produce the pigment that is primarily responsible for skin colour in health and disease, there are only a handful of pigmentary disorders which can be diagnosed based on abnormalities in the components of the pigment system, i.e. melanocytes and melanin.

Authors are employees of the Government of India

R. Bhatia · M. Ramam (✉)
Department of Dermatology and Venereology,
All India Institute of Medical Sciences, New Delhi,
Delhi, India

© Government of India 2018
P. Kumarasinghe (ed.), *Pigmentary Skin Disorders*, Updates in Clinical Dermatology,
https://doi.org/10.1007/978-3-319-70419-7_2

Dermal Melanocytosis

The finding of dendritic melanocytes in the dermis is a characteristic feature of this group of disorders. These melanocytes are believed to be derived from precursor cells that failed to migrate from the neural crest to the epidermis during embryogenesis. The dermal location of melanin within melanocytes lends a bluish-greyish colour to macules due to the Tyndall phenomenon. These disorders vary in the age of onset, evolution and sites of predilection.

Nevus of Ota/Nevus Fuscoceruleus Ophthalmomaxillaris

Biopsy reveals pigmented melanocytes with long dendritic processes, often accompanied by melanophages (Fig. 2.1a). A histopathological classification of nevus of Ota according to its depth has been found to be useful in predicting the outcome of treatment with Q-switched alexandrite laser, with the superficial type responding better than the deeper type [1, 2]. This classification describes five histopathological variants of nevus of Ota according to the depth and the pattern of involvement, which are superficial, deep, diffuse, superficial dominant and deep dominant. Also, the colour (blue, grey, brown) varies according to the depth of involvement. If required, dermal melanocytes can be identified using immunohistochemical stains such as Melan-A, MART-1 and GP-100. Electron microscopy reveals an extracellular fibrous sheath around dermal melanocytes. There is thickening of this sheath as the age of the lesion advances [3].

Clinically, patients present with a roughly triangular patch on one cheek that has a deep blue-grey colour, involving the area innervated by first and second branches of the trigeminal nerve (Fig. 2.1b). It is commoner in females and in Asians. Pigmentation is present at birth but becomes obvious in early childhood or puberty. In darkly pigmented patients, the blueness of the cutaneous component of the nevus may be obscured by the brown colour of melanin in the lower epidermis. Scleral pigmentation is common and has a more obvious blue colouration

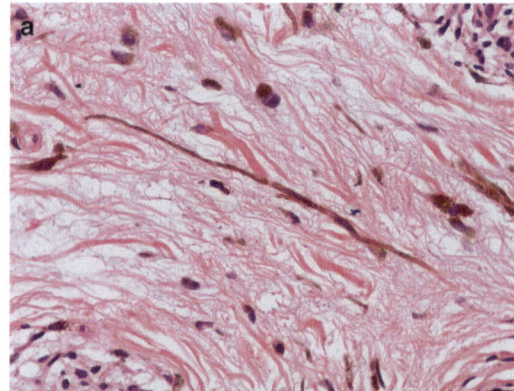

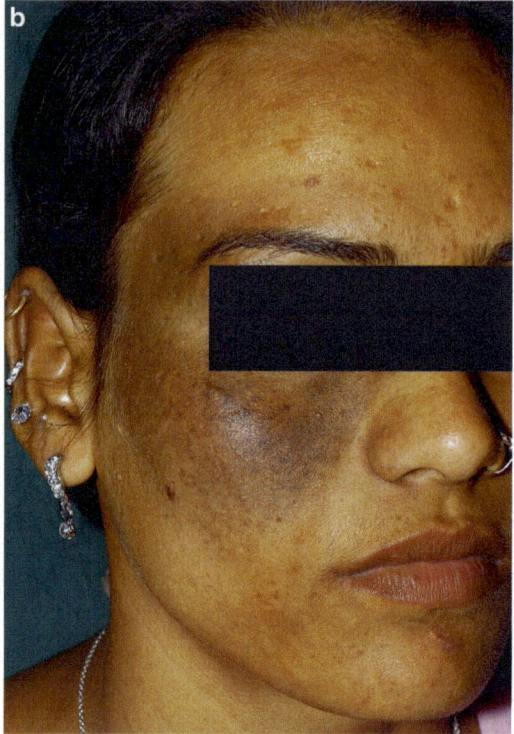

Fig. 2.1 Nevus of Ota. (**a**) Melanocytes with long pigmented dendritic processes in the upper dermis (H&E, X400). (**b**) Grey-blue mottled pigmentation on the right cheek with scleral pigmentation

because of the transparency of the overlying conjunctiva. Less frequently, there may be bluish pigmentation of the ipsilateral palatal and buccal mucosa, and rarely it can involve nasal mucosa, external auditory canal, tympanic membrane, meninges and the brain [4, 5]. Rarely, nevus of Ota may be bilateral [6].

Identical histopathological changes are seen in the nevus of Ito which presents on the acromio-clavicular area.

Acquired Dermal Melanocytosis

There are two types of acquired dermal melanocytosis: *Sun's nevus* is acquired unilateral nevus of Ota and *Hori's nevus* is acquired bilateral nevus of Ota-like macules or ABNOM [7, 8]. This is a condition that is seen mainly in people of Asian origin and is commoner in women than in men. It has an adult onset and does not involve the mucosae, unlike nevus of Ota. However, mucosal involvement has been described in a single case of Hori's nevus recently [9]. The histopathological findings are the same as in nevus of Ota.

Mongolian Spot

Elongated dendritic melanocytes containing melanin are present in the lower half of the dermis [10]. It presents as slate-grey macules classically located in the lumbo-sacral area, at or soon after birth (Fig. 2.2). Less frequently it affects the buttocks and scalp. It usually involutes in early childhood but may persist into adulthood in a small proportion of people.

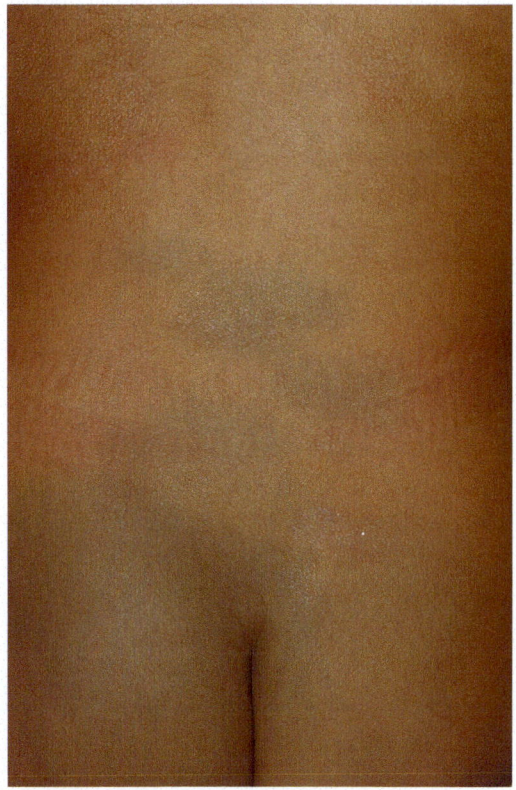

Fig. 2.2 Mongolian spot. Ill-defined bluish macules on the lower back and buttocks

Other Melanocytic Proliferations

Lentigines present as dark, pigmented macules that show mild acanthosis and an increased number of melanocytes particularly around the bases and sides of rete pegs [11]. Other melanocytic neoplasms, benign nevi and malignant melanoma, are beyond the scope of this chapter as they are not macules.

Halo Nevi

Depigmented macules may develop around melanocytic nevi which are then known as halo nevi. The epidermis of depigmented macules shows a loss of melanin and melanocytes, analogous to vitiligo. Lymphocytes may be seen close to melanocytes in developing lesions. The loss of melanocytes was also confirmed electron microscopically [12].

The central nevus shows a junctional or, more commonly, intradermal nested proliferation of cells accompanied by a dense inflammatory infiltrate of lymphocytes and histiocytes in the dermis.

Melanosome Synthesis and Transport Disorders

The genetic disorders characterized by pigmentary dilution of the skin, hair and eyes include Hermansky-Pudlak syndrome, Chédiak-Higashi syndrome, Elejalde syndrome and Griscelli syndrome. Griscelli syndrome is an example of a disease which can be diagnosed based on the morphological appearance of melanocytes.

Biopsies from the skin of these patients show enlarged, darkly pigmented melanocytes in the basal layer of the epidermis (Fig. 2.3a). The adjacent keratinocytes are pale indicating the lack of melanin transfer which is the pathogenesis of the skin changes in this disorder [13].

Griscelli syndrome is an autosomal recessive disorder caused by mutations in one of three genes that are associated with pigment granule transfer, *MYO5A*, *RAB27A* and *MLPH* [14, 15]. All three varieties manifest with pale skin and silvery hair. However, in Griscelli syndrome types 1 and 2, there are additional defects of the nervous system and immune system, respectively, while Griscelli syndrome type 3 only shows pigment dilution of the skin and hair [13, 15, 16].

Hair microscopy reveals irregular clumps of melanin granules along the hair shaft (Fig. 2.3b). Silvery grey hair is also seen in Chédiak-Higashi syndrome and Elejalde syndrome. However, in Chédiak-Higashi syndrome, pigment clumps are small and uniformly distributed along the

hair shaft and granulocytes show giant granules on peripheral blood smear examination. In Elejalde syndrome, in addition to the silvery grey hair and bronze-coloured skin, there is profound dysfunction of the central nervous system and a normal immune system. It is now recognized that Elejalde syndrome is identical to Griscelli syndrome type 1 [17].

Vitiligo

Let us turn from melanocytes to melanin. As stated above, using the quantum of melanin to make a diagnosis of hypo- or hyperpigmentation is not easy. Established vitiligo (Fig. 2.4a) is fairly simple to diagnose, particularly if a biopsy of normal skin from the same patient is available for

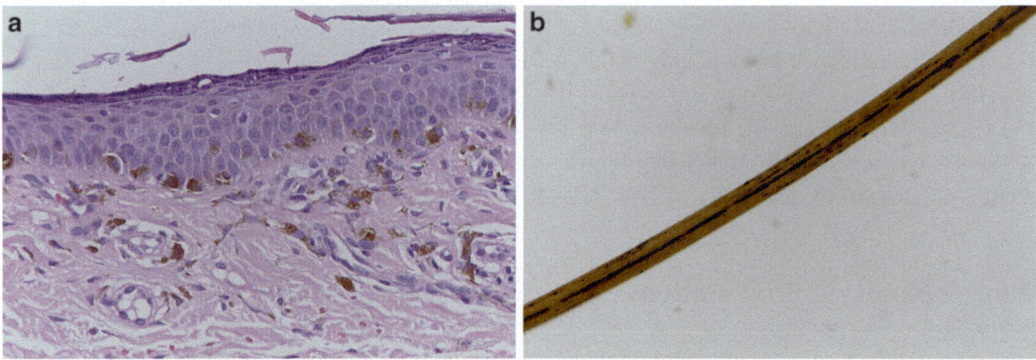

Fig. 2.3 Griscelli syndrome. (**a**) Enlarged melanocytes in basal layer of the epidermis and melanophages in the upper dermis (H&E, x200). (**b**) Irregular clumps of pigment in scalp hair (x200)

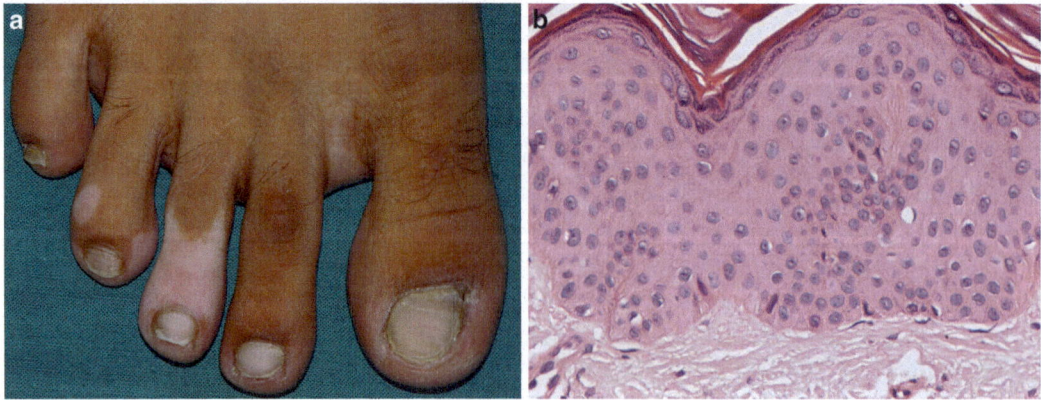

Fig. 2.4 Vitiligo. (**a**) Depigmented macules on the toes. (**b**) 'Washed-out' epidermis with absent melanocytes and melanin (H&E, X400)

comparison. The epidermis in biopsies from vitiligo has a washed-out look as they lack melanin
within keratinocytes. In addition, there is a paucity or complete absence of melanocytes in the
basal layer [18] (Fig. 2.4b). However, biopsies are
hardly ever performed for the diagnosis of fully
developed vitiligo. Early vitiligo can resemble
other hypopigmented disorders and may present a clinical diagnostic dilemma. Unfortunately,
there are no good histopathological criteria to
diagnose early vitiligo and differentiate it from
other disorders of hypopigmentation with which
it might be confused. A mild, superficial lymphocytic infiltrate has been described along with
some epidermotropism [19]. Melanocytes are
usually preserved at this stage of disease and
can be easily visualized, both using haematoxy-
lin and eosin (H&E) and immunohistochemical
stains. Inflammatory vitiligo is vanishingly rare,
but biopsies from the inflammatory margin are
reported to show a few melanocytes along with
lymphocytes in the upper dermis. A lichenoid
and superficial perivascular infiltrate of lymphocytes and histiocytes with dermal oedema is also
seen. Normal-appearing adjacent skin may also
show focal basal vacuolization with a moderate
mononuclear infiltrate [20]. T cells were seen in
the dermo-epidermal junction of uninvolved skin
in patients with active vitiligo, followed by disap-
pearance of melanocytes in the same area [21].
Ultramicroscopically, in the outer margin of vitiligo macules, melanocytes are often larger, vacuo-
lated, with long dendritic processes [22]. Electron
microscopy study of 15 biopsies showed vacuolar
degeneration of keratinocytes along with extracellular granular deposits in apparently normal skin
up to 15 cm away from the vitiligo macule [23].

Leucoderma secondary to chemicals toxic to
melanocytes such as phenols and catechols can be
difficult to distinguish from vitiligo as both have a
similar clinical and histopathological appearance.

Carbon Baby

Universal acquired melanosis (familial progressive hypermelanosis) is a rare disorder in which
neonates show prominent darkening of the skin

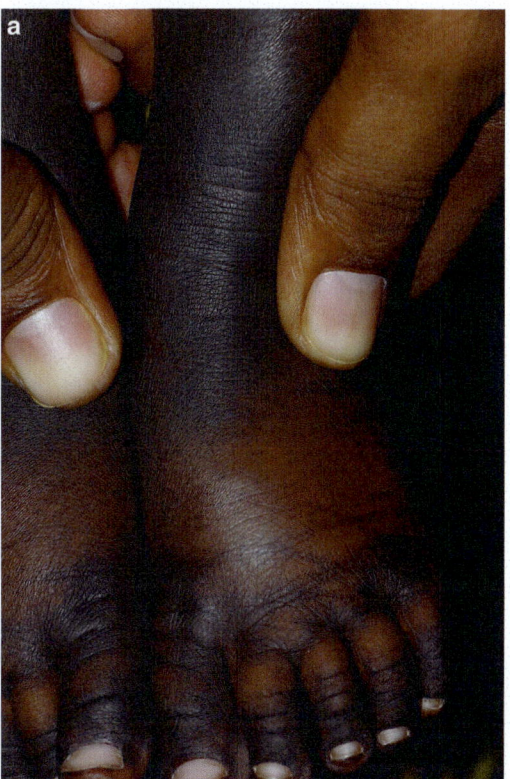

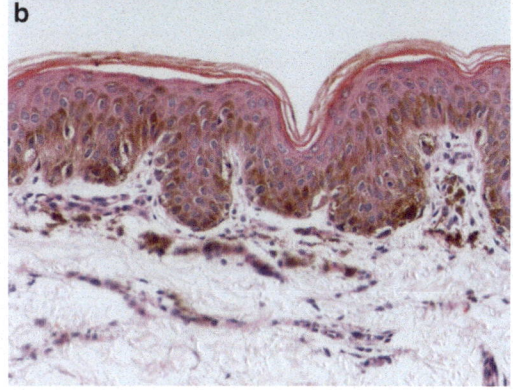

Fig. 2.5   Carbon baby. (**a**) Darkly pigmented skin in an
infant. Note the contrast with the skin colour of the father.
(**b**) Intense melanization of all layers in the epidermis and
melanophages in the upper dermis (H&E, X200)

over the first several months of life, unassoci-
ated with any other abnormalities (Fig. 2.5a).
These babies are much darker than their parents
and siblings and have been referred to as 'carbon babies' [24].

Skin biopsy shows marked basal and suprabasal   pigmentation   in   the   epidermis   with

melanin extending into the upper layers of the epidermis and the stratum corneum [24] (Fig. 2.5b). This represents a condition where an excess of melanin is by itself sufficient to suggest the diagnosis.

II Clues: Non-melanin Pigments

As we have seen in the previous section, quantitative changes in pigment are difficult to identify except at significant levels of excess or depletion. However, when the pigmentary disorder is due to a pigment other than melanin, detection of the causative agent is a helpful diagnostic clue even when it is present in small quantities.

Tattoo

Tattoos are an obvious example of non-melanin pigment leading to a pigmentary change in the skin. They may be traumatic or decorative (Fig. 2.6a).

Biopsy reveals pigment deposits in the dermis (Fig. 2.6b). The pigment appears dark on microscopy irrespective of its colour in vivo except some red and yellow tattoo dyes which appear coloured in biopsies, too [25]. Small and larger irregular aggregates of fine granules are present around vessels, within macrophages and between collagen bundles (Fig. 2.6c). With most tattoos, a biopsy is not necessary for diagnosis, but in the oral mucosa, the finding of granules and frag-

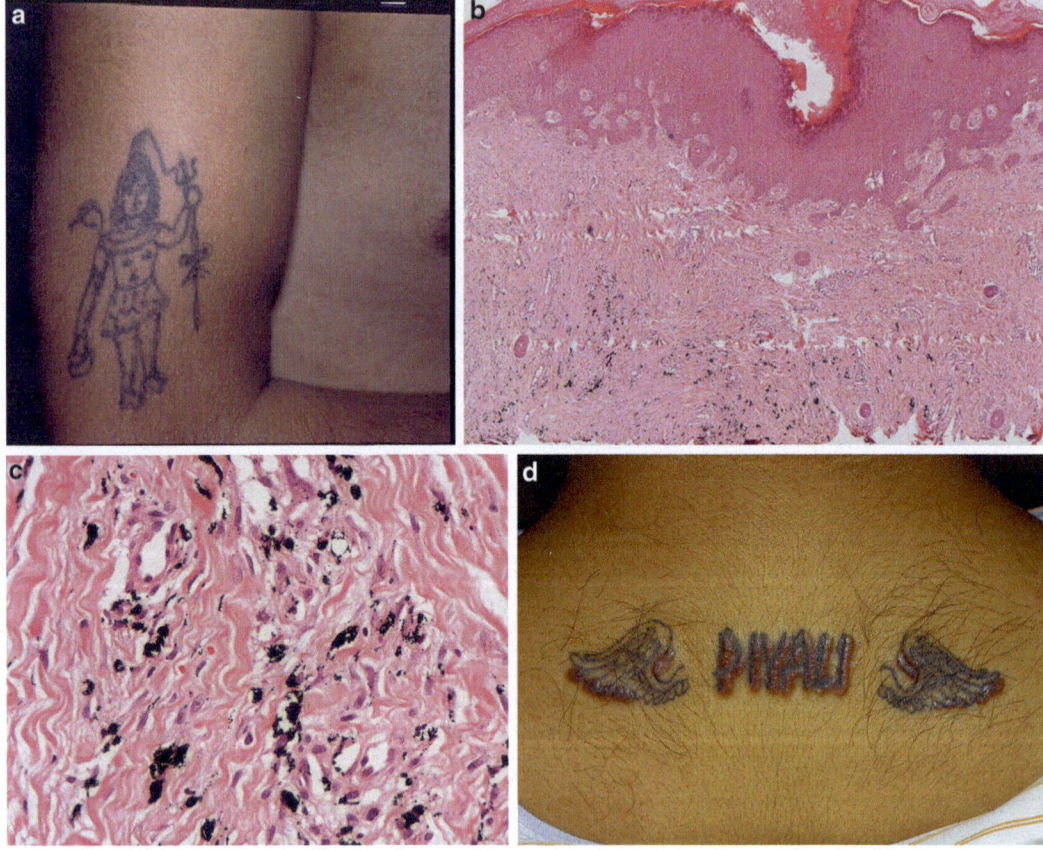

Fig. 2.6 Tattoo. (**a**) Blue-black tattoo depicting Lord Shiva. (**b**) Tattoo pigment in the dermis (H&E, X100). (**c**) Small and larger aggregates of fine pigment granules between thickened collagen bundles (H&E, x400). (**d**) Infiltrated papules at the sites of red tattoo dye

ments of pigment may help to establish a diagnosis of amalgam tattoo and allay concerns about mucosal melanosis or melanoma. The intensity of pigment in a tattoo decreases as it becomes older. Non-inflamed tattoos usually show little infiltrate. However, when there is a tattoo reaction clinically, there may be a variable inflammatory response (Fig. 2.6d). A wide variety of reaction patterns including lichenoid, sarcoidal, granuloma annulare-like, pseudolymphomatous, psoriasiform, morphoeaform and vasculitic have been described [26]. Importantly, the infiltrate may obscure the pigment in biopsies from inflamed tattoos, and this may lead to misdiagnosis unless the dermatopathologist is alerted to the clinical setting.

Electron microscopy findings are variable. Granular, fine, moderately dense material due to organic dyes; large, highly dense, annular aggregates of mercury; and cytoplasmic semi-crystalline membrane-bound particles of iron were observed in a study of patients with tattoos of different colours [27].

Drug-Induced Pigmentation

The deposition of some drugs in the skin leads to hyperpigmentation, chiefly minocycline, amiodarone, antimalarials and clofazimine [28–30]. The pigmentation is hardly ever due to the drug itself but occurs due to differing combinations of melanin, in the epidermis and within melanophages, haemosiderin and lipofuscin. The identification of these pigments is a clue to the diagnosis.

Patients present with diffuse or localized pigmentation. Some drugs produce particular colours such as orange-red due to clofazimine (Fig. 2.7a) and yellow due to amiodarone and mepacrine [30, 31]. Other drugs lead to brown-black hyperpigmentation. The pigmentation due to clofazimine is due to two types of pigments: redox dye, that is accumulated in the skin during the early period, and lipofuscin, that gets deposited around 6 months later, leading to reversible hyperpigmentation [30]. Deposition of lipofuscin in dermal macrophages is also described in amiodarone-induced hyperpigmentation [31]. Minocycline-induced pigmenta-

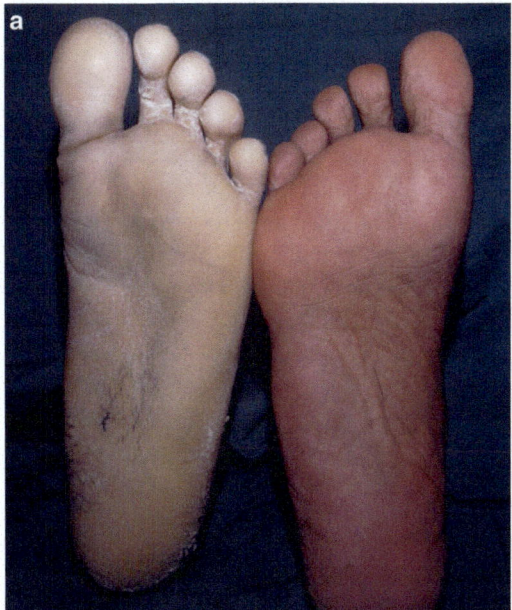

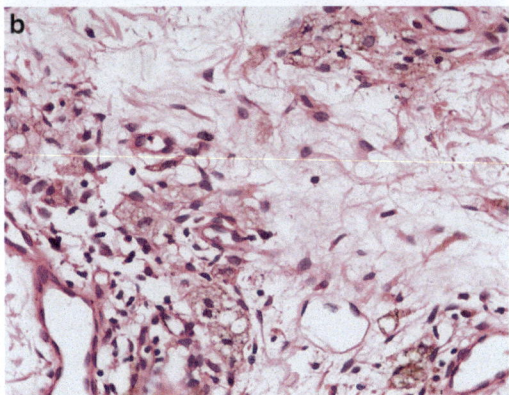

Fig. 2.7 Clofazimine pigmentation. (**a**) Orange-red discolouration of the sole. The control foot (L) is of a person of similar skin colour not taking the drug. (**b**) Brownish pigment within foamy macrophages (H&E, x400)

tion has been classified into three types: type I, bluish-grey pigmentation in old scars; type II, bluish-grey pigmentation of apparently normal skin; and type III, brownish pigmentation of photo-exposed areas [32].

Biopsies show some increase in epidermal melanin. There are pigmented macrophages around vessels and appendages in the dermis which contain melanin, haemosiderin or lipofuscin (Fig. 2.7b). These pigments can be identified by appropriate stains. Clofazimine-induced lipofuscin pigment stains positively with Mallory's haemofuscin stain [30]. Minocycline-induced pigment deposits stain positively with Masson-Fontana in all three types and with Perl's stain in types I and II [32]. The yellow-brown pigment induced by antimalarial drugs stains weakly with Perl's stain. Amiodarone-induced yellow-brown pigment granules in the macrophages are stained with periodic acid-Schiff (PAS) stain [31]. The relative depth of pigment deposits has been used to type the pigmentation caused by minocycline [32]. Electron microscopy in minocycline-induced bluish-grey hyperpigmentation shows electron-dense particles both within and outside macrophages [32]. In amiodarone-induced hyperpigmentation, there are intra-cytoplasmic lysosomal membrane-bound bodies, also known as 'myelin bodies' [31].

Heavy Metal-Induced Pigmentation

Deposits of heavy metals such as gold, silver and bismuth produce a slate-grey skin pigmentation that is usually more pronounced in sun-exposed areas and is long lasting. Of these rare diseases, silver deposits or argyria is most likely to present to a dermatologist. It is caused by local or systemic exposure to silver salts. Localized exposure occurs at the sites of contact with silver-containing topical medication and jewellery, while systemic exposure occurs due to the ingestion of silver in medication or food. There is a wide individual variation in the quantum and duration of exposure required to produce argyria. Following systemic intake, argyria results in an ashy to blue-black, diffuse pigmentation that affects both the skin (Fig. 2.8a) and mucosae. The slate-blue colour is due to both silver salts and increased melanin [33].

Biopsies from argyric skin appear normal at first glance apart from some increase in epidermal melanin content. On higher magnification, there are several, distinctive, uniformly sized, tiny black dots in vessel walls, around eccrine glands and in the connective tissue sheaths around hair follicles (Fig. 2.8b). In addition, smaller numbers may be seen lying free in the dermis [33].

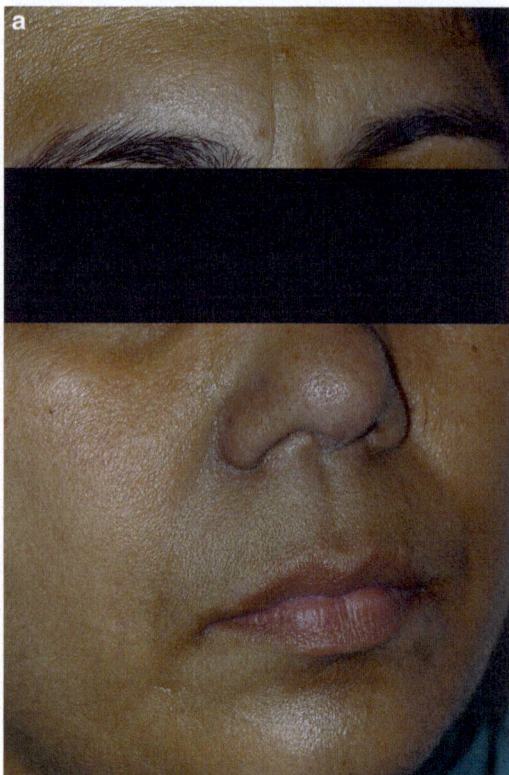

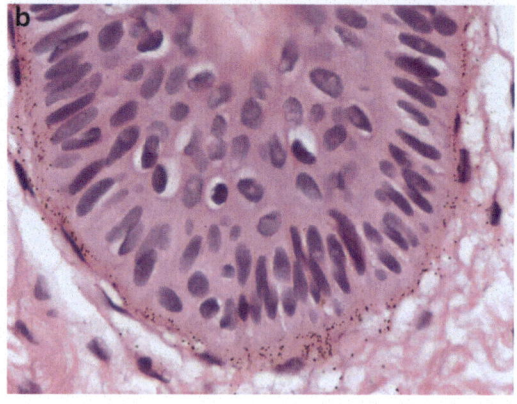

Fig. 2.8 Argyria. (**a**) Faint greenish discolouration of the face, most prominent on the nose and lip. (**b**) Fine pigment granules in the fibrous sheath of a hair follicle (H&E, x1000) (courtesy of Dr Asha Kubba)

Cutaneous silver deposits are also detectable using dark-ground microscopy and electron microscopy, which may be useful in cases where no findings are seen on light microscopy. The appearance of silver deposits on dark-ground microscopy is also known as 'stars in heaven' pattern [34]. Electron dense deposits measuring around 100–500 nm are seen on electron microscopy [35].

In chrysiasis (gold-induced pigmentation), round black granules are deposited in macrophages around blood vessels in the dermis. These are larger than silver granules and are not deposited in membranes, unlike silver deposits. Orange-red birefringence of gold deposits on fluorescent microscopy is observed [36]. Bismuth gets deposited as small granules in the dermis, including in membranes [37].

Talon Noir

This condition, also known as black heel, presents with dark spots of recent origin usually on the soles of the feet [38] (Fig. 2.9a). Lesions are usually bilateral and there is a history of jogging or prolonged walking. When the clinical diagnosis is not suspected, eruptive nevi, lentigines and acral nevi/melanoma may be considered. If a biopsy is undertaken, the histopathological findings are confined to the stratum corneum which shows intracorneal haemorrhage [38] (Fig. 2.9b). Depending on how old the haemorrhage is, one can see RBCs or an orange-yellow stained crust. This material stains negatively with Perl's stain for haemosiderin but often stains positively with benzidine for haemoglobin [39].

Once the pigmentation is confirmed to be due to blood, the diagnosis is proved and other conditions can be safely excluded. Lesions resolve spontaneously in a few days but may recur.

Pigmented Purpuric Dermatoses

This is a group of disorders manifesting as brown macules on the lower extremities in young adults, accompanied by purpuric macules that may be difficult to discern in brown skin. Six variants are described: Schamberg's disease (Fig. 2.10a), purpura annularis telangiectodes of Majocchi, lichen aureus, itching purpura of pigmented purpuric dermatitis of

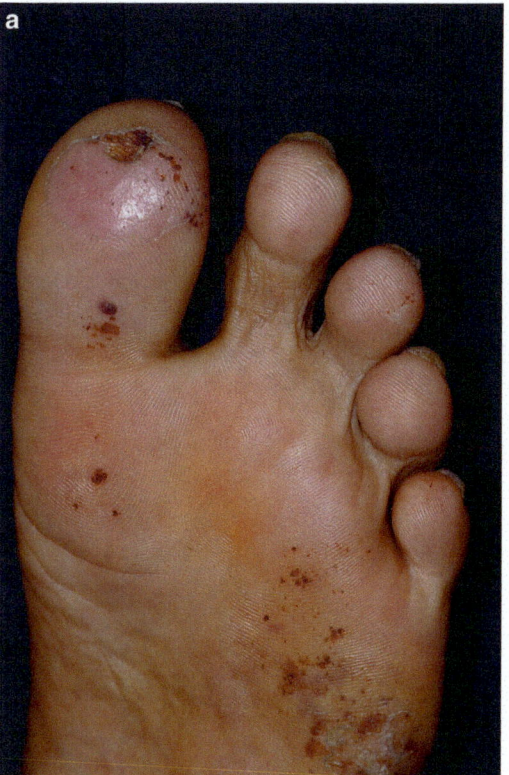

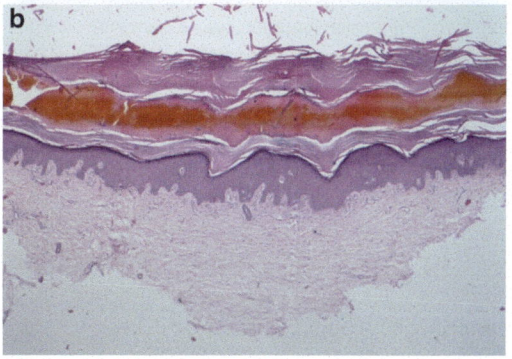

Fig. 2.9 Talon noir. (**a**) Scattered small, irregular, reddish-brown macules on the sole. (**b**) Intracorneal haemorrhage (H&E, X40)

Gougerot and Blum, eczematid-like purpura of Kapetanakis and granulomatous pigmented purpura. Histopathologically, a band-like infiltrate of lymphocytes and histiocytes is seen in the upper dermis accompanied by extravasation of RBCs admixed with siderophages (Fig. 2.10b). A Perl's stain highlights the presence of haemosiderin (Fig. 2.10c) [40].

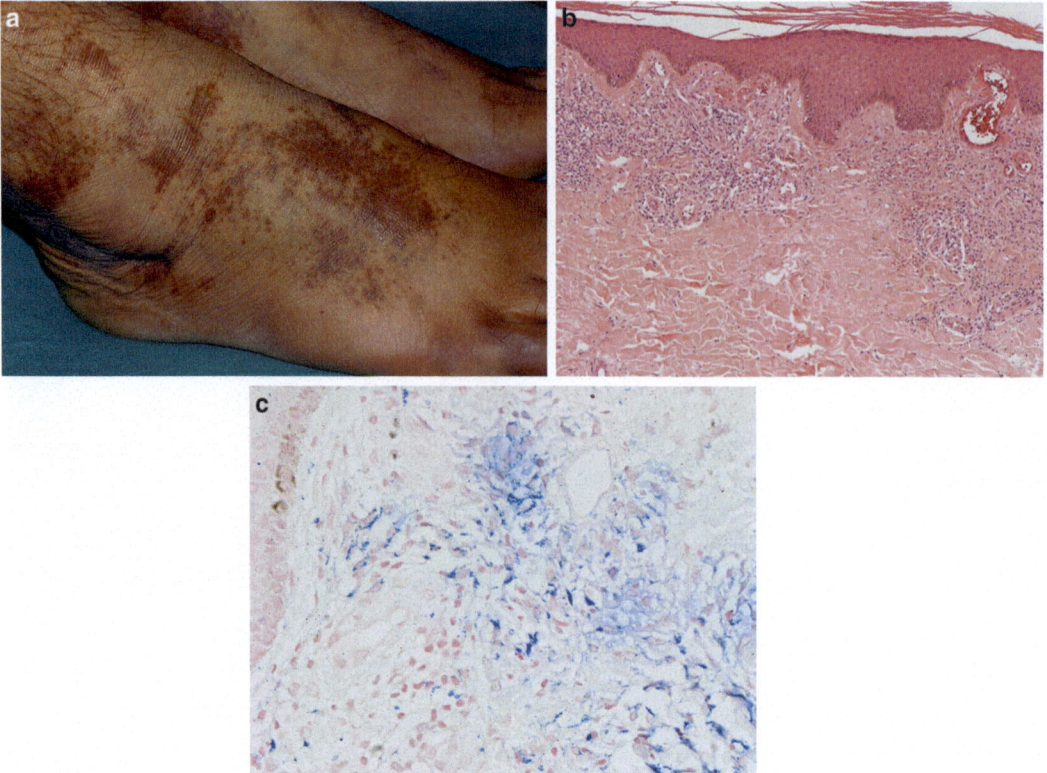

Fig. 2.10 Pigmented purpuric dermatosis. (**a**) Brown tiny macules becoming confluent at places on the feet and lower legs. (**b**) Band-like infiltrate of lymphocytes and histiocytes with extravasated RBCs and dilated capillaries in upper dermis (H&E, X200). (**c**) Haemosiderin (Perl's stain, X40)

Ochronosis

In ochronosis, the superficial dermis reveals clumps of golden brown, crescentic and fragmented collagen fibres [41] (Fig. 2.11a). In addition, pigment may be present free in the dermis or within sweat glands or vessels [42]. Methylene blue stains the fibres a dark blue-black colour. Ultrastructurally, electron-dense deposits are found in the elastic fibres and interstitium. An identical histopathological appearance is seen in alkaptonuria [43]. Clinically, the condition usually presents in a patient with melasma or another hyperpigmented disorder who has been applying hydroquinone as a prescription or over-the-counter skin lightening cream for long without significant benefit [44] (Fig. 2.11b). The development of reticulation and darkening of pigment has been identified as an early clue to exogenous

ochronosis. Unfortunately, in some patients, this leads to a more vigorous use of higher strengths of hydroquinone and perpetuates the process. In established disease, there is bilaterally symmetrical involvement of malar areas and temples with blue-grey speckled pigmentation and pinpoint 'caviar-like' papules and, less commonly, nodules. Dermoscopic features are irregular annular, arciform and globular structures on a background of diffuse hyperpigmentation. Recently curvilinear worm-like structures were described [45]. In some African countries, hydroquinone use is far more widespread with creams being applied all over the body for months and years [42].

Alkaptonuria has a similar histopathological appearance but a different clinical presentation [43]. The disease occurs due to the accumulation of homogentisic acid in tissues due to the inherited deficiency of the enzyme homogentisate

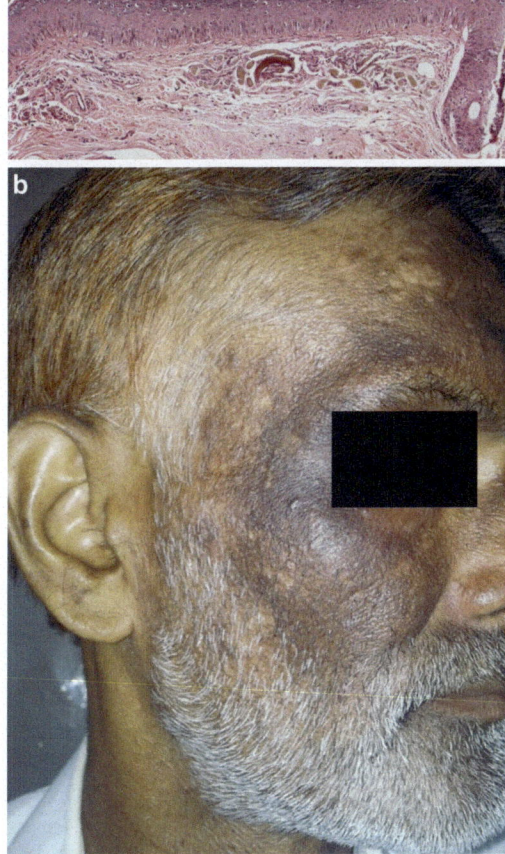

Fig. 2.11 Ochronosis. (**a**) Golden brown crescentic and globular pigment deposits in upper dermis (H&E, X200) (courtesy Dr Avninder Singh). (**b**) Confluent brownish-black pigmentation with confetti-like hypopigmented macules at the periphery (courtesy Dr Kanika Sahni)

1,2-dioxygenase (HGO). Patients present with arthritis and discolouration of sclera and ear cartilage in the fourth decade of life. In some patients, there is pigmentation of plaques on the palms and soles. However, staining of diapers and dark colouration of urine on standing may be noticed from early childhood.

III Clues: Additional Histopathological Findings

In a number of different conditions, clues to the histopathological diagnosis of a pigmentary disorder come from the presence of findings not related to the pigmentary system. In some cases, there is a pathogenetic connection between the histopathological process and the clinical manifestation of pigmentation. For example, a lichenoid tissue reaction leads to basal cell damage and pigment incontinence producing the pigmentary changes seen in lichen planus pigmentosus. In other instances, such as macular amyloidosis and lichen sclerosus, the pathogenetic connection is obscure, but the histopathological findings are distinctive and help to confirm the diagnosis.

Lichen Planus Pigmentosus

This is an idiopathic condition of uncertain pathogenesis which presents with ashy pigmentation predominantly on the exposed skin of the face, neck and arms (Fig. 2.12a) [46]. Pigmentation usually begins as asymptomatic, small macules that enlarge in size and become confluent. In some patients, pigmentation is more prominent in flexures such as the antecubital fossae, axillae and inframammary and neck folds. The hyperpigmentation is usually uniform, but in some patients, it may be vaguely reticular [46]. Other patterns described are blotchy and perifollicular. Combinations of different distributions and types of pigmentation may occur in the same patient. Unilateral and linear variants have been described [47, 48]. In a small proportion of patients, papular and mucosal lichen planus has been noted [49]. A gradual increase in extent and intensity of pigmentation is common but may be followed in several months by fading and complete clearance.

Biopsies show numerous melanophages in the superficial dermis as a constant feature. This may be the only finding in the majority of biopsies from this condition. Early in disease, an upper dermal lichenoid infiltrate of lymphocytes is seen with basal cell damage in the overlying epidermis [50] (Fig. 2.12b). Biopsies taken at an intermediate stage show colloid bodies and a mild infiltrate in the papillary dermis as evidence of a subsiding lichenoid process (Fig. 2.12c). In combination with the clinical picture, this provides evidence

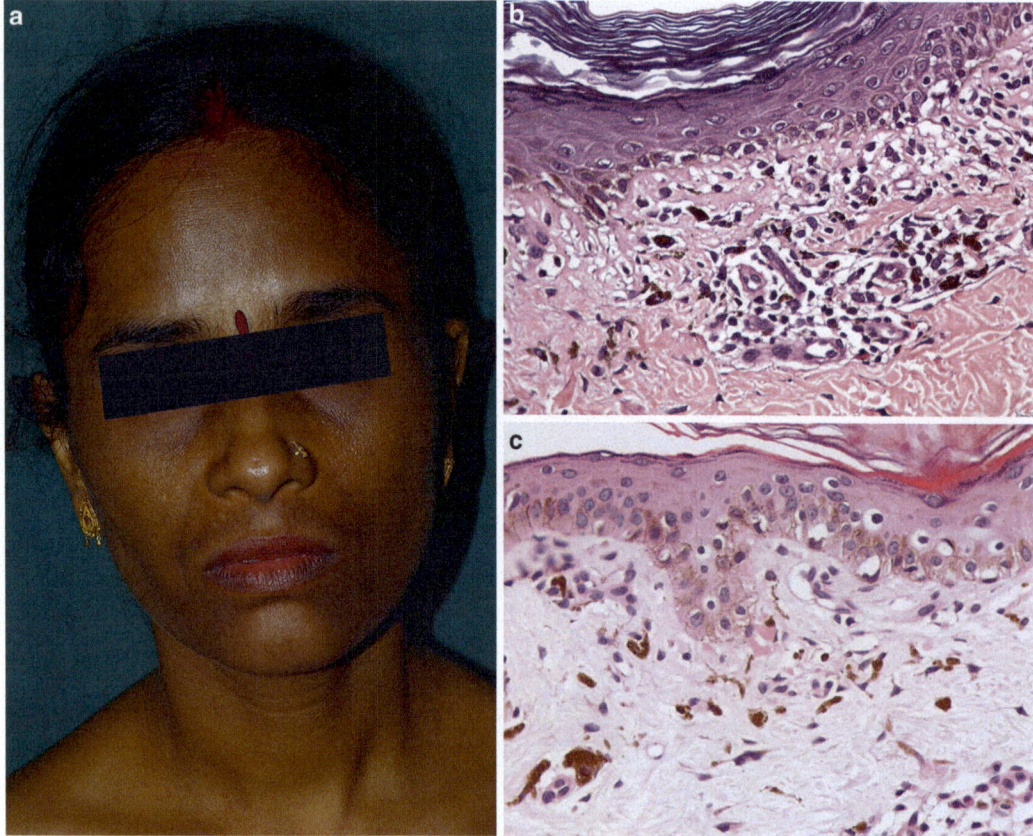

Fig. 2.12 Lichen planus pigmentosus. (**a**) Ashy pigmentation on the face relatively sparing the neck. (**b**) Basal layer vacuolization with a moderate upper dermal infiltrate and pigment incontinence (H&E, x400). (**c**) Pigment incontinence with a few colloid bodies in the papillary dermis (H&E, x200)

for a diagnosis of lichen planus pigmentosus. In a study of 65 patients of lichen planus pigmentosus, basal cell degeneration was reported in 78.5% of patients with melanophages in the upper dermis in 63% and a band-like lichenoid infiltrate in 18% [51]. However, in an unpublished series of 40 cases recently seen in our department, we found melanophages in all biopsies and basal cell degeneration in only three (7.5%) cases.

Ashy dermatosis and erythema dyschromicum perstans probably represent the same disease. The term lichen planus pigmentosus should not be used to describe the persistent, dark brown pigmentation that follows the subsidence of lichen planus and the papular/plaque form of lichenoid eruption.

Dowling-Degos Disease and Reticulate Acropigmentation of Kitamura

Dowling-Degos disease, also known as reticulate pigmentary anomaly of the flexures, manifests pigmented macules which, in spite of the name, show a mottled rather than a truly reticulate appearance (Fig. 2.13a). These macules are noted in the skin flexures and beyond them. Some patients show pigmented follicular pits and papules in addition, and in some, this is a prominent finding. Hypopigmented macules may be noted on the trunk in a subset of patients [52]. Follicular Dowling-Degos disease is a recently described variant with folliculocentric hyperpigmented macules, comedones and pitted

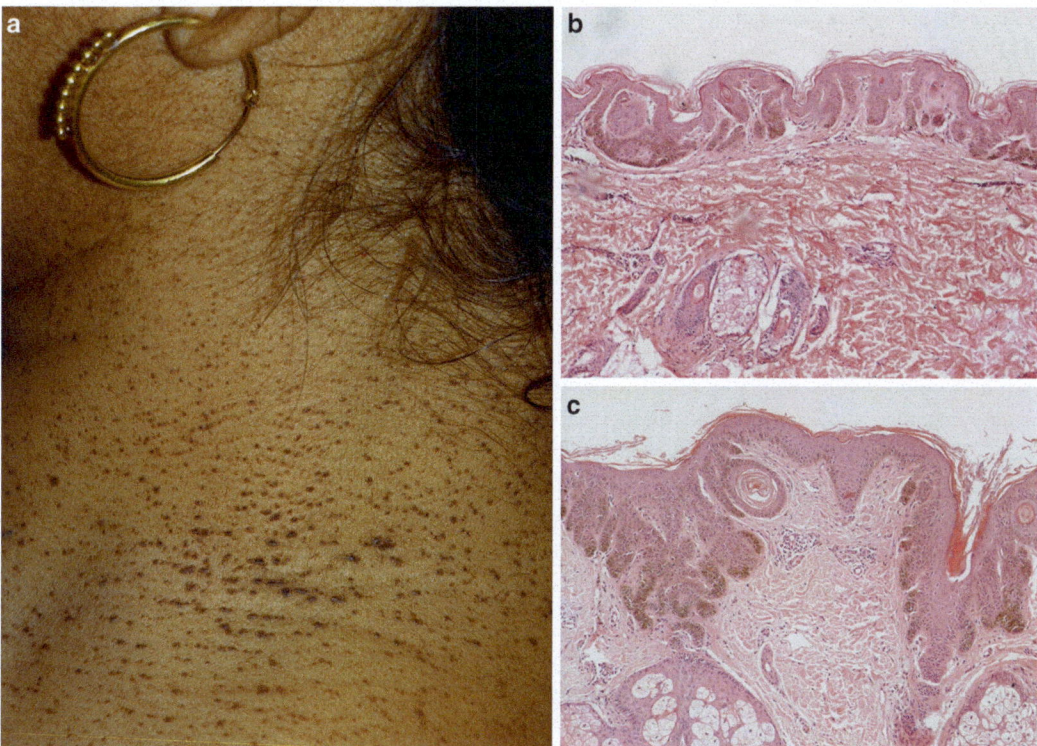

Fig. 2.13 Dowling-Degos disease. (**a**) Brownish macules and follicular papules in a mottled pattern on the neck. (**b**) Elongated, finger-like rete pegs with increased pigmenta- tion at the tips (H&E, x100). (**c**) These changes are limited to the follicular epithelium in follicular Dowling-Degos disease (H&E, X200)

scars that lacks the classical mottled flexural pig- mentation [53].

Reticulate acropigmentation of Kitamura presents with small, brown, angulated, slightly depressed macules on the sides of the forehead and face and on the hands and feet. Palmar der- matoglyphics show breaks [54].

Because of the overlap in clinical features, it was believed that Dowling-Degos disease was in a continuum with Kitamura's reticulate acropigmen- tation with some members of an affected family showing one disease, while some members showed the other and some patients show clinical features of both diseases [55].However, studies have revealed distinct genes underlying these diseases: KRT5 gene on chromosome 12q13 in Dowling- Degos disease and ADAM10 gene on chromosome 15q21 in Kitamura's reticulate acropigmentation.

Biopsy shows slender prolongations of rete pegs that extend into the dermis and interconnect with each other. These rete pegs show melaniza- tion that is notably greater than within the surface epidermis and adjacent, normal rete [52] (Fig. 2.13b). Similar epidermal prolongations are seen from follicular epithelium. Pseudo-horn cysts and comedo-like features are seen in some cases.

In follicular Dowling-Degos, these changes are confined to the hair follicle with the interven- ing interfollicular epithelium showing mild or no change [53] (Fig. 2.13c).

When the histopathological changes of Dowling-Degos disease are accompanied by acantholysis, the condition is termed Galli-Galli disease [56]. The clinical appearance is identical to that of patients who show no acantholysis.

Reticulate acropigmentation of Kitamura shows elongated thin rete pegs with increased pigmentation at the tips and epidermal thinning.

Melanosomes within keratinocytes and melanocytes are increased in number on electron microscopy [57].

Indeterminate Leprosy

Indeterminate leprosy usually presents in children and young adults with ill-defined hypopigmented macules showing variable hypoesthesia (Fig. 2.14a), and patients may seek medical advice for the pigmentary change [58]. It may be difficult to document the loss of sensation as children find it difficult to provide clear responses during sensory testing. Occasionally, one of the unnamed sensory nerve twigs supplying the affected area may be thickened and can be palpated as a thread-like structure in the vicinity of the patch. Regional nerve thickening is absent, as are macules in other areas of the body. This is a difficult clinical diagnosis to make even in endemic areas, and the differential diagnoses include pityriasis alba, early vitiligo and postinflammatory hypopigmentation.

Biopsies from indeterminate leprosy show mild, superficial and deep dermal infiltrates of lymphocytes and a few histiocytes (Fig. 2.14b) arranged around vessels and nerve twigs (Fig. 2.14c). Stain for acid fast bacilli is usually negative. These findings, in the appropriate clinical context, constitute evidence for a diagnosis of indeterminate leprosy.

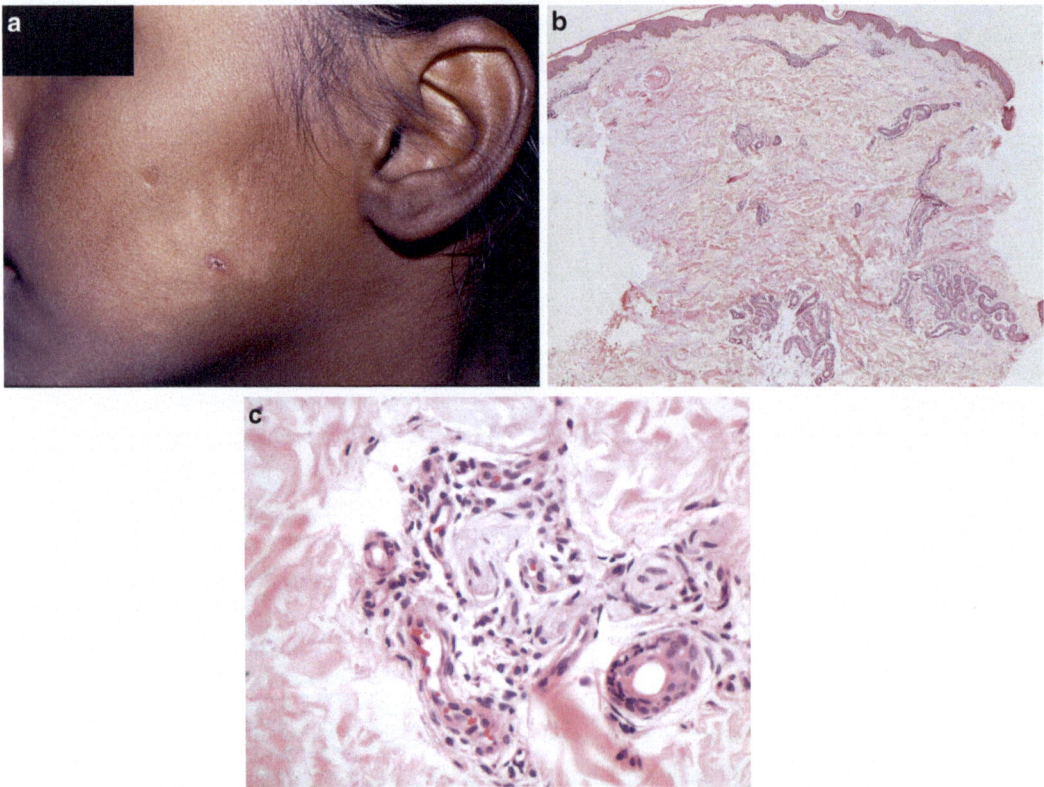

Fig. 2.14 Indeterminate leprosy. (**a**) Ill-defined hypopigmented macule on the cheek. (**b**) Superficial and deep mild infiltrates inflammatory (H&E, X100). (**c**) Perineural infiltrate of lymphocytes and histiocytes (H&E, x400)

Pityriasis Alba: 'Hypopigmenting Dermatitis'

Pityriasis alba presents as ill-defined, hypopigmented, finely scaly macules on the face in children (Fig. 2.15a). Macules come and go over several weeks and months. In this classical presentation, the disease is easily recognized and hardly ever biopsied.

However, a condition that is probably similar causes greater diagnostic difficulty when it occurs on the trunk and extremities in young adults. These macules tend to be larger, about 5–7 cm in size, more hypopigmented and better defined. Fine scaling may be associated. Hair loss is frequently noted (Fig. 2.15b). Since a combination of hypopigmentation and hair loss is common in leprosy, some of these patients are labelled macular tuberculoid leprosy even though cutaneous sensations over the patches are invariably normal. Some also receive antileprosy treatment, to no avail.

We have studied biopsies of some of these patients and noted mild to moderate spongiotic changes in the follicular infundibulum along with lymphocyte exocytosis (Fig. 2.15c), a feature that has also been reported in pityriasis alba [59]. Importantly, none of them have the superficial and deep, perivascular and perineural lymphocytic infiltrates of indeterminate leprosy. In reporting these biopsies, it is important to take sufficient sections to include the follicular epithelium and to mention the absence of features of leprosy, since this is frequently the clinical concern that prompted the biopsy.

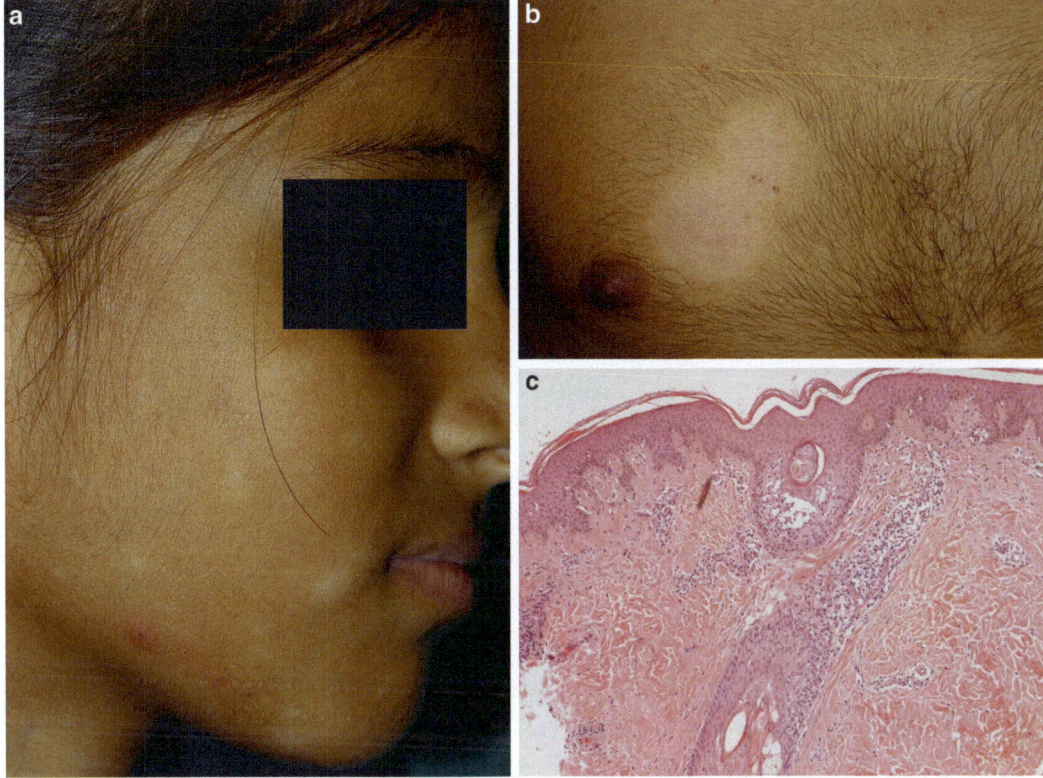

Fig. 2.15 Pityriasis alba. (**a**) Multiple, ill-defined hypopigmented macules in a child (**b**) Hypopigmented, well-defined macule with hair loss. (**c**) Hair follicle showing spongiosis and lymphocyte exocytosis (H&E, x200)

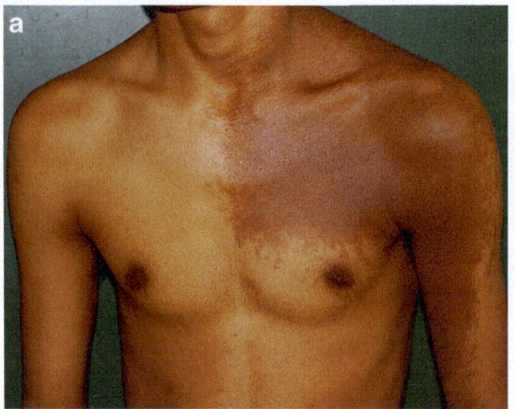

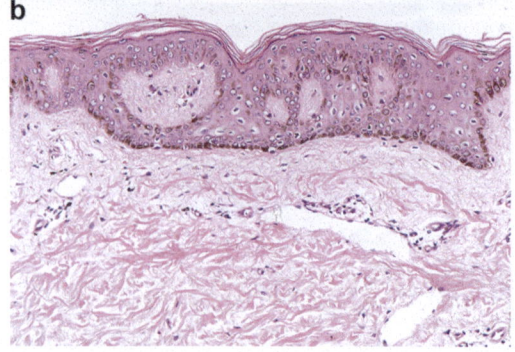

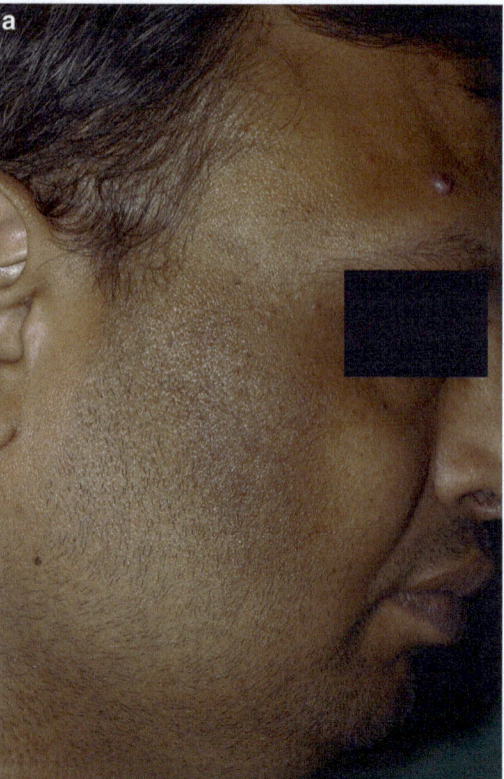

Fig. 2.16 Becker's nevus. (**a**) Unilateral dark brown pigmented macule with splashed margins in a checkerboard pattern. (**b**) Flattening and fusion of the bases of pigmented rete pegs (H&E, X400)

Becker's Nevus

Becker's nevus, a pigmented hairy epidermal nevus, classically manifests as a single, sharply demarcated, unilateral, tan-coloured macule with splashed margins over the shoulder or pectoral area usually presenting at adolescence. It is seen more frequently in men [60] (Fig. 2.16a). Multiple Becker's nevi have been described [61]. Rarely it can occur at atypical sites such as the legs [62]. It is rarely associated with ipsilateral developmental anomalies, known as the Becker's nevus syndrome [63].

Biopsy shows mild papillomatosis, acanthosis and increased basal layer pigmentation. The enlarged rete pegs are squared off, with a flat lower edge (Fig. 2.16b). Ultrastructural studies reveal an increase in the number and size of melanosomes in the stratum basale and spinosum.

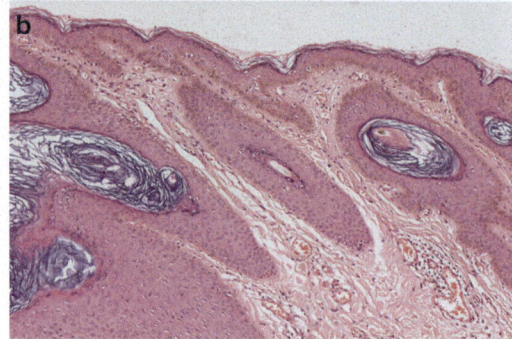

Fig. 2.17 Acanthosis nigricans. (**a**) Ill-defined brownish patches on side of the face. (**b**) Papillomatosis, acanthosis and prominent basal layer pigmentation (H&E, x200) (courtesy Dr Avninder Singh)

Acanthosis Nigricans

Acanthosis nigricans may present as facial pigmentation. Typically, the sides of the face are affected, not the front or the butterfly area (Fig. 2.17a). As disease progresses, there is further darkening and a mild, thickening of the skin. Obesity is commonly associated, and hyperinsulinemia has been documented in these patients

[64]. The usual, recognizable appearance of acanthosis nigricans as velvety, papillomatous skin occurs only in late disease, and many of these patients receive skin lightening creams for hyperpigmentation. If the diagnosis is suspected, evidence to corroborate the diagnosis may be found in axillary acanthosis nigricans which is frequently present concomitantly. Acanthosis nigricans of the neck folds develops late.

Biopsies from these cases of subtle acanthosis nigricans show subtle changes of hyperkeratosis and papillomatosis [64] (Fig. 2.17b). These findings become more obvious as disease advances.

Joshi et al. described a condition characterized histologically by 'pigmented papillomatosis' that they labelled idiopathic eruptive macular pigmentation [65]. The disease presents with brown-black, velvety, round and oval macules and thin plaques on the trunk and proximal extremities, usually starting in adolescence. Skin biopsy shows findings similar to acanthosis nigricans of which it probably represents an eruptive variant.

Solar Lentigo/Flat Seborrheic Keratosis

This presents as sharply demarcated brown-black flat macules and plaques on sun-exposed skin in the elderly (Fig. 2.18a). When flat, early seborrheic keratosis can cause diagnostic confusion with other macular pigmentary disorders. Histopathologically, rete ridges are bulbous and sometimes fused, with increased basilar pigmentation which may be accompanied by an increased number of melanocytes and solar elastosis (Fig. 2.18b) [66].

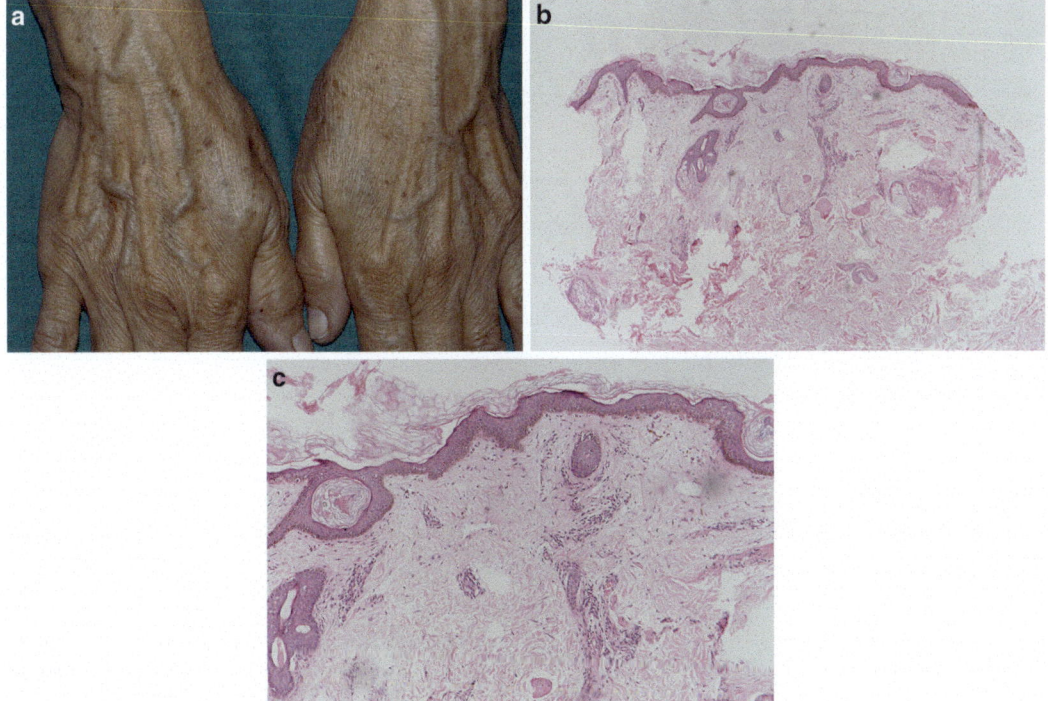

Fig. 2.18 Solar lentigo. (**a**) Symmetrical brownish macules on dorsa of hands in an elderly man. (**b**) Acanthosis and horn cysts (H&E, x40). (**c**) Prominent basal layer pigmentation (H&E, x200)

Macular Amyloidosis

Macular amyloidosis presents as brown-black hyperpigmentation on the extensors of the forearms and the legs (Fig. 2.19a) and on the upper back [67]. Some patients are itchy and have scratched their skin with their fingernails or other objects, but many have not. A helpful clinical clue is the presence of a rippled pattern to the pigmentation. Long-standing disease usually shows confluent pigmentation in the main, but areas of rippled pigmentation may be noted in some areas and assist in making the diagnosis.

Biopsy shows little under low power. Closer examination reveals small deposits of amyloid in the dermal papillae [67] (Fig. 2.19b). These are appreciated better with special stains for amyloid such as Congo red (Fig. 2.19c), crystal violet,

methyl violet and pagoda red. Apple-green birefringence is seen with Congo red stain. Diligence and some luck are required to find amyloid in macular amyloidosis. In patients who have both macular and papular cutaneous amyloidosis, referred to as 'biphasic amyloidosis', the chances of making a specific diagnosis are strengthened if a papule is chosen for biopsy [68].

Amyloidosis Cutis Dyschromica

The histopathological appearance of amyloidosis cutis dyschromica is indistinguishable from macular amyloidosis. However, the clinical appearance is rather different.

Patients present with an asymptomatic, mottled hypo- and hyperpigmentation that begins in

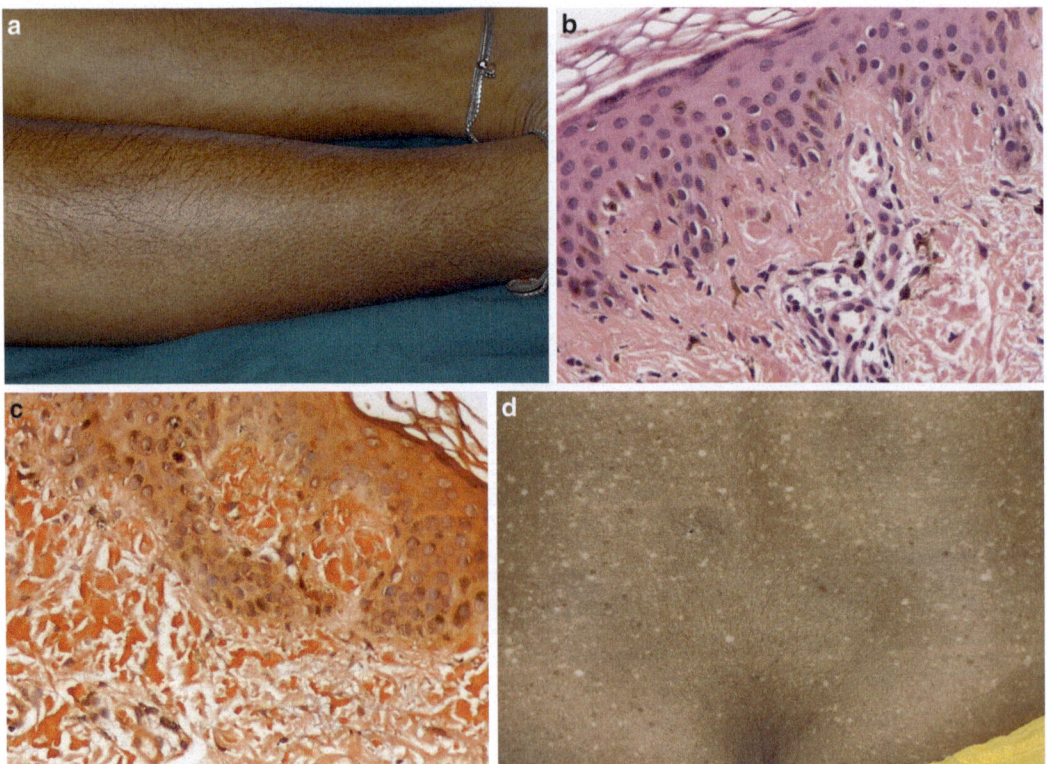

Fig. 2.19 Cutaneous amyloidosis. (**a**) Brownish, barely elevated macules arranged in a rippled pattern. (**b**) Eosinophilic globular deposits in the papillary dermis (H&E, X400). (**c**) Orange-reddish deposits of amyloid in the upper dermis (Congo red, x400). (**d**) Multiple, guttate, hypopigmented and hyperpigmented macules on a background of diffuse hyperpigmentation in amyloidosis cutis dyschromica

childhood (Fig. 2.19d). In some patients, papules are also associated. Ripple patterned hyperpigmentation may be seen in some areas [69]. Biopsies from both hypopigmented and hyperpigmented macules show amyloid deposits in the papillary dermis. As in macular amyloidosis, the amyloid is derived from keratinocytes and is not associated with systemic amyloidosis.

Hypopigmented Mycosis Fungoides

Mycosis fungoides may present as hypopigmentation in people with brown skin. This variant is commoner in children and young adults and presents with hypopigmented, irregularly shaped, small- and medium-sized macules that begin on the covered areas such as the buttocks (Fig. 2.20a). Clinically, hypopigmented mycosis fungoides can appear similar to pityriasis alba and indeterminate leprosy, and there are a number of reports describing vitiligo-like mycosis fungoides [70, 71]. This variant of mycosis fungoides behaves even more indolently than the classical type and progression to lymph node, and visceral disease is extremely uncommon.

Skin biopsy reveals a large number of lymphocytes in the epidermis without significant spongiosis [72] (Fig. 2.20b). As is usual in early mycosis fungoides, lymphocyte atypia is not seen. A papillary dermal infiltrate of lymphocytes between wiry collagen bundles may be noted.

Lichen Sclerosus

On dark skin, lichen sclerosus is hypo- or depigmented and can create genuine diagnostic difficulty on genital skin (Fig. 2.21a). It can be virtually impossible to tell genital vitiligo from early lichen sclerosus as both conditions present with depigmentation [73]. If disease is present at other sites, the morphology at the non-genital location may be helpful in making a diagnosis, but often this is the only site affected.

A skin biopsy shows sclerosis of the upper dermis with flattening of the overlying epidermis, follicular plugs (Fig. 2.21b) and basal cell damage. Colloid bodies or telangiectasias may also be seen. If the biopsy is taken before sclerosis is obvious, one notes aggregates of lymphocytes present between and around wiry bundles of collagen in the papillary dermis. These findings contrast sharply with those noted in vitiligo (see above). Scanning electron microscopy demonstrates homogenized collagen in the upper dermis and round structures corresponding to aggregates of immune complexes and matrix proteins along collagen fibres [74].

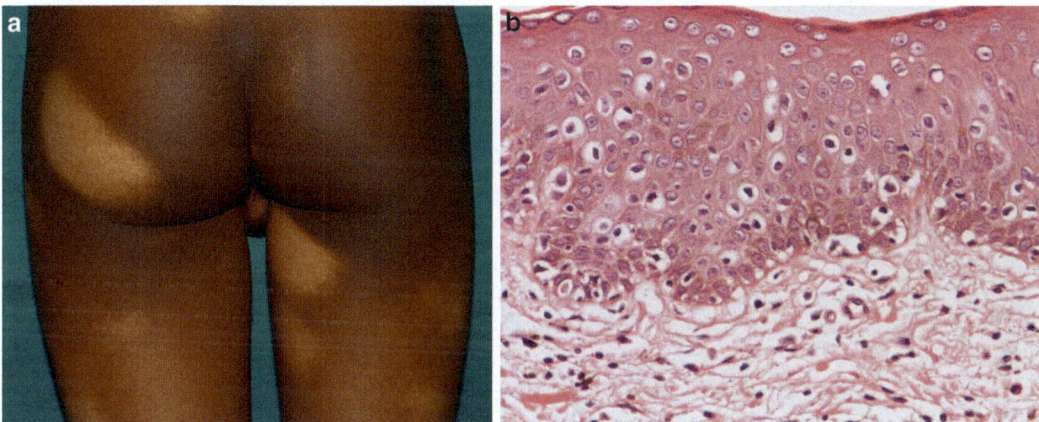

Fig. 2.20 Hypopigmented mycosis fungoides. (**a**) Hypopigmented macules on sun-protected sites. (**b**) Haloed lymphocytes in the epidermis larger than lymphocytes in the dermis (H&E, X400)

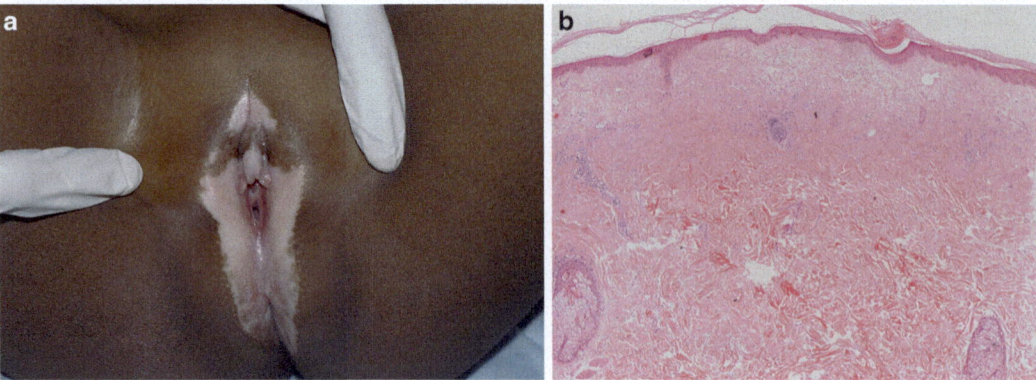

Fig. 2.21 Lichen sclerosus. (**a**) Well-defined depigmented macule on the labia majora. (**b**) Follicular plugging in the epidermis and pallor of the upper dermis (H&E, x200)

Morphoea, Atrophoderma of Pasini and Pierini

Morphoea is characterized by indurated plaques with ivory coloured or hypopigmented macules in the centre. While induration is striking in active morphoea, burnt-out morphoea shows only pigmentary alteration and a subtle change in skin texture. Hyperpigmentation is commoner than hypopigmentation. Dermal and subcutaneous atrophy may be clinically discernible. Skin biopsy at this stage of morphoea shows homogenization of collagen fibres in the dermis with mild perivascular lympho-plasmacytic infiltrates. Atrophoderma of Pasini and Pierini has a similar clinical and histopathological appearance. Polarized microscopy has been used to highlight the homogenized collagen bundles [75].

Connective Tissue Disease-Associated Pigmentary Changes

Diffuse hyperpigmentation and depigmented macules on a background of hyperpigmentation, 'salt and pepper pigmentation', can occur in systemic sclerosis. Some reports of its occurrence in isolation, preceding development of other cutaneous features such as bound-down skin, suggest its usefulness as an indicator of developing systemic sclerosis [76]. In a recent unpublished study on the histopathological spectrum of pig-

mentary changes in systemic sclerosis undertaken in our department, we found fairly uniform basal layer melanization and pigment incontinence in biopsies from hyperpigmented areas, while the areas with 'salt and pepper' pigmentation showed a variegation in basal layer pigmentation. Interestingly, more melanophages were noted beneath the pale, less pigmented basal layer than the more pigmented portion.

Poikiloderma, a combination of hyper- or hypopigmentation, epidermal atrophy and telangiectasias, is a characteristic feature of dermatomyositis. It may or may not be accompanied by myositis. The violaceous colour and distribution in periorbital areas (heliotrope rash) and extensors of limbs, which may accompany poikiloderma in some cases, are characteristic and distinguish it from poikilodermatous changes in other dermatological disorders including cutaneous T-cell lymphoma. Skin biopsy shows vacuolar alteration of the epidermis, epidermal atrophy, dilated capillaries in upper dermis and a mild perivascular infiltrate of lymphocytes and histiocytes in the upper dermis. These histopathological changes are indistinguishable from those of lupus erythematosus [77].

Epidermodysplasia Verruciformis

The pityriasis versicolour-like lesions of epidermodysplasia verruciformis appear as hypopigmented

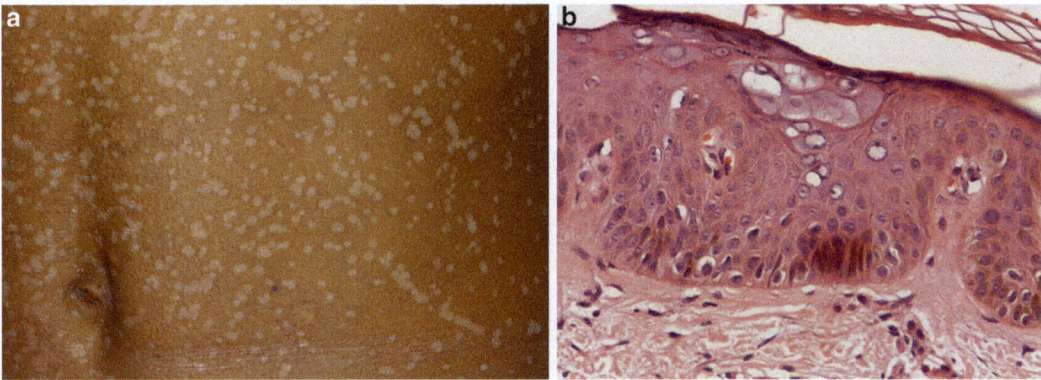

Fig. 2.22 Epidermodysplasia verruciformis. (**a**) Multiple hypopigmented macules with koebnerization. (**b**) Large keratinocytes with abundant pale blue cytoplasm arranged discretely and in nests in the epidermis (H&E, x400)

macules [78] (Fig. 2.22a). When these are the major clinical manifestation, the patient may present with what appears to be a pigmentary disorder.

Skin biopsy reveals some acanthosis with focal aggregates of large keratinocytes in the upper epidermis. These keratinocytes have abundant pale blue cytoplasm, enlarged nuclei and prominent nucleoli (Fig. 2.22b). The keratohyalin granules in these cells are coarse and large. Koilocytes are not seen. Ultrastructurally, papova virus particles and antigens have been observed in the stratum spinosum and stratum granulosum in lesional biopsy scrapings [79].

Plane wart-like lesions in epidermodysplasia verruciformis have the same clinical and histopathological features as ordinary plane warts. There are slightly elevated hyperpigmented or skin-coloured small papules [78]. Histopathological changes are subtle, unlike common warts. Mild acanthosis and papillomatosis are accompanied by koilocytic changes in the upper stratum spinosum.

Superficial Pigmented Mycoses

Superficial mycoses are commonly seen in tropical climates. Pityriasis versicolour presents as flat hypo- or hyperpigmented, round and oval macules with mild branny scaling seen on seborrheic sites, particularly the upper back and shoulders.

Hypopigmentation is ascribed to the melanocyte inhibitory effects of dicarboxylic acids of the causative fungus, *Malassezia furfur*. Skin biopsy shows hyperkeratosis, mild acanthosis and parakeratosis along with short septate hyphae and budding yeasts in the stratum corneum [80]. Tinea nigra is caused by *Hortaea werneckii* and usually affects young children. It presents as brown, well defined, small macules on the palm or sole that may be confused with acral melanocytic nevus or melanoma [80]. Skin biopsy shows compact hyperkeratosis and brown septate hyphae and spores in the stratum corneum. Diamond-shaped spaces in the cornified layer are described. Periodic acid-Schiff (PAS) staining helps to delineate fungal elements.

Hairy Pigmented Macules in Neurofibromatosis

In neurofibromatosis, café-au-lait macules are present in large numbers. In addition, patients may have hairy pigmented macules (Fig. 2.23a); the colour of these macules tends to be darker brown than café-au-lait macules but the resemblance is close enough to cause confusion. These hairy macules represent early plexiform neurofibromas. A biopsy of adequate depth shows pale fascicles of spindle cells at the junction of the dermis and subcutis [81] (Fig. 2.23b, c).

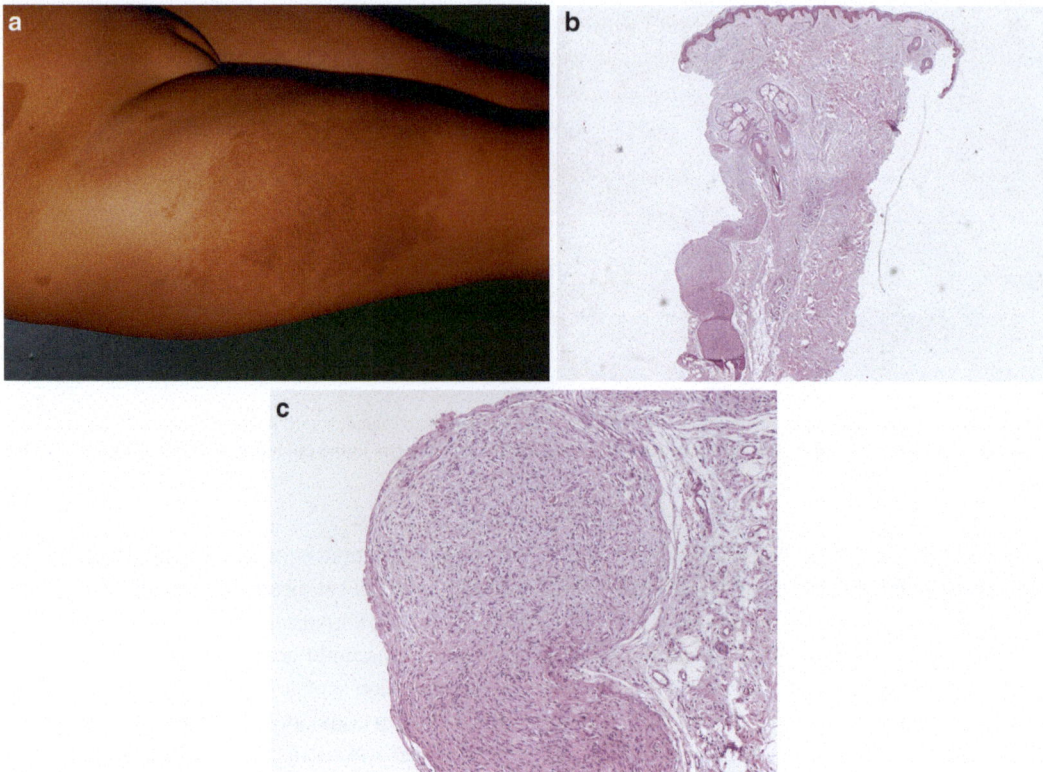

Fig. 2.23 Plexiform neurofibroma. (**a**) Hairy hyperpigmented macule with a splashed irregular border on the thigh. (**b**) Lower dermis shows a spindle cell proliferation on the left edge of the biopsy (H&E, x40). (**c**) The spindle cell proliferation consists of cells with elongated, slender, wavy nuclei (H&E, X200)

Leucoderma Syphiliticum

This is a rare manifestation of early or late secondary syphilis, usually seen as hypopigmented macules following healing of papules of secondary syphilis or rarely, as a primary manifestation [82, 83]. The macules usually develop around 6 months after onset of disease. Depigmented macules on the back and lateral portion of neck are known as the 'necklace of Venus'.

Histopathologically, there is a mild infiltrate, limited to the superficial perivascular areas. Plasma cells and the endarteritis obliterans of syphilis are usually not seen in these macules. These biopsy findings are not pathognomonic and need to be interpreted in conjunction with the appropriate clinical setting along with the results of serological tests. However, there are two reports of an intense lympho-plasmacytic infiltrate in perivascular areas and a band-like pattern in biopsies taken from depigmented macules [82, 84]. Ultrastructural studies have shown normal melanocytes in leucoderma syphiliticum, and depigmentation is attributed to an abnormality in melanin transfer [85].

Clear Cell Papulosis

This is an exceedingly rare condition affecting children in the age group of 1–4 years. It is considered to be a benign counterpart of extramammary Paget's disease. Affected patients present with hypopigmented macules and papules on the anterior chest and abdomen, usually along the milk line [86].

Biopsy from involved skin shows acanthosis and 'clear cells' which are large keratinocytes mainly found in the basal layer of the epidermis and in lesser numbers in the upper layers. These cells contain abundant mucin. Focal clustering and nuclear grooving of these cells have been observed by some authors [86, 87]. The cells closely resemble Toker cells in the nipple as well as Paget cells but can be differentiated by the presence of intra-cytoplasmic mucin in clear cell papulosis, which is not seen in Toker cells [87]. The immunohistochemical profile of these cells suggests an eccrine origin as they stain with carcinoembryonic antigen, cytokeratin CK-7, epithelial membrane antigen and IKH-4 antibody and do not stain or stain weakly with gross cystic disease fluid protein (GCDFP) antigen [88]. Paget cells, on the other hand, stain strongly with gross cystic disease fluid protein antigen, suggesting an apocrine origin. The clinical features, age of onset and immunohistochemistry are helpful in differentiating clear cell papulosis from other conditions with clear cells in the epidermis including extra-mammary Paget's disease, pagetoid squamous cell carcinoma, sebaceous carcinoma and pagetoid melanoma. The hypopigmentation may be due to a defect in melanogenesis as suggested by a report of reduced melanin pigment in the areas of the epidermis occupied by clear cells [87].

Hypopigmented Acantholytic Disorders

Confetti-like hypopigmented macules are described in Darier's disease and Grover's disease, more apparent in darkly pigmented skin. These may occur in isolation or along with the classical clinical manifestations. Disseminated and unilateral segmental variants are known (Fig. 2.24a) [89]. Biopsy from hypopigmented macules shows subtle suprabasal acantholysis with dyskeratotic keratinocytes (Fig. 2.24b). These findings are considerably less prominent than in keratotic papules. Electron microscopy in hypopigmented macules of Grover's disease reveals a decrease in melanocyte number and variation in size of keratinocytes, with condensed tonofilaments and vacuoles in the cytoplasm limited to the lower layers of the epidermis [90]. On the contrary, hypopigmentation in Darier's dis-

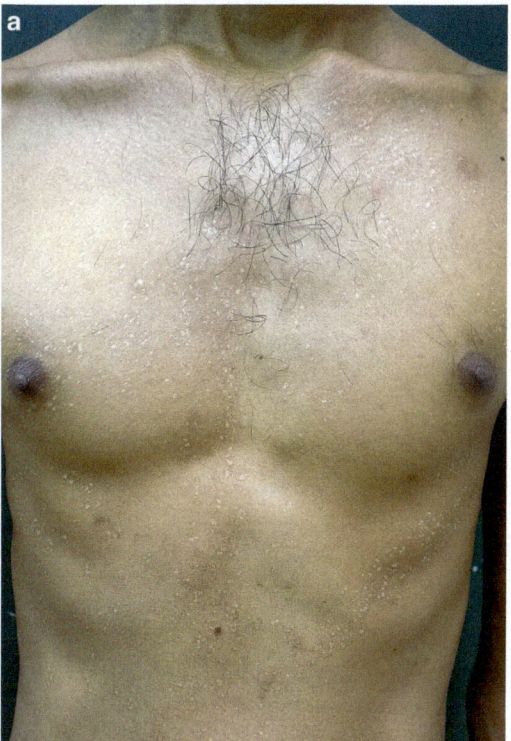

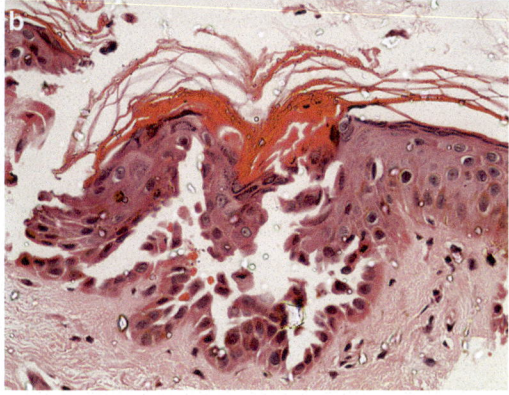

Fig. 2.24 Darier's disease. (**a**) Multiple guttate depigmented macules in a blaschkoid pattern. (**b**) The epidermis shows suprabasal acantholysis with dyskeratotic keratinocytes (H&E, 400)

ease was attributed to abnormal melanosomes on the basis of electron microscopy studies [90].

Urticaria Pigmentosa

Accumulation of mast cells in the skin can present either as hyperpigmented macules (urticaria

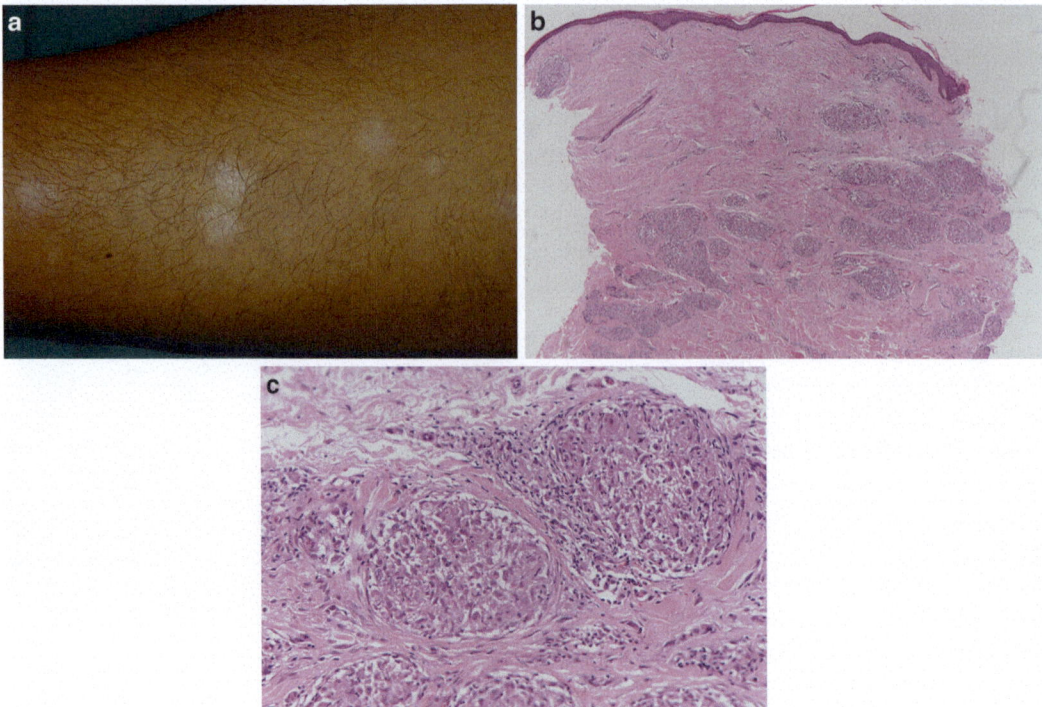

Fig. 2.25 Hypopigmented sarcoidosis. (**a**) Multiple, hypopigmented, mildly erythematous, oval plaques on the forearm. (**b**) The dermis shows multiple discrete granulo- mas with a tendency to coalesce (H&E, x40). (**c**) The granulomas consist of epithelioid cells with no necrosis (H&E, X200)

pigmentosa), erythematous macules (TMEP/ telangiectasia macularis eruptiva perstans), pap- ules and nodules (mastocytoma) or infiltrated plaques (diffuse cutaneous mastocytosis) [91]. Urticaria pigmentosa is usually seen in children as self-resolving brown round and oval macules on the trunk that may develop wheals on stroking (Darier's sign). An infiltrate of mast cells is seen in the upper dermis, with higher numbers around blood vessels. Mast cells are appreciated as cells with amphophilic granular cytoplasm and a cen- tral nucleus that has a 'fried egg'-like appearance. Eosinophils can be seen in some cases. Giemsa, chloroacetate esterase and toluidine blue stains are used to highlight the granules [91].

Hypopigmented Sarcoidosis

A rare variant of sarcoidosis can present with hypopigmented, mildly elevated, infiltrated plaques with a rim of erythema usually affecting

the trunk. Clinically it resembles hypopigmented plaques seen in Hansen's disease and post-kala- azar dermal leishmaniasis (Fig. 2.25a). Skin biopsy is diagnostic of sarcoidosis with non- caseating discrete granulomas in the dermis with- out any alteration in melanin or melanocytes (Fig. 2.25b) [92].

Tumour of Follicular Infundibulum

Hypopigmented macules or flat papules occurring on the head and neck are a feature of the eruptive variant of tumour of follicular infundibulum. These may be confused with hypopigmented macules in other disorders such as vitiligo and lichen sclerosus. Ackerman defined four histopathological criteria for diagnosing tumours of follicular infundibulum: a distinctive silhou- ette with a horizontal proliferation of keratino- cytes, epithelial cells with small monomorphic nuclei and abundant pink cytoplasm and thin columns of cells interconnected with bulkier aggregations [93]. Peripheral palisading may be seen in well-developed lesions. PAS and orcein stains are used to highlight glycogen in cells and elastic fibres at the tumour periphery, respectively. Decreased melanin is observed in the lesional epidermis.

References

1. Hirayama T, Suzuki T. A new classification of Ota's naevus based on histopathological features. Dermatologica. 1991;183:169–72.
2. Kang W, Lee E, Choi GS. Treatment of Ota's nevus by Q-switched alexandrite laser: therapeutic outcome in relation to clinical and histopathological findings. Eur J Dermatol. 1999;9:639–43.
3. Hori Y, Ouhara K, Miimura M, et al. Electron microscopy: ultrastructural observations of the extracellular sheath of dermal melanocytes in nevus of Ota. Am J Dermatopathol. 1982;4:245–51.
4. Page DG, Swirsky JA, Kaugars GE. Nevus of Ota with associated palatal involvement. Oral Surg Oral Med Oral Pathol. 1985;59:282–4.
5. Wilcox JC. Melanomatosis of skin and central nervous system. Am J Dis Child. 1939;57:391.
6. Rathi SK. Bilateral nevus of ota with oral mucosal involvement. Indian J Dermatol Venereol Leprol. 2002;68:104.
7. Sun CC, Lü YC, Lee EF, Nakagawa H. Naevus fusco-caeruleus zygomaticus. Br J Dermatol. 1987; 1:545–53.
8. Hori Y, Kawashima M, Oohara K, Kukita A. Acquired, bilateral naevus of Ota-like macules. J Am Acad Dermatol. 1984;10:961–4.
9. Bhat RM, Pinto HP, Dandekeri S, Ambil SM. Acquired bilateral nevus of ota-like macules with mucosal involvement: a new variant of Hori's nevus. Indian J Dermatol. 2014;59:293–6.
10. Barnhill RL. Dermal melanocytoses, blue nevi, and related conditions. In: Barnhill RL, editor. Pathology of melanocytic nevi and melanoma. Boston: Butterworth-Heinemann; 1995. p. 131–52.
11. Kerl H, Massi D. Melanotic macules, simple lentigo and lentiginous melanocytic naevus. In: Leboit PE, editor. Pathology and genetics of skin tumours. Lyon: IARC; 2006. p. 103–4.
12. Wayte DM, Helwig EB. Halo nevi. Cancer. 1968;22: 69–90.
13. Menasche G, Ho CH, Sanal O, Feldmann J, Tezcan I, Ersoy F, et al. Griscelli syndrome restricted to hypopigmentation results from a melanophilin defect (GS3) or a MYO5A F-exon deletion (GS1). J Clin Invest. 2003;112:450–6.
14. Menasche G, Feldmann J, Huodusse A, Desaymard C, Fischer A, Goud B, et al. Biochemical and functional characterization of Rab27a mutations occurring in Griscelli syndrome patients. Blood. 2003;101:2736–42.
15. Pastural E, Barrat FJ, Dufoureq-Lagelouse R, Certain S, Sanal O, Jabade N, et al. Griscelli disease maps to chromosome 15q21 and is associated with mutations in the myosin Va gene. Nat Genet. 1997;16:289–92.
16. Griscelli C, Durandy A, Guy Grand D, Daguillard F, Herzog C, Prunieras M. A syndrome associating partial albinism and immunodeficiency. Am J Med. 1978;65:691–702.
17. Sanal O, Yel L, Kucukali T, Gilbert-Barnes E, Tardieu M, Texcan I, et al. An allelic variant of Griscelli disease: presentation with severe hypotonia, mental-motor retardation, and hypopigmentation consistent with Elejalde syndrome (neuroectodermal melanolysosomal disorder). J Neurol. 2000;247:570–2.
18. LePoole IC, Van den Wijingaard RM, Westerhof W, Dutrieux RP, Das PK. Presence or absence of melanocytes in vitiligo lesions: an immunohistochemical investigation. J Invest Derma. 1993;100:816–22.
19. Sharquie KE, Mehenna SH, Naji AA, Al-Azzawi H. Inflammatory changes in vitiligo: stage I and II depigmentation. Am J Dermatopathol. 2004;26:108–12.
20. Attili VR, Attili SK. Lichenoid inflammation in vitiligo--a clinical and histopathologic review of 210 cases. Int J Dermatol. 2008;47:663–9.
21. Wańkowicz-Kalińska A, van den Wijngaard RM, Tigges BJ, Westerhof W, Ogg GS, Cerundolo V, et al. Immunopolarization of CD4+ and CD8+ T cells to Type-1-like is associated with melanocyte loss in human vitiligo. Lab Investig. 2003;83:683–95.
22. Yaghoobi R, Omidian M, Bagherani N. Vitiligo: a review of the published work. J Dermatol. 2011;38: 419–31.
23. Moellmann G, Klein-Angerer S, Scollay DA, Nordlund JJ, Lerner AB. Extracellular granular material and degeneration of keratinocytes in the normally pigmented epidermis of patients with vitiligo. J Invest Dermatol. 1982;79:321–30.
24. Ruiz-Maldonado R, Tamayo L, Fernandez-Diaz J. Universal acquired melanosis: the carbon baby. Arch Dermatol. 1978;114:775–8.
25. Abdallah MA, Abdallah MMA, Abdallah MA-R. Foreign body reactions. In: Bolognia JL, Jorizzo JL, Schaffer JV, editors. Dermatology. 3rd ed. England: Saunders Elsevier; 2012. p. 1573–83.
26. Ploysangam T, Breneman DL, Mutasim DF. Cutaneous pseudolymphomas. J Am Acad Dermatol. 1998;38:877–95.
27. Slater DN, Durrant TE. Tattoos: light and transmission electron microscopy studies with x-ray microanalysis. Clin Exp Dermatol. 1984;9:1365–2230.
28. Angeloni VL, Salasche SJ, Ortiz R. Nail, skin, and scleral pigmentation induced by minocycline. Cutis. 1987;40:229–33.
29. Dereure O. Drug-induced skin pigmentation. Epidemiology, diagnosis and treatment. Am J Clin Dermatol. 2001;2:253–62.

30. Job CK, Yoder L, Jacobson RR, Hastings RC. Skin pigmentation from clofazimine therapy in leprosy patients: a reappraisal. J Am Acad Dermatol. 1990;23:236–41.
31. Trimble JW, Mendelson DS, Fetter BF, Ingram P, Gallagher JJ, Shelburne JD. Cutaneous pigmentation secondary to amiodarone therapy. Arch Dermatol. 1983;119:914–8.
32. Argenyi ZB, Finelli L, Bergfeld WF, Tuthill RJ, McMahon JT, Ratz JL, et al. Minocycline-related cutaneous hyperpigmentation as demonstrated by light microscopy, electron microscopy and X-ray energy spectroscopy. J Cutan Pathol. 1987;14:176–80.
33. Johansson EA, Kanerva L, Niemi KM, Lakomaa EL. Generalised argyria with low ceruloplasmin and copper levels in the serum. A case report with clinical and microscopic findings and a trial of penicillamine treatment. Clin Exp Dermatol. 1982;7:169–76.
34. Pariser RJ. Generalized Argyria clinicopathologic features and histochemical studies. Arch Dermatol. 1978;114:373–7.
35. Hori Y, Miyazawa S. Argyria: electron microscope and x-ray microanalysis. J Electron Microsc (Tokyo). 1977;26:193–201.
36. al-Talib RK, Wright DH, Theaker JM. Orange-red birefringence of gold particles in paraffin wax embedded sections: an aid to the diagnosis of chrysiasis. Histopathology. 1994;24:176–8.
37. Zala L, Hunziker T, Braathen LR. Pigmentation following long-term bismuth therapy for pneumatosis cystoides intestinalis. Dermatology. 1993;187:288–9.
38. Crissey JT, Peachy JC. Calcaneal petechiae. Arch Dermatol. 1961;83:501.
39. Hafner J, Haenseler E, Ossent P, et al. Benzidine stain for the histochemical detection of hemoglobin in splinter hemorrhage (subungual hematoma) and black heel. Am J Dermatopathol. 1995;17:362–7.
40. Cox NH, Piette WW. In: Burns DA, Breathnach SM, Cox NH, Griffiths C, editors. Textbook of dermatology, vol. 3. 8th ed. Oxford: Blackwell Scientific Publications; 1998. p. 2327–77.
41. Zawar VP, Mhaskar ST. Exogenous ochronosis following hydroquinone for melasma. J Cosmet Dermatol. 2004;3:234–6.
42. Phillips JI, Isaacson C, Carman H. Ochronosis in black South Africans who used skin lighteners. Am J Dermatopathol. 1986;8:14–21.
43. Albers SE, Brozena SJ, Glass LF, Fenske NA. Alkaptonuria and ochronosis: case report and review. J Am Acad Dermatol. 1992;27:609–14.
44. Findlay GH, Morrison JGL, Simson IW. Exogenous ochronosis and pigmented colloid milium from hydroquinone bleaching creams. Br J Dermatol. 1975;93:613–22.
45. Khunger N, Kandhari R. Dermoscopic criteria for differentiating exogenous ochronosis from melasma. Indian J Dermatol Venereol Leprol. 2013;79:819–21.
46. Bhutani LK, Bedi TR, Pandhi RK, Nayak NC. Lichen planus pigmentosus. Dermatologica. 1974;149:43–50.
47. Seo JK, Lee HJ, Lee D, Choi JH, Sung H-S. A case of linear lichen planus pigmentosus. Ann Dermatol. 2010;22:323–5.
48. Kumar YH, Babu AR. Segmental lichen planus pigmentosus: an unusual presentation. Indian Dermatol Online J. 2014;5:157–9.
49. Laskaris GC, Papavasiliou SS, Bovopoulou OD, Nicolis GD. Lichen planus pigmentosus of the oral mucosa: a rare clinical variety. Dermatologica. 1981;162:61–3.
50. Vega ME, Waxtein L, Arenas R, Hojyo T, Dominguez-Soto L. Ashy dermatosis and lichen planus pigmentosus: a clinicopathologic study of 31 cases. Int J Dermatol. 1992;31:90–4.
51. Kanwar AJ, Dogra S, Handa S, Parsad D, Radotra BD. A study of 124 Indian patients with lichen planus pigmentosus. Clin Exp Dermatol. 2003;28:481–5.
52. Kim YC, Davis MD, Schanbacher CF, Su WP. Dowling-Degos disease (reticulate pigmented anomaly of the flexures): a clinical and histopathologic study of 6 cases. J Am Acad Dermatol. 1999;40:462–7.
53. Singh S, Khandpur S, Verma P, Singh M. Follicular Dowling Degos disease: a rare variant of an evolving dermatosis. Indian J Dermatol Venereol Leprol. 2013;79:802–4.
54. Kanwar AJ, Kaur S, Rajagopalan M. Reticulate acropigmentation of Kitamura. Int J Dermatol. 1990;29:217–9.
55. Lestringant GG, Masouyé I, Frossard PM, Adeghate E, Galadari IH. Co-existence of leukoderma with features of Dowling-Degos disease: reticulate acropigmentation of Kitamura spectrum in five unrelated patients. Dermatology. 1997;195:337–43.
56. Hanneken S, Rütten A, Pasternack SM, Eigelshoven S, El Shabrawi-Caelen L, Wenzel J, et al. Systematic mutation screening of KRT5 supports the hypothesis that Galli-Galli disease is a variant of Dowling-Degos disease. Br J Dermatol. 2010;163:197–200.
57. Grosshans E, Geiger JM, Hanau D, Jelen G, Heid E. Early pigmentary changes in dowling-degos' disease. J Cutan Pathology. 1984;7:77–87.
58. Fajardo TT. Indeterminate leprosy: a 3 year study, clinical observations. Int J Lepr. 1971;39:94–5.
59. Vargas-Ocampo F. Pityriasis alba: a histologic study. Int J Dermatol. 1993;32:870–3.
60. Copeman PWM, Wilson-Jones EWJ. Pigmented hairy epidermal nevus (Becker). Arch Dermatol. 1965;92:249–51.
61. Khaitan BK, Manchanda Y, Mittal R, Singh MK. Multiple Becker's naevi: a rare presentation. Acta Derm Venereol. 2001;81:374–5.
62. Alhusayen R, Kanigsberg N, Jackson R. Becker nevus on the lower limb: case report and review of the literature. J Cutan Med Surg. 2008;12:31–4.
63. Angelo C, Grosso MG, Stella P, et al. Becker's nevus syndrome. Cutis. 2001;68:123–4.
64. Matsuoka LY, Wortsman J, Goldman J. Acanthosis nigricans. Clin Dermatol. 1993;11:21–5.

65. Joshi R. Idiopathic eruptive macular pigmentation with papillomatosis: report of nine cases. Indian J Dermatol Venereol Leprol. 2007;73:402–5.
66. Weedon D, Haneke E, Martinka M, et al. Acanthomas. In: Leboit PE, editor. Pathology and genetics of skin tumours. Lyon: IARC; 2006. p. 39–47.
67. Kurban AK, Malak JA, Afifi AK, Mire J. Primary localized macular cutaneous amyloidosis: histochemistry and electron microscopy. Br J Dermatol. 1971;85:52–60.
68. Brownstein MH, Hashimoto K, Greenwald G. Biphasic amyloidosis: link between macular and lichenoid forms. Br J Dermatol. 1973;88:25–9.
69. Moriwaki S, Nishigori C, Horiguchi Y, Imamura S, Toda K, Takebe H. Amyloidosis cutis dyschromica: DNA repair reduction in the cellular response to UV light. Arch Dermatol. 1992;128:966–70.
70. Ngo JT, Trotter MJ, Haber RM. Juvenile-onset hypopigmented mycosis fungoides mimicking vitiligo. J Cutan Med Surg. 2009;13:230–3.
71. Das JK, Gangopadhyay AK. Mycosis fungoides with unusual vitiligo-like presentation. Indian J Dermatol Venereol Leprol. 2004;70:304–6.
72. Werner B, Brown S, Ackerman AB. Hypopigmented mycosis fungoides is not always mycosis fungoides! Am J Dermatopathol. 2005;27:56–67.
73. Attili VR, Attili SK. Vitiligoid lichen sclerosus: a reappraisal. Indian J Dermatol Venereol Leprol. 2008;74:118–21.
74. Almeida HL Jr, Bicca Ede B, Breunig Jde A, Rocha NM, Silva RM. Scanning electron microscopy of lichen sclerosus. An Bras Dermatol. 2013;88:247–9.
75. Elbendary A, Valdebran M, Parikh K, et al. Polarized microscopy in lesions with altered dermal collagen. Am J Dermatopathol. 2016;38:593–7.
76. De Villiers WJ, Jordaan HF, Bates W. Systemic sclerosis sine scleroderma presenting with vitiligo-like depigmentation and interstitial pulmonary fibrosis. Clin Exp Dermatol. 1992;17:127–31.
77. Smith ES, Hallman JR, DeLuca AM, Goldenberg G, Jorizzo JL, Sangueza OP. Dermatomyositis: a clinicopathological study of 40 patients. Am J Dermatopathol. 2009;31:61.
78. Lutzner MA, Blanchet-Bardon C, Orth G. Clinical observations, virologic studies, and treatment trials in patients with epidermodysplasia verruciformis, a disease induced by specific human papillomaviruses. J Invest Dermatol. 1984;83:18s–25s.
79. Yabe Y, Sadakane HJ. The virus of epidermodysplasia verruciformis: electron microscopic and fluorescent antibody studies. J Invest Dermatol. 1975;65:324–30.
80. Elewski BE, Hughey LE, Sobera JO, Hay R. Fungal diseases. In: Bolognia JL, Jorizzo JL, Schaffer JV, editors. Dermatology. 3rd ed. England: Saunders Elsevier; 2012. p. 1251–84.
81. Landau M, Krafchik BR. The diagnostic value of café-au-lait macules. J Am Acad Dermatol. 1999;40:877–90.
82. Pandhi RK, Bedi TR, Bhutani LK. Leucoderma in early syphilis. Br J Vener Dis. 1977;53:19–22.
83. Fiumara NJ, Cahn T. Leukoderma of secondary syphilis: two case reports. Sex Transm Dis. 1982;9:140–2.
84. Miranda MF, Bittencourt Mde J, Lopes Ida C, Cumino Sdo S. Leucoderma syphiliticum: a rare expression of the secondary stage diagnosed by histopathology. An Bras Dermatol. 2010;85:512–5.
85. Frithz A, Lagerholm B, Kaaman T. Leukoderma syphiliticum: ultrastructural observations on melanocyte function. Acta Derm Venereol. 1982;62:521–5.
86. Kuo TT, Chan HL, Hsueh S. Clear cell papulosis of the skin. A new entity with histogenetic implications for cutaneous Paget's disease. Am J Surg Pathol. 1987;11:827–34.
87. Kumarasinghe SPW, Chin GY. Clear cell papulosis of the skin a case report from Singapore. Arch Pathol Lab Med. 2004;128:e149–52.
88. Kim YC, Mehregan DA, Bang D. Clear cell papulosis: an immunohistochemical study to determine histogenesis. J Cutan Pathol. 2002;29:11–4.
89. Gupta V, Bhatia R, Ramam M, Khanna N. Hypopigmented macules and papules following the lines of Blaschko: a novel variant of Darier's disease. Int J Dermatol. 2016;55:e623–5.
90. Rowley MJ, Nesbitt LT Jr, Carrington PR, Espinoza CG. Hypopigmented macules in acantholytic disorders. Int J Dermatol. 1995;34:390–2.
91. Tharp MD. Mastocytosis. In: Bolognia JL, Jorizzo JL, Schaffer JV, editors. Dermatology. 3rd ed. England: Saunders Elsevier; 2012. p. 1993–2002.
92. Clayton R, Breathnach A, Martin B, Feiwel M. Hypopigmented sarcoidosis in the negro. Report of eight cases with ultrastructural observations. Br J Dermatol. 1977;96:119–25.
93. Ackerman AB, De Viragh PA, Chonchitnant N. Neoplasms with follicular differentiation. Philadelphia: Lea&Febiger; 1995. p. 553.

Measurements of Skin Colour

3

Deepani Munidasa, Gerrit Schlippe, and Sharnika Abeyakirthi

Introduction

The Skin Colour Spectrum

Variation in skin colour is one of the most striking aspects of human phenotypic variability. Skin pigmentation shows vast differences among continental populations. The distribution of pigmentation according to a latitudinal gradient probably stems from a strong influence of natural selection and sexual selection as supported by recent genetic evidence [1, 2].

The human skin colour also depends on ethnic origin, gender and age among other factors [3] (Figs. 3.1 and 3.2). At individual level, a person's natural skin colour at non-sun-exposed sites is lighter than at exposed sites (Fig. 3.3). The former, as seen in the inner upper arm or buttock region of a person, is known as the constitutive skin colour [4].

The Fitzpatrick skin phototype classification system is a widely used clinical tool that classifies human skin into phototypes I–VI based on a person's skin colour (constitutive) and responses to sun exposure in terms of self-reported erythema, burning and tanning ability [5, 6] (Table 3.1). Originally created for Caucasian skin, the Fitzpatrick skin type classification has been shown to be less well applicable to some other populations including Asians and African Americans [7–9].

Another classification system known as the individual typology angle (ITA)-based skin colour classification system shows better physiological relevance across different geographical regions and ethnicities. This classification is based on colorimetric data obtained from skin measurements (described later in the chapter) and classifies skin colour types into six groups from very light to dark [10, 11] (Table 3.2).

Why Do We Measure Skin Colour?

Many disease processes directly or indirectly affecting the skin result in localized or generalized changes in skin pigmentation: melasma (Fig. 3.4), facial melanoses, lichen planus pigmentosus, vitiligo (Fig. 3.5) and progressive macular hypomelanosis to name a few.

D. Munidasa
Department of Dermatology, Anuradhapura Teaching Hospital, Anuradhapura, Sri Lanka
e-mail: deepanimunidasa@yahoo.com

G. Schlippe (✉)
Dermatest GmbH, Münster, Germany
e-mail: dr.schlippe@dermatest.de

S. Abeyakirthi
Department of Dermatology, Panadura Base Hospital, Panadura, Sri Lanka
e-mail: sharnikaabeyakirthi@yahoo.com

© Springer International Publishing AG, part of Springer Nature 2018
P. Kumarasinghe (ed.), *Pigmentary Skin Disorders*, Updates in Clinical Dermatology,
https://doi.org/10.1007/978-3-319-70419-7_3

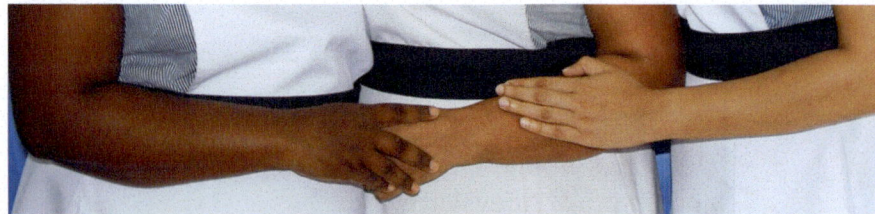

Fig. 3.1 Sri Lankan nurses of Fitzpatrick phototypes III, IV and V

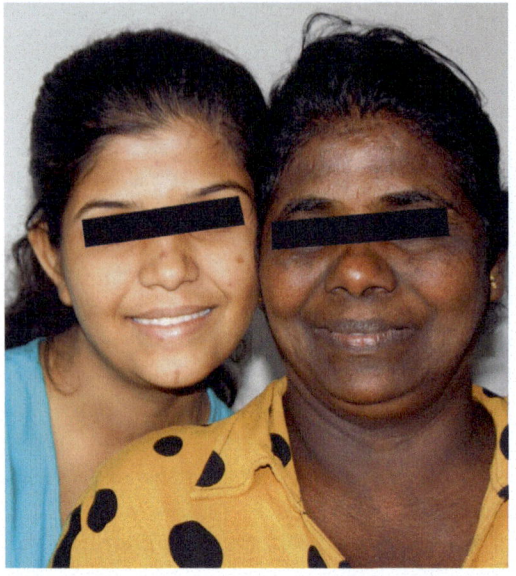

Fig. 3.2 Biological mother and daughter of skin phototypes IV and VI

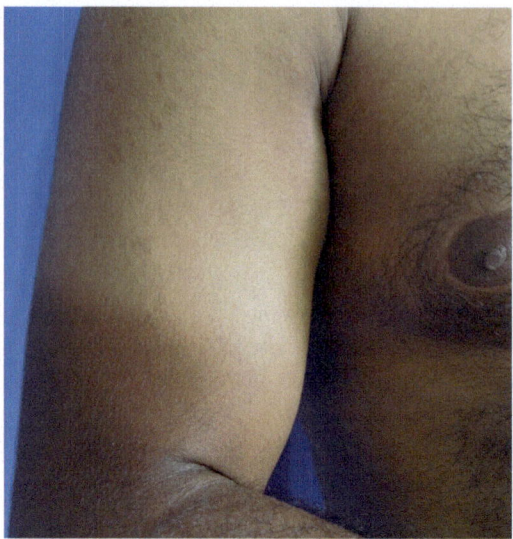

Fig. 3.3 Profuse tanning of sun exposed skin in a phototype IV subject

In the fields of clinical dermatology and cosmetology, the accurate measurement of skin pigmentation and reliable reproducibility are important key factors. In situ objective skin colour measurements are necessary for the correct documentation and monitoring of the treatment response in pigmentary disorders, testing the efficacy of depigmenting or hyperpigmenting agents, etc.

What Gives the Skin Its Colour?

The skin colour that we perceive depends on the way the skin, particularly the epidermis, interacts with ambient light and the presence of chromophores in the skin.

Four to six percent of a photon of visible light (400–700 nm) incident on the skin gets reflected from the skin surface at the air-skin interface (regular reflectance). The remainder penetrates and scatters diffusely within the skin due to inhomogeneities of the tissue constituents. Some of these waves are absorbed by the main chromophores: melanin in keratinocytes and oxyhaemoglobin and deoxyhaemoglobin in the dermal capillaries [13, 14]. The remainder gets scattered and backscattered out of the skin mostly by dermal components like collagen fibres (dermal remittance) [13].

Melanin absorbs all wavelengths of visible light and produces a brown to black colour. With heavy pigmentation as in Fitzpatrick type V/VI skin, it masks the red colour produced by haemoglobin.

Table 3.1 Fitzpatrick's skin phototypes [5, 6]

Skin phototype	Constitutive skin colour	Response to sun exposure
I	Ivory white	Burns easily, never tans
II	White	Burns easily, tans minimally with difficulty
III	Cream white	Burns moderately, tans moderately
IV	Olive, brown	Burns minimally, tans easily
V	Dark brown	Burns very rarely, tans easily
VI	Black	Never burns, tans profusely

Table 3.2 The ITA° (individual typology angle)-based skin colour classification [10, 11]

Individual typology angle	Skin classification
ITA > 55	Very light
41 < ITA < 55	Light
28 < ITA < 41	Intermediate
10 < ITA < 28	Tan
−30 < ITA < 10	Brown
ITA < −30	Dark

All non-invasive instrumental measurements of skin pigmentation are based on the ability of melanin to attenuate light [14].

Haemoglobin shows maximum light absorption in the green spectral band with minimal absorption in the red spectral band of the visual light spectrum. Oxyhaemoglobin in the dermal capillaries produces a bright red colour, while deoxyhaemoglobin in the venules gives the skin a blue hue. Accordingly, the skin colour tends to be reddish in inflammatory conditions leading to vasodilatation and in areas of the body with an increased blood flow, such as the face. Ischaemia and vasoconstriction impart a bluish colour [4].

Thus, skin colour is primarily a product of skin pigmentation (melanin) and erythema. However, other externally acquired chromophores like carotenoids, when taken in large amounts, and some drugs may also contribute to skin colour.

Drug-induced skin pigmentation is either caused by accumulation of the drug or its metabolites in the skin (psychotropic drugs), accumulation

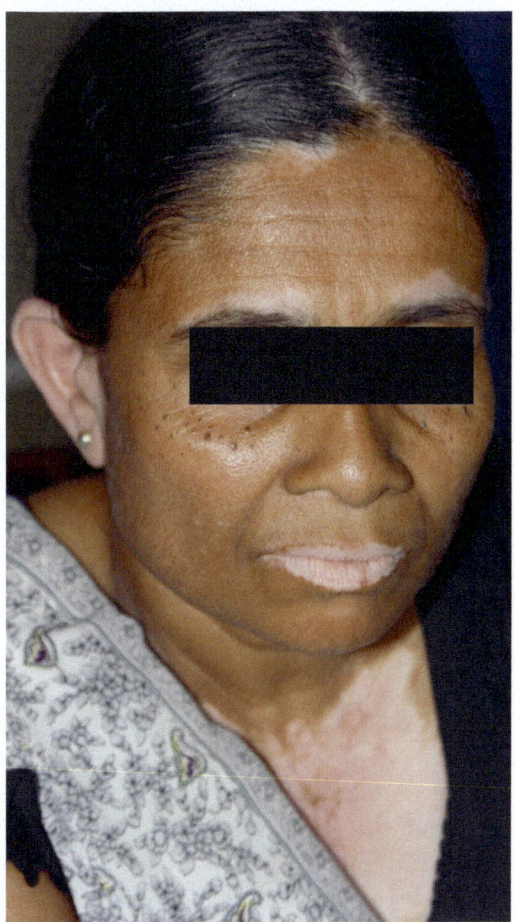

Fig. 3.4 Vitiligo causing depigmentation in a phototype V person

of melanin in the dermal macrophages (antimalarials), synthesis of special pigments under the direct influence of the drug (lipofuscin synthesis with clofazimine) or a combination of these mechanisms [12]. Drug-induced pigmentation could interfere with skin colour measurements.

Measurements of Skin Colour

Human perception of skin colour is complex and highly subjective. Although we can perceive changes in skin colour, accurate quantification is difficult. In practice, dermatologists and other clinicians use several clinical scoring systems and skin colour charts to overcome this problem.

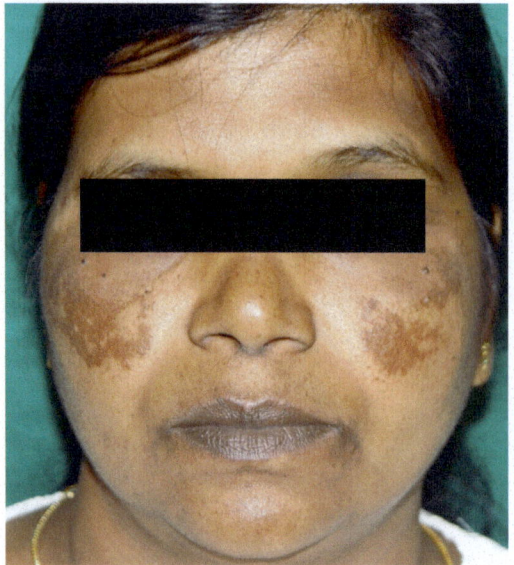

Fig. 3.5 Melasma

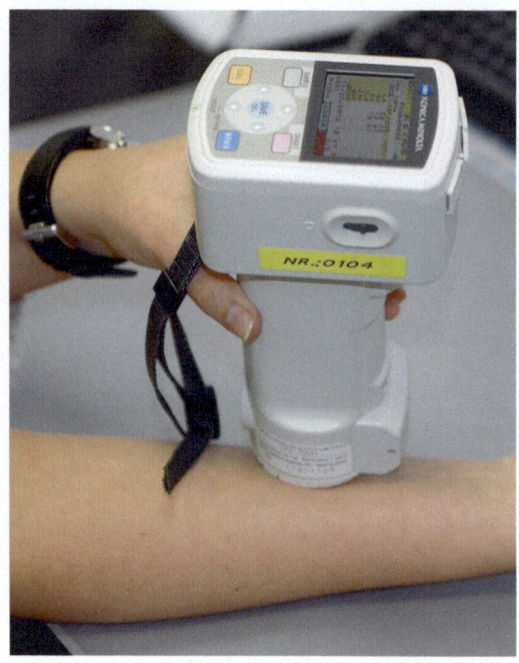

Fig. 3.6 Konica Minolta Spectrophotometer

Some schemes have been standardized and validated [3]. Although useful in the clinical setting, these methods have their own limitations in terms of low reliability and reproducibility due to inter-/intra-observer errors.

With the advances in modern optoelectronic engineering, several instruments are available today to obtain objective and fairly accurate measurements of skin colour [15, 16].

Instruments

The instruments for measuring skin colour (pigmentation and erythema) are designed based on two main principles: reflectance spectrophotometry and tristimulus colorimetry. The light reflectance data from the skin, as described earlier in the chapter, are converted into indices or colorimetric values for the estimation of chromophores in the skin.

In reflectance spectrophotometry, either broadband or selected narrowband wavelengths of visible light are used with measurement of absorbance and reflectance. Scanning reflectance spectrophotometers utilize a broad band of wavelengths to provide detailed information about physical skin colour properties. These instru-

ments are expensive and often rather cumbersome to use in routine clinical work as they are bulky. They are mainly used for fundamental laboratory research [18, 19]. However, new-generation spectrophotometric devices such as the Konica Minolta Spectrophotometer CM-700d are more compact and portable (Fig. 3.6).

Narrowband reflectance spectrophotometers (such as Mexameter MX 18, Courage-Khazaka) rely on the difference in absorption between melanin and haemoglobin of visible light at well-chosen wavelengths [20–22]. They analyse reflectance data of three colour channels (red, green, blue) and compute erythema and melanin indices. These instruments are commonly used in dermatological research and clinical practice (Fig. 3.7).

Antera 3D is a new camera device which uses reflectance mapping of seven different light wavelengths and provides measurements of skin texture in addition to erythema and pigmentation [23].

Colorimetric instruments (e.g. Minolta Chroma Meter CR-400) are less expensive and are used in clinical/research work. They function based on the measurements of reflected light at specific wavelengths corresponding to the spec-

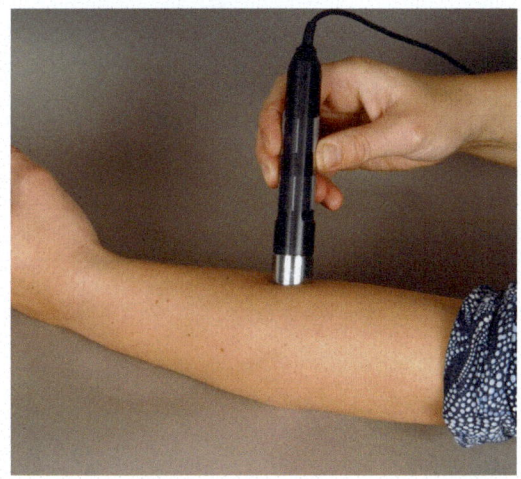

Fig. 3.7 Mexameter MX 18, Courage-Khazaka

The ITA° (Individual Typology Angle)- Based Skin Colour Classification

The ITA° is considered an objective parameter of skin colour quantification. Once the L* and b* values are determined, the ITA° is calculated with the formula: ITA° = [arc tan(L*−50)/b*] 9180/3.14159. Based on the ITA° value, skin colour types are classified into six groups, from very light to dark skin. The lighter the skin, the higher the ITA°. Increased browning of the skin is indicated by a rising b* value and a falling L* value and ITA°. Conversely, lightening of the skin is indicated by a falling b* value and rising L* value and ITA° [11, 25] (Table 3.2).

trum of visible light. The skin surface is illuminated by a pulse xenon arc lamp, and the reflected light is collected via built-in colour filters for tristimulus colour analysis at the wavelengths of 450, 560 and 600 nm [18]. The results are expressed in accordance with the CIELAB colour system as defined by the Commission International de l'Eclairage (CIE) in 1976.

Overall, despite their usefulness, it has been shown that the repeatability of skin measurements may vary depending on the instrument type as well as with ethnicity and body location [24].

The CIE Colour Space

The CIE colour space ("CIELAB" or CIE 1976 L *a*b*) is a widely accepted system used to describe colour and utilizes a combination of three colour values (L *(white-black, brightness), a* (red-green) and b* (blue-yellow)) that are plotted on a 3D space [17].

The skin colour is an admixture of the L*a* b* values. When these values are combined, they can reproduce any colour that the human eye can perceive [19]. With darkening of skin colour (due to pigmentation or erythema), the L * value decreases. The a* value increases with erythema. With pigmentation, the b* value becomes more positive [18, 19].

Factors Affecting Skin Colour Measurements

To obtain accurate measurements of erythema or pigmentation in any study, it is most important to follow the established guidelines [18]. It is equally important to be thorough with the operating instructions provided for the instrument in terms of calibration, application of the probe to the test area, etc. The measuring probes of most spectrophotometric devices have a wide contact surface, and it is important that accurate contact is made between the actual measuring area of the probe head and the skin by careful, correct placement over the site of interest.

The optimal ambient temperature for making measurements is 19–23 °C, to avoid variations in skin vasoactivity. Direct sunlight should be avoided. Before commencing any measurement, it is recommended that the subject should rest for approximately 20 min to acclimatize. Test sites should be exposed and kept motionless for at least 5 min before obtaining readings.

In making a measurement, the instrument (probe) should be held perpendicular to the skin in a steady manner exerting very light pressure. Three measurements in rapid succession are often made within the same test site to calculate the mean value for better accuracy [18].

Table 3.3 Factors affecting skin colour measurements [18]

Individual-related variables	Environment-related variables	Instrument-related variables
Age: Aged skin may be less pigmented	Ambient temperature: Changes in local skin temperature and core temperature cause changes in erythema by means of vasoconstriction or dilatation	Intra- and inter-instrumental variability
Sex: Erythema may be greater in male skin	Ambient light: Avoid false light by keeping probe perpendicular to the skin surface	Physical contact and pressure of probe on the skin
Race: Visual estimation of erythema in pigmented skin can be misleading		
Anatomical site: Erythema indices and a* values are higher in the face, neck palms and soles. Melanin indices and b* values are higher in sun-exposed sites		
Skin surface properties: Scaling, hairs, topical applications and cosmetics can affect measurements		
Diurnal variation: Erythema increases during the course of the day		
Physical and mental activity: Exercise increases blood flow and erythema. Mental stress induces adrenergic vasoconstriction of peripheral blood vessels causing pallor		
Medication, nicotine, alcohol: Vasoactive medication affects erythema. Alcohol causes vasodilatation. Nicotine vasoconstricts		

Several pitfalls in making measurements, transfer of data and acceptance of data could result in invalid values. For example, negative values in a* and b* are measurable but do indicate that the measurement should be repeated after thorough calibration of the measuring instrument. For all instruments measuring skin pigmentation or inflammation, it would be important to have accurate instructions that denote the range of L*, a*, b* values compatible with the particular panel used.

Table 3.3 summarizes the factors affecting skin colour measurements.

References

1. Parra EJ. Human pigmentation variation: evolution, genetic basis, and implications for public health. Am J Phys Anthropol. 2007;(Suppl 45):85–105.
2. Aoki K. Sexual selection as a cause of human skin colour variation: Darwin's hypothesis revisited. Ann Hum Biol. 2002;29(6):589–608.
3. De Rigal J, Abella ML, Giron F, Caisey L, Lefebvre MA. Development and validation of a new skin colour chart. Skin Res Technol. 2007;13:101–9.
4. Holm EA. Skin colour and pigmentation. In: Fluhr JW, editor. Practical aspects of cosmetic testing. Berlin, Heidelberg: Springer; 2011. p. 175–81.
5. Fitzpatrick TB, Pathak MA, Parrish JA. Protection of human skin against the effects of the sunburn ultraviolet (290–302 nm). In: Fitzpatrick TB, Pathak MA, Harber LC, Seiji M, Kukita A, editors. Sunlight and man. Tokjo: University of Tokyo Press; 1974. p. 751.
6. Sachdeva S. Fitzpatrick skin typing: applications in dermatology. Indian J Dermatol Venereol Leprol. 2009;75:93–6.
7. Rampen FH, Fleuren BA, de Boo TM, et al. Unreliability of self-reported burning tendency and tanning ability. Arch Dermatol. 1988;124:885–8.
8. Rawlings AV. Ethnic skin types: are there differences in skin structure and function? Int J Cosmet Sci. 2006;28:79–93. 15
9. Pichon LC, Landrine H, Corral I, et al. Measuring skin cancer risk in African Americans: is the Fitzpatrick skin type classification scale culturally sensitive? Ethn Dis. 2010;20:174–9.
10. Chardon A, Cretois I, Hourseau C. Skin colour typology and suntanning pathways. Int J Cosmet Sci. 1991;13:191–208.

11. Del Bino S, Bernerd F. Variations in skin colour and the biological consequences of ultraviolet radiation exposure. Br J Dermatol. 2013;169(Suppl 3):33–40.
12. Dereure O. Drug-induced skin pigmentation. Epidemiology, diagnosis and treatment. Am J Clin Dermatol. 2001;2(4):253–62.
13. Anderson RR, Parrish JA. The optics of human skin. J Invest Dermatol. 1981;77(1):13–9.
14. Stamatas GN, Zmudzka BZ, KolliasN BJZ. Non-invasive measurements of skin pigmentation in situ. PigmentCell Res. 2004;17:618–26.
15. Taylor S, Westerhof W, Im S, Lim J. Non-invasive techniques for the evaluation of skin color. J Am Acad Dermatol. 2006;54(5 Suppl 2):S282–90.
16. Kollias N, Stamatas GN. Optical non-invasive approaches to diagnosis of skin diseases. J Investig Dermatol Symp Proc. 2002;7(1):64–75.
17. Robertson AR, The CIE. Colour difference formulas. Colour Research and Application. 1976;1977(2):7–11.
18. Fullerton A, Fischer T, Lahti A, Wilhelm KP, Takiwaki H, Serup J. Guidelines for measurement of skin colour and erythema. A report from the Standardization Group of the European Society of Contact Dermatitis. Contact Dermatitis. 1996;35(1):1–10.
19. Takiwaki H. Measurement of skin color: practical application and theoretical considerations. J Med Investig. 1998;44(3–4):121–6.
20. Clarys P, Alewaeters K, Lambrecht R, Barel AO. Skin color measurements: comparison between three instruments: the Chromameter(R), the DermaSpectrometer(R) and the Mexameter(R). Skin Res Technol. 2000;6(4):230–8.
21. Baquié M, Kasraee B. Discrimination between cutaneous pigmentation and erythema: comparison of the skin colorimeters Dermacatch and Mexameter. Skin Res Technol. 2014;20(2):218–27.
22. Dornelles S, Goldim J, Cestari T. Determination of the minimal erythema dose and colorimetric measurements as indicators of skin sensitivity to UV-B radiation. Photochem Photobiol. 2004;79(6):540–4.
23. Matias AR, Ferreira M, Costa P, Neto P. Skin colour, skin redness and melanin biometric measurements: comparison study between Antera(®) 3D, Mexameter(®) and Colorimeter(®). Skin Res Technol. 2015;21(3):346–62.
24. Wang M, Xiao K, Wuerger S, Cheung V, Luo MR. Measuring human skin colour. In: Proceedings of 23rd colour and imaging conference. Colour science, systems and applications (CIC23), 19–23 Oct 2015, Darmstadt, Germany. IS&T: Society for imaging science and technology, p. 230–234(5). ISBN 978-0-89208-319-0.
25. COLIPA Guideline. Guideline for the colorimetric determination of skin colour typing and prediction of the Minimal Erythemal Dose (MED) without UV exposure. Brussels: European Toiletry and Perfumery Association; 2007.

Dermoscopy of Melanoma

4

Benjamin Carew and James Muir

Introduction

Dermoscopy is a technique using a hand-held magnification device (a dermatoscope) to visualise morphologic structures in the skin not visible to the naked eye [1]. It was developed as a tool for assessing pigmented skin lesions, especially melanoma. In the 2008 evidence-based Clinical Practice Guidelines for the Management of Melanoma in Australia and New Zealand, dermoscopy was recommended for clinicians routinely examining pigmented lesions [2]. The dermatoscope has been described as the equivalent of a physician's stethoscope. A survey of dermatology trainees in Australia supports this statement reporting that 96% of trainees think a dermatoscope is an essential tool [3]. Currently the two primary care training providers in Australia, Royal Australian College of General Practitioners (RACGP) and the Australian College of Rural and Remote Medicine (ACRRM), include training in dermoscopy as a part of the curriculum for trainees. Over time the usefulness of dermoscopy has expanded from pigmented lesions to non-melanoma skin cancer (NMSC), to hair disorders (trichoscopy) and to

vgeneral dermatoses of the skin. This chapter primarily discusses dermoscopy in relation to melanoma, whereas Chapter 5 describes dermoscopy of other pigmented lesions.

Optics of Dermoscopy

Light is either reflected, dispersed or absorbed by the stratum corneum because of its refraction index and its optical density [4]. Dermoscopy utilises magnification combined with either fluid emersion or polarised light systems, to reduce optical reflectance from the stratum corneum. By reducing reflectance the clinician is able to visualise superficial and deeper structures including pigment and vascular structures.

The Dermoscopic Language

The language and terms used in dermoscopy have evolved over time. Many dermoscopic terms are descriptive metaphors; some examples of metaphoric terms and their associations include the 'strawberry' pattern (in actinic keratosis), 'cerebriform' pattern (in seborrhoeic keratosis) and 'spoke-wheel' areas (in basal cell carcinoma). Supporters of the metaphoric terms suggest that the visual analogies are colourful and memorable. A criticism of this language however is that the metaphors can be ambiguous [5].

B. Carew (✉) · J. Muir
Department of Medicine (Dermatology), Mater Hospital South Brisbane, Brisbane, QLD, Australia
e-mail: info@qlddermgroup.com.au

© Springer International Publishing AG, part of Springer Nature 2018
P. Kumarasinghe (ed.), *Pigmentary Skin Disorders*, Updates in Clinical Dermatology,
https://doi.org/10.1007/978-3-319-70419-7_4

An alternative descriptive approach, using elements of pattern analysis, aims to make description simple, logical and reproducible. The descriptive terminology relates to five elements, i.e. lines, dots, clods, circles and pseudopods. These are the elements of revised pattern analysis [6]. A criticism of this descriptive approach is that complex structures that can be described succinctly with a visual analogy may require complicated descriptive terms [7].

At the third consensus meeting of the International Dermoscopy Society in 2016, 23.5% of participants preferentially used descriptive terminology, 20.1% used metaphoric terminology, and 56.5% used both [5]. The consensus group devised definitions of both the descriptive and metaphoric terms with a view to review and update this dictionary every 5 years.

Dermoscopic Approaches for the Diagnosis of Melanoma on the Body

In this chapter, we will outline the two main approaches used for dermoscopic analysis of melanoma. These are the two-step algorithm and pattern analysis.

Two-Step Algorithm

In 2001 a consensus meeting of the International Dermoscopy Society agreed on using the two-step algorithm for classification of pigmented lesions [8].

The first step of this algorithm is used to classify the lesion as either melanocytic or non-melanocytic [9] (see Fig. 4.1). The second step is to evaluate

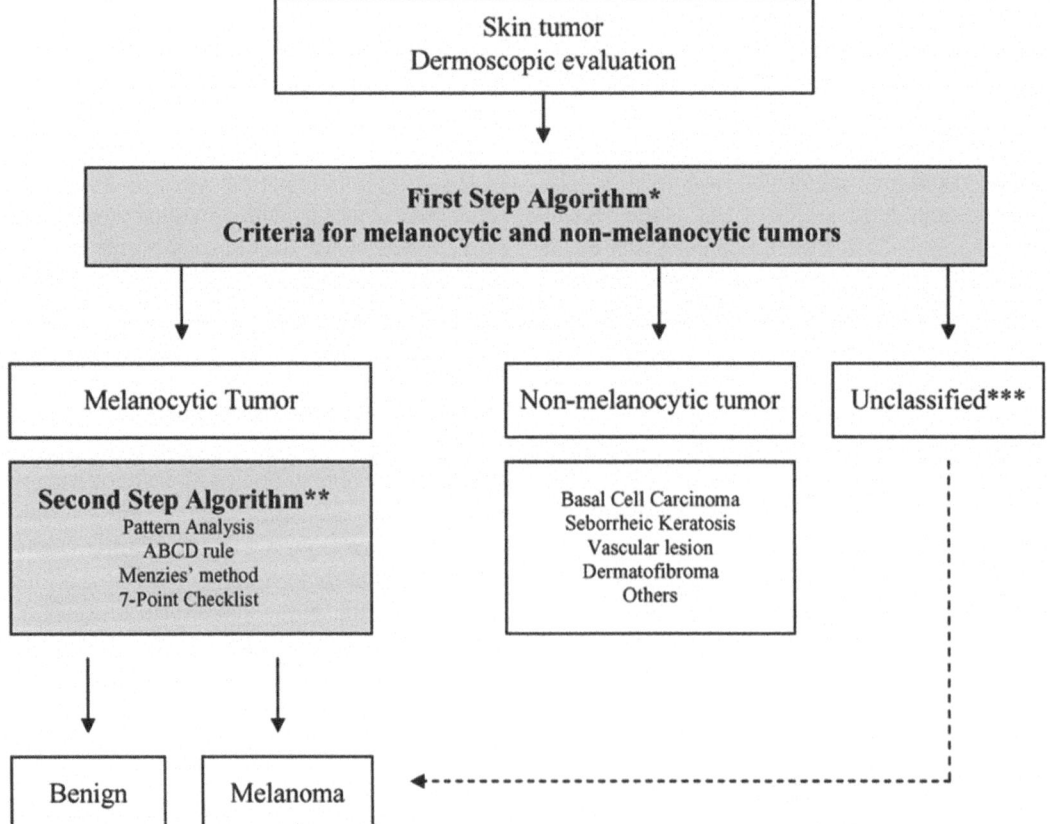

Fig. 4.1 The two-step method as defined by the Consensus Net Meeting on dermoscopy. *, first step: discrimination between melanocytic and non-melanocytic lesions. **, second step: discrimination between benign melanocytic lesions and melanomas. ***, in the case of nonspecific criteria or indeterminate pattern, possibility of melanoma exists and should be in differential diagnosis (Reproduced with permission. Malvehy et al. [9])

melanocytic lesions to determine if they are benign or a potential melanoma. The outcome of the assessment will determine management with excision/biopsy or no treatment required.

A revision to this two-step approach was suggested to improve the evaluation of structureless and amelanotic/hypomelanotic lesions [10].

First Step of the Revised Two-Step Algorithm

The first step of the evaluation process is summarised below (1–4):

1. The lesion is evaluated for melanocytic features:
   - True network
   - Pseudonetwork (face)
   - Branched streaks
   - Streaks
   - Aggregated globules
   - Homogenous blue pigmentation
   - Parallel pattern (palms, soles, mucosa)

Examples of melanocytic features can be seen in Fig. 4.2.

There are some exceptions to this step, such as lesions that appear melanocytic but are benign and may be identified by other key dermoscopic features (Fig. 4.3).

2. If a lesion is determined to be non-melanocytic, it is then specifically examined for features of dermatofibroma, seborrhoeic keratosis, blue naevus, basal cell carcinoma (BCC) and haemangioma/angiokeratoma. Features of BCC include (Fig. 4.4):
   - Arborising blood vessels
   - Leaf-like areas
   - Large blue-grey ovoid nests
   - Large blue-grey globules
   - Spoke wheel-like areas

Features of seborrhoeic keratoses include (see Fig. 4.5):

- Milia-like cysts
- Comedo-like openings

- Crypts
- Moth-eaten borders
- Network-like structures
- Fat fingers or light brown fingerprint structures
- Fissures and ridges (also known as gyri and sulci) giving a brain-like/cerebriform appearance

Features of haemangioma include (see Fig. 4.6):

- Red maroon or red blue to black
- Lacunae (lagoon-like structures)

3. If not readily able to be classified as one of the lesions outlined above, the lesion is then examined for:

   Vascular features in some non-melanocytic lesions:
   - Glomerular vessels seen in intraepidermal carcinoma (IEC) (Fig. 4.7)
   - Crown vessels (sebaceous hyperplasia (Fig. 4.8), molluscum contagiosum)
   - Blood vessels arranged "like a string of pearls" or "serpiginous" (clear-cell acanthoma (Fig. 4.9))

     Hairpin vessels surrounded by a whitish halo (keratinising tumours, e.g. keratoacanthoma and seborrhoeic keratosis (Fig. 4.10)).

   Vascular features in some melanocytic lesions:

   - Comma-like vessels (intradermal naevi (Fig. 4.11)).
   - Dotted, linear irregular, atypical hairpin (serpentine), corkscrew or tortuous (melanoma) (Fig. 4.12).
   - Polymorphous = more than one type of vascular pattern.
   - Multiple shades of pink (milky red areas).
   - Note: the most common vascular polymorphous combination is dotted and linear.

4. If the lesion is found to be featureless/structureless (unclassifiable) after the previous steps, it should be viewed as suspicious and biopsy considered.

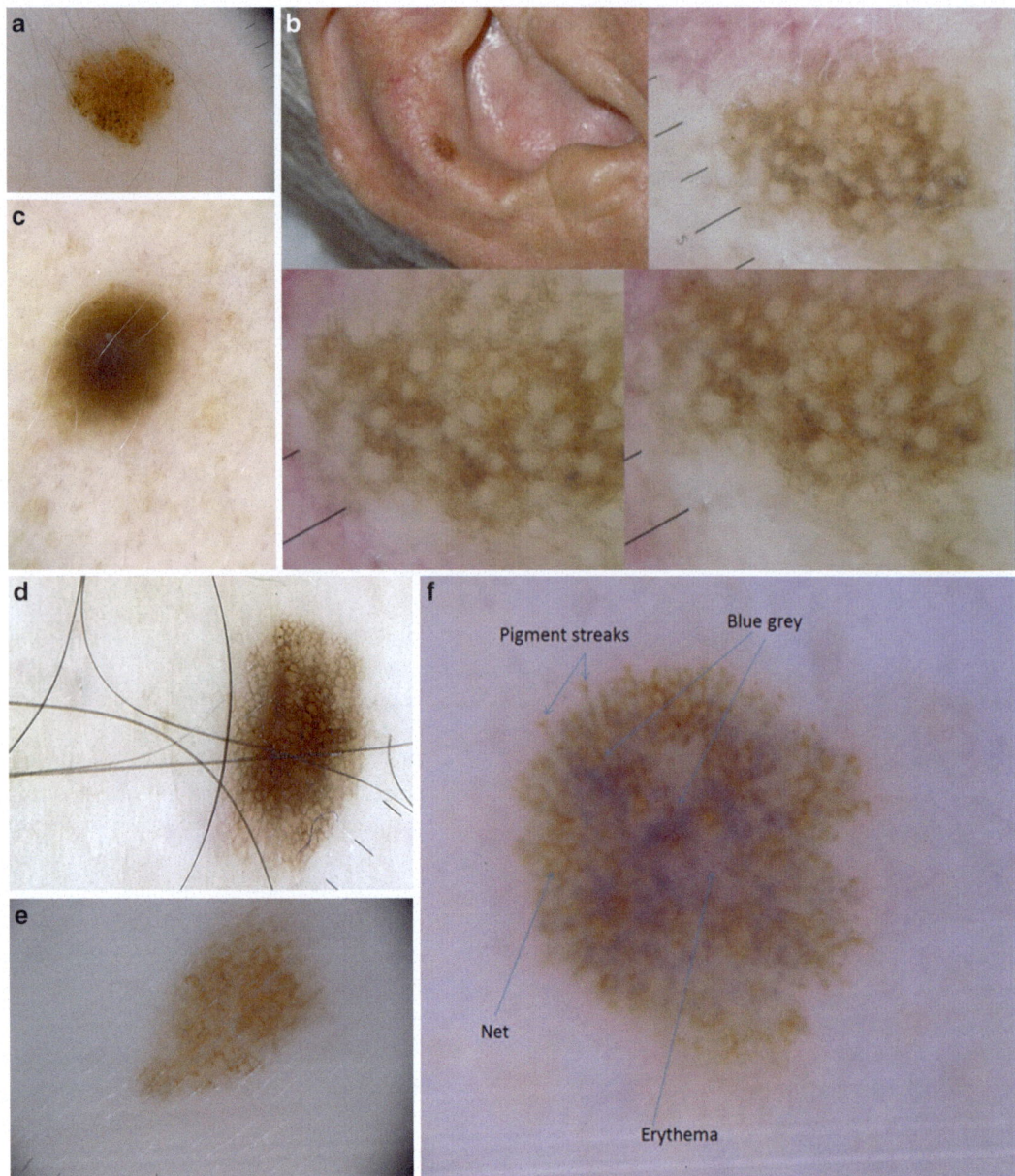

Fig. 4.2 Examples of melanocytic features. (**a**) Globules; (**b**) pseudonetwork; (**c**) homogenous pattern; (**d**) reticular pattern; (**e**) acral parallel pattern; (**f**) streaks

Second Step of the Revised Two-Step Algorithm

Once a lesion is identified as melanocytic, the next step is for the clinician to decide whether the lesion is benign or potentially a melanoma. To aid this decision, there are various algorithms available. These scoring systems involve assessment of lesions for the presence of features seen commonly in melanoma. Carrera et al. [11] outline in depth the various common features of the scoring algorithms. In Table 4.1 we have pre-

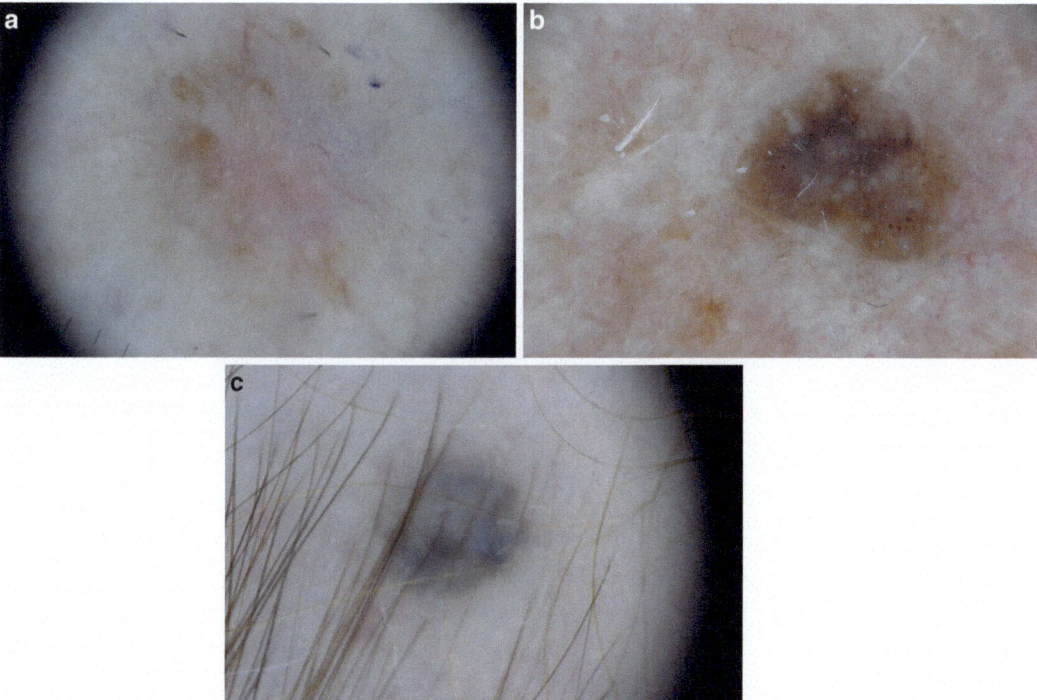

Fig. 4.3 Lesions that appear melanocytic but are benign and may be identified by other key dermoscopic features. (**a**) Dermatofibroma: peripheral network with a central scar-like area. (**b**) Seborrhoeic keratosis: faint network and pseudonetwork can be seen. Other typical seborrhoeic keratosis features allow discrimination. (**c**) Blue naevus: homogenous pigmentation (steel blue)

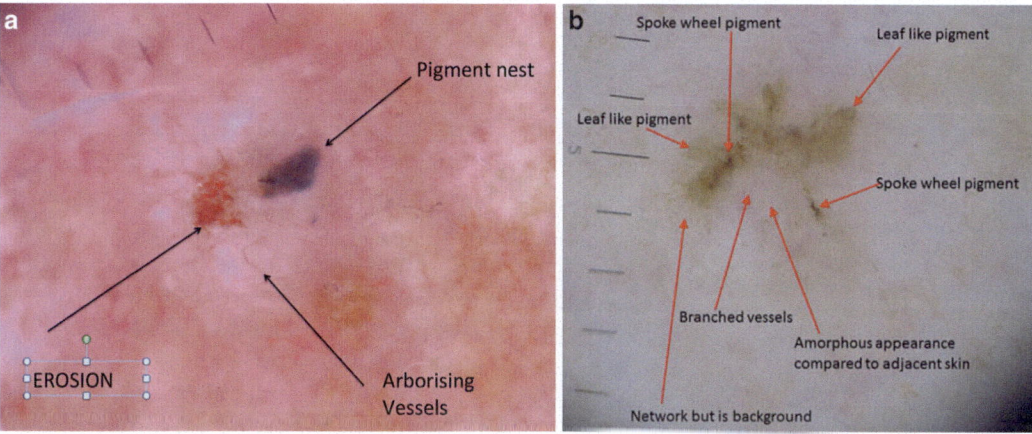

Fig. 4.4 (**a**, **b**) Features of BCC

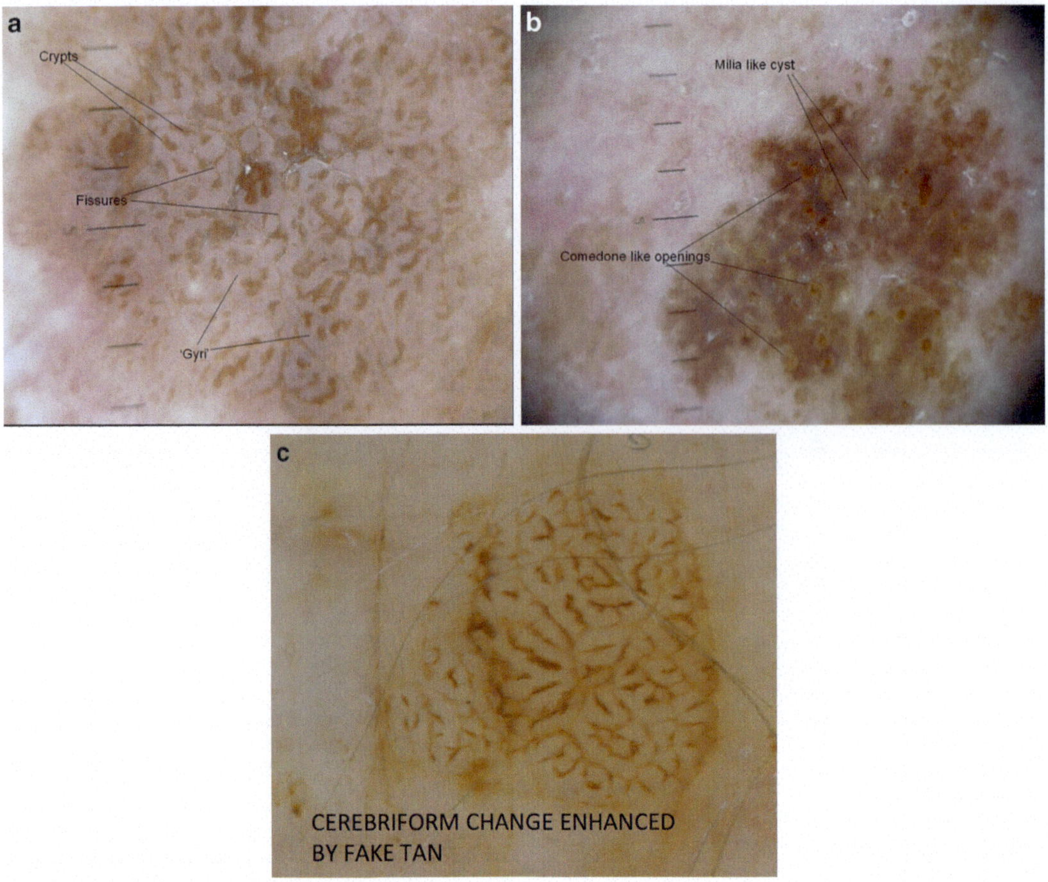

a
Crypts

Fissures

'Gyri'

b
Milia like cyst

Comedone like openings

c
CEREBRIFORM CHANGE ENHANCED
BY FAKE TAN

Fig. 4.5 (a, b, c) Features of seborrhoeic keratoses

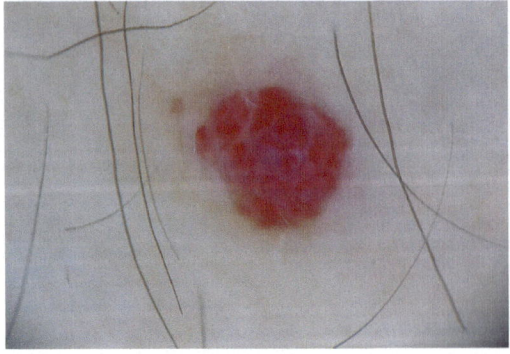

Fig. 4.6 Features of haemangioma

sented an abbreviated comparison of some commonly used algorithms and the dermoscopic criteria they employ. This demonstrates some common elements between the methods. These scoring algorithms have been criticised for being too simplistic in comparison to comprehensive pattern analysis [12]. Aside from accuracy of diagnosis however, the ease of use and training are important factors in choosing an algorithm. Many of the algorithms have been reported as effective methods adopted by novice dermoscopists in the primary care setting [13, 14].

Limitations of the Two-Step Algorithm

A potential failing of the two-step algorithm is the first step decision (melanocytic vs non-melanocytic). A failure at this step leads to failure overall and incorrect diagnosis. This algorithm is not perfect, but it has been shown to have high diagnostic accuracy, i.e. 93% with a sensitivity of

Fig. 4.7 Intraepidermal carcinoma

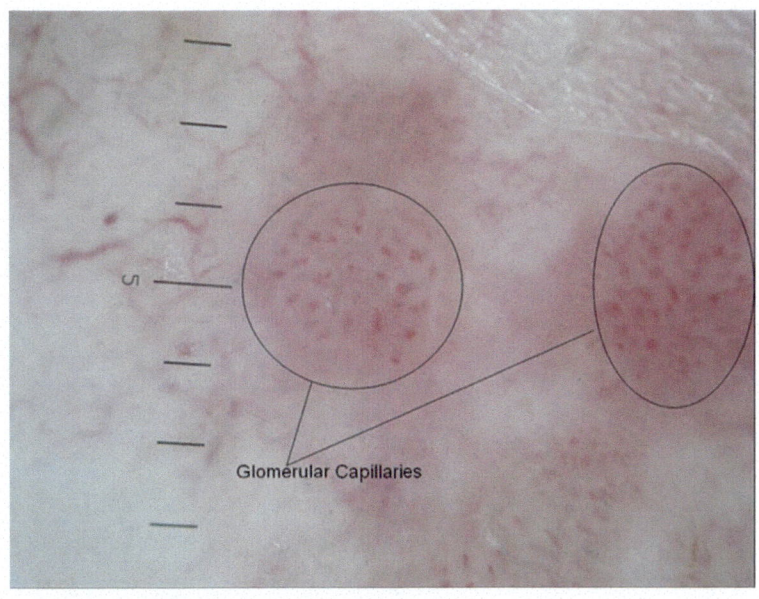

Glomerular Capillaries

Fig. 4.8 Sebaceous hyperplasia

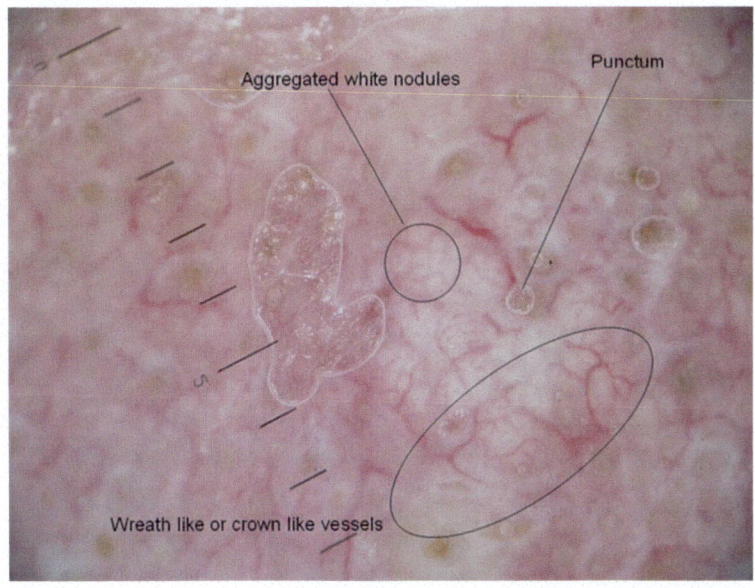

Aggregated white nodules

Punctum

Wreath like or crown like vessels

85% and a specificity of 94% [15]. The first step has been shown to be less accurate in populations with high sun exposure and a large number of solar lentigines [16]. In recognition of these pitfalls, all clinically indeterminate lesions (i.e. lesions that have insufficient features to be definitively called melanocytic or non-melanocytic) are classified as melanocytic and potential melanoma. There are some sites on the body, such as the mucosa and acral surfaces, where some scoring algorithms may not be useful.

Pattern Analysis and Melanoma

In 1987 Pehamberger, Steiner and Wolff [17, 18] published the first analytical method to distinguish between the primary types of pigmented

Fig. 4.9 Clear cell acanthoma

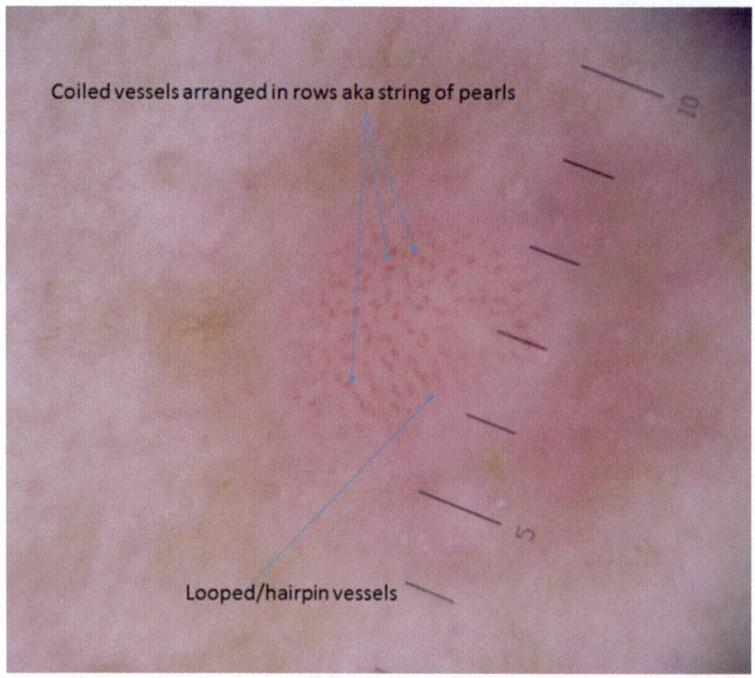

Coiled vessels arranged in rows aka string of pearls

Looped/hairpin vessels

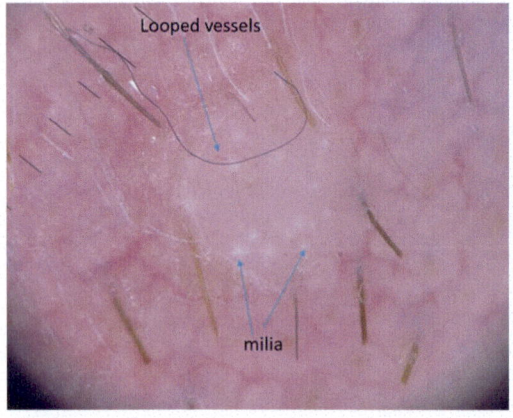

Looped vessels

milia

Fig. 4.10 Seborrhoeic keratosis

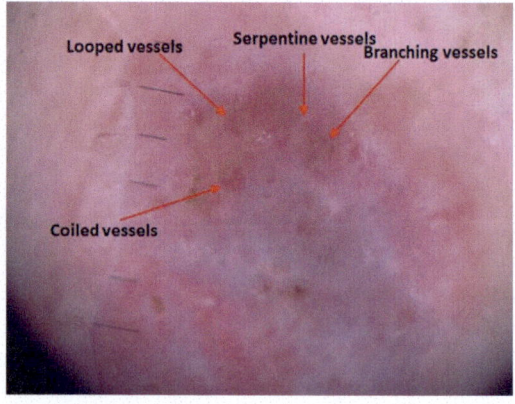

Looped vessels   Serpentine vessels   Branching vessels

Coiled vessels

Fig. 4.12 Melanoma

Fig. 4.11 Intradermal naevi

skin lesions. The method relied on pattern analysis, i.e. recognition of a number of dermatoscopic structures which form reproducible patterns characteristic of known pigmented lesions. The revised pattern analysis involves application of standard, agreed descriptors to define lesions [6].

Using this information a diagnosis is made and a decision regarding treatment is made. This is in contrast to the two-step algorithm where the objective is to make a decision between benign

Table 4.1 Dermoscopic algorithms and shared criteria

Criterion	Menzies method	7-point checklist	3-point checklist	Chaos and clues
Symmetry in colour or structure	x		x	x
Scoring of specific colours, i.e. black, grey, blue, dark brown, tan and red	x			
Blue/white veil *or* any blue/white colour	x	x	x	x
Atypical dots/globules	x	x		x
Regression	x	x	x	x
Streaks	x	x		x
Atypical network	x	x	x	x
Atypical vessels		x		x
Irregular blotches		x		x

Adapted from a more comprehensive summary table by Carrera et al. [11]

lesion and possible melanoma, to determine management with biopsy/excision. Advantages of pattern analysis include avoidance of ambiguous metaphoric terms and the ability to perform analysis in locations such as the face, mucosa and acral surfaces where other scoring algorithms may not be useful. Due to the large number of criteria to be considered, pattern analysis may be considered more difficult and demanding for the novice dermoscopist than the simple scoring systems used in the two-step algorithm. Chaos and clues is an algorithm developed using revised pattern analysis principles to identify pigmented lesions (melanocytic and non-melanocytic) that require further investigation [19, 20]. Table 4.2 outlines the process of pattern analysis.

Patterns

Kitler et al. [6] defined five elements in revised pattern analysis, i.e. lines, dots, clods, circles and pseudopods. There are also five patterns formed by lines (reticular, branched, parallel, radial and curved), and patterns may also be formed by the other elements, i.e. aggregated dots, clods, circles and pseudopods. An area where there is no predominant pattern is referred to as structureless. Combinations of patterns are possible. An important feature in dermoscopy is symmetry of pattern. Symmetry exists when the lesion's pattern can be mirrored in any axis. Symmetry is independent of the outline/shape of the lesion; it is assessed on internal pattern (see Fig. 4.13). The more numerous the patterns, the greater is the likelihood of their being asymmetrical. Asymmetry of pattern (structure) is a key feature of melanoma in the chaos and clues algorithm [21]. Asymmetry is a common feature of the two-step algorithms. Carrera et al. [11] found that architectural disorder, pattern asymmetry and contour asymmetry were the criteria most associated with melanoma and had the highest interobserver agreement.

Colour

A pigmented lesion may be composed of one or many colours. As is true for pattern, colour in a lesion may be arranged symmetrically or asymmetrically (see Fig. 4.13) . The appearance of pigment is affected by its location within the skin (see Table 4.3). Asymmetry of colour is another key risk factor for melanoma in the chaos and clues algorithm [19].

Clues

In pattern analysis clues are the dermoscopic features that favour one diagnosis over another.

Table 4.2 Steps involved in pattern analysis

1. Recognize patterns and arrangement.
2. Recognize colours and arrangement.
3. Look for characteristic clues.
4. From the above information, make a specific diagnosis.
5. Depending on the diagnosis, decide whether to treat or not.

Table 4.4 lists the dermatoscopic clues found in melanoma according to revised pattern analysis [6].

Examples of dermoscopic features found in melanoma can be found in Fig. 4.14a–c.

AN EXPLANATION OF SYMMETRY/ASYMMETRY

SYMMETRICAL LESIONS

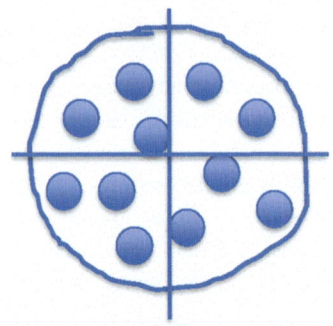 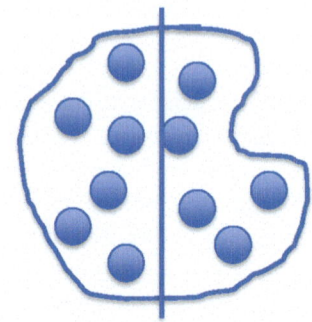

ASYMMETRICAL LESIONS

Asymmetry of colour

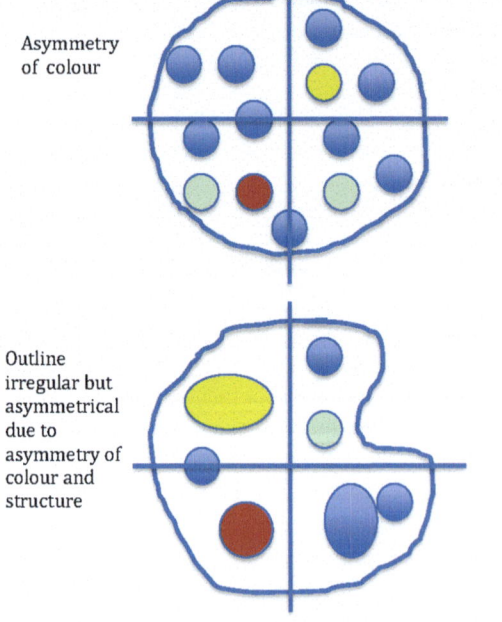 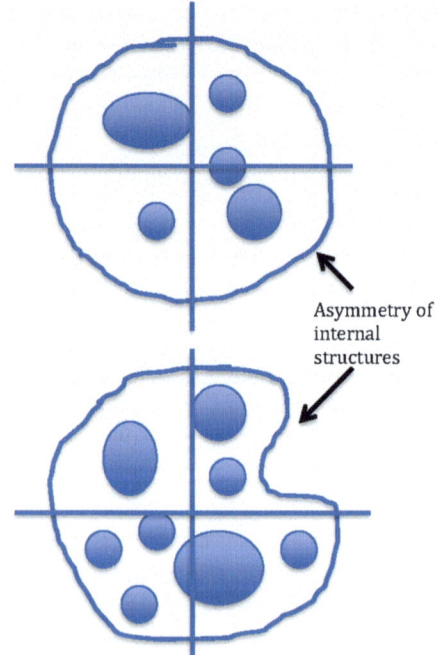

Asymmetry of internal structures

Outline irregular but asymmetrical due to asymmetry of colour and structure

Fig. 4.13 Visual explanation of asymmetry in structure/colour. Image by Claire Palmer

Table 4.3 Pigment colour

Location of Pigment	Colour of pigment	
Stratum corneum	Black	
Basal epidermis	Brown	
Papillary dermis	Grey	
Reticular dermis	Blue	

Table 4.4 Dermoscopic Clues for Melanoma

1. Eccentric structureless zones of any colour (except when skin coloured)
2. Grey circles, lines, dots or clods
3. Black dots or clods at the periphery
4. Pseudopods or radial lines at the periphery, which do not occupy the entire circumference
5. White lines
6. Thick reticular lines
7. Polymorphous vessels
8. Parallel lines on the ridge

Adapted from Kittler et al. [6]

Dermoscopy of Melanoma in Special Sites

Facial Pigmented Lesions

Assessment of pigmented facial lesions is complicated because facial lentigo maligna, pigmented actinic keratosis, solar lentigo and seborrhoeic keratosis may show overlapping features [22–24]. When reviewing a pigmented facial lesion, it is recommended that clinicians focus on the follicular unit for early signs of lentigo maligna. Lallas et al. determined the most potent predictors of lentigo maligna were grey rhomboid structures, nonevident follicles and intense pigmentation [24]. In contrast white circles, scales and red colour are correlated with pigmented actinic keratoses [24].

A scoring system for facial pigmented lesions has been proposed (not yet validated) by Lallas et al. [24] to help clinicians decide on management of pigmented facial lesions (see Table 4.5).

Examples of pigmented facial lesions can be seen in Fig. 4.15.

Acral Melanoma

Acral melanoma is the most prevalent type of malignant melanoma in non-Caucasian populations [25]. There are three major dermoscopic patterns in acral naevus: the parallel furrow, lattice-like and fibrillar patterns. In the benign acral naevi, the parallel furrow pattern is the most common. In this pattern there is linear pigmentation along the sulci of the surface skin markings (dermatoglyphic grooves). Histopathologically, the parallel furrow pattern is caused by melanin columns in the cornified layer derived from nests located in the crista profunda limitans situated under the surface furrow [25].

The typical dermoscopic appearance of pigmented acral melanoma is the parallel ridge pattern with pigmentation of the surface skin markings. This is in complete contrast to the parallel furrow pattern. The sensitivity and specificity of this parallel ridge pattern are high for both in situ and advanced acral melanoma (sensitivity 86%, specificity 99%) [25]. The furrow ink test is a useful test to identify the location of pigmentation in acral skin [26, 27]. In this test the skin is wet and a whiteboard marker applied to the edge of the lesion. The skin is then wiped. The *remaining ink will be located in the furrows*. Another dermoscopic pattern seen in acral melanoma is irregular, diffuse pigmentation. In this pattern, pigmentation is structureless with areas of diffuse, brownish-black pigmentation (variable shades) and occasional grey tone. Sensitivity and specificity of the irregular diffuse pigmentation are 69% and 97% in acral melanoma in situ and 94% and 97% in invasive melanoma [28].

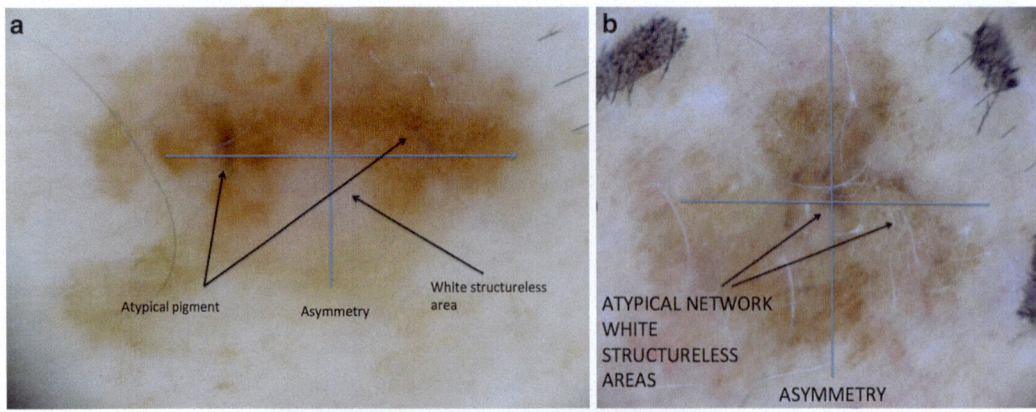

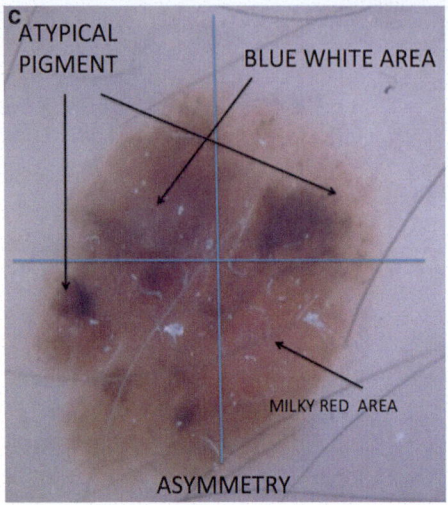

Fig. 4.14 (a–c) Examples of dermoscopic features found in melanoma

Table 4.5 Lallas et al. proposed scoring scheme for pigmented facial lesions

Criterion	Score
Grey rhomboidal lines	+2
Nonevident follicles	+1
Grey circles	+1
Pigmentation intensity (heavy)	+1
White circles	−2
Scaly surface	−1
Total score in our sample (range)	−3 to +5

A total score ≥ 1 is suggestive of lentigo maligna with a specificity of 55.4% and a sensitivity of 92.9%

1. If the lesion shows the parallel ridge pattern, biopsy regardless of size.
2. If the lesion does not show a parallel ridge pattern, then check for typical benign dermoscopic patterns, i.e. typical parallel furrow, typical lattice-like or regular fibrillar pattern. If the lesion shows a typical benign pattern, there is no need for further follow-up.
3. If the lesion does not show typical dermoscopic patterns, measure the maximum diameter.
   - >7 mm recommend biopsy
   - 7 mm or less, periodic clinical and dermoscopic follow-up

Koga et al. [29] have proposed a revised three-step algorithm for evaluation of acquired acral naevi. The steps in this algorithm include:

Examples of acral pigment pattern can be seen in Fig. 4.16.

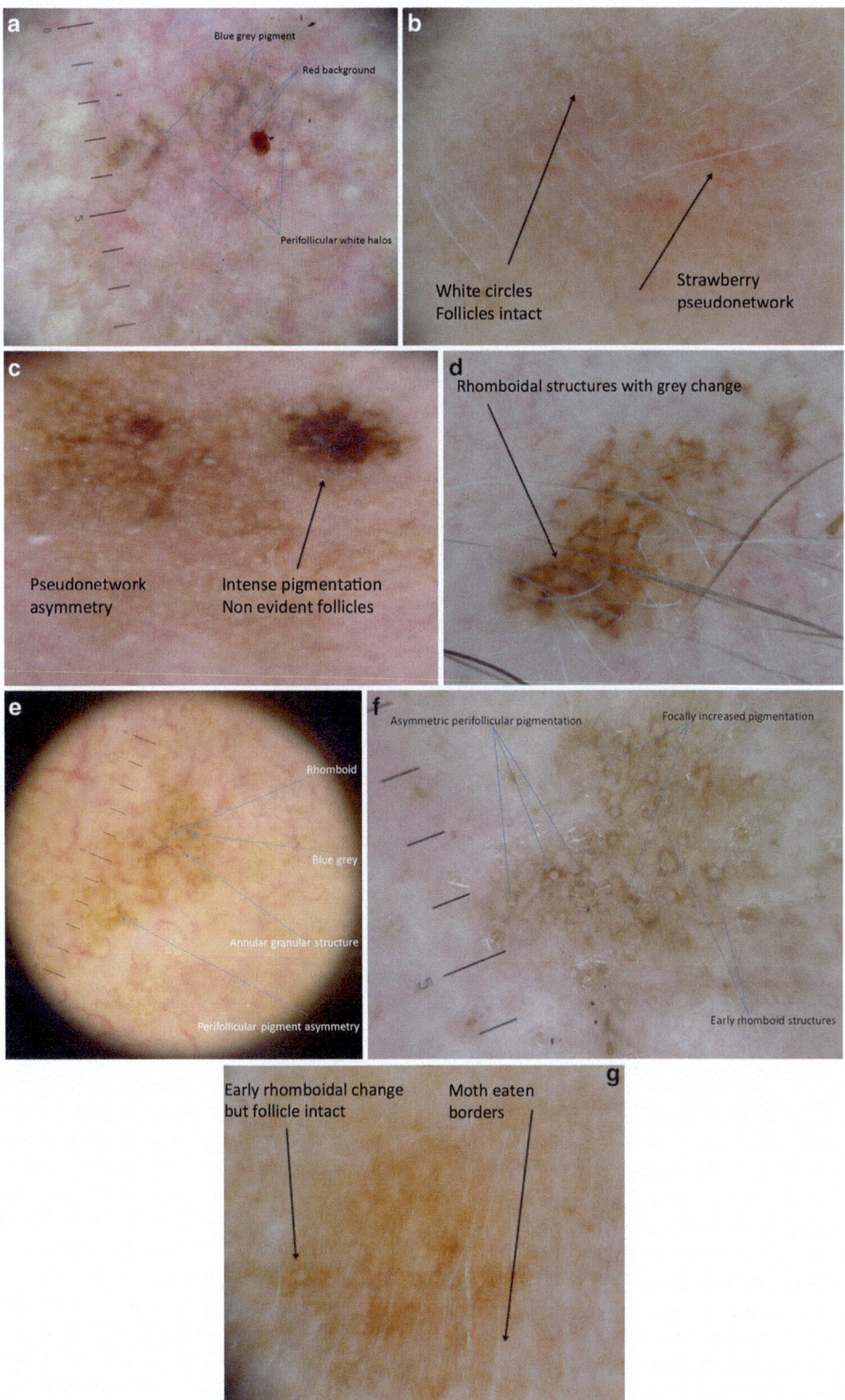

Fig. 4.15 Examples of pigmented facial lesions. (**a**, **b**) Pigmented actinic keratosis; (**c**, **d**, **e**) lentigo maligna; (**f**, **g**) solar lentigo/seborrhoeic keratosis

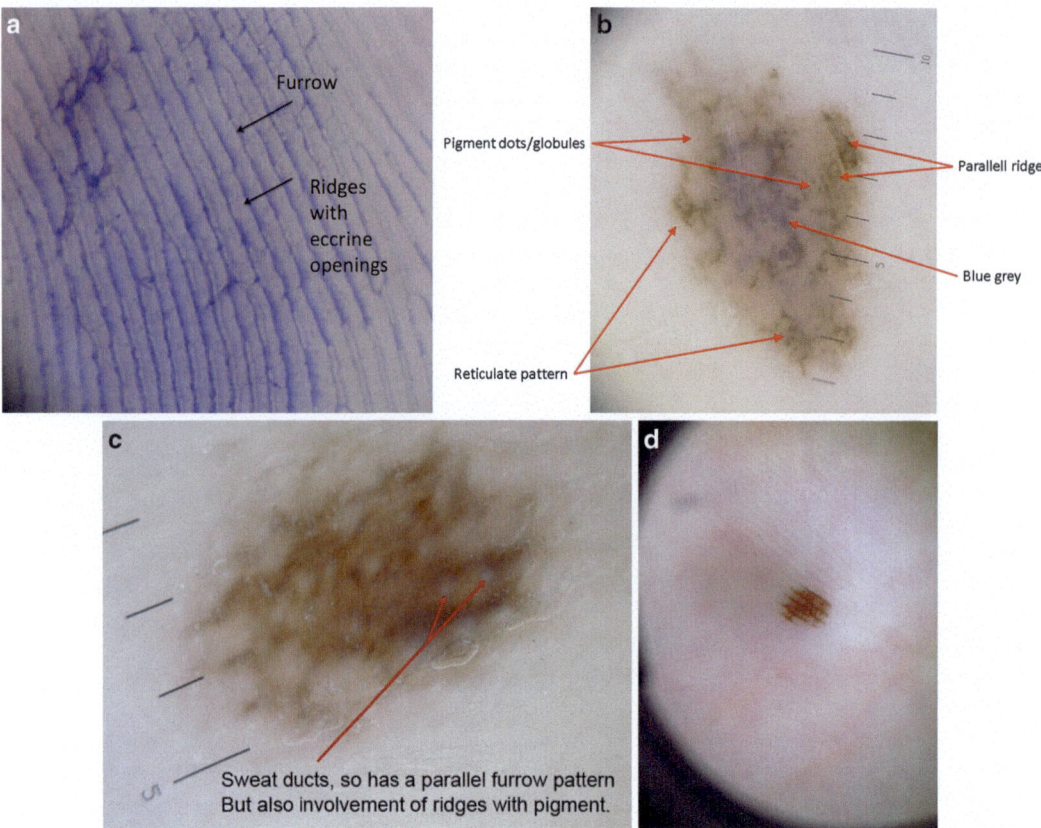

Fig. 4.16 Examples of acral pigment pattern. (**a**) Furrow ink test; (**b**) dysplastic acral naevus; (**c**) benign acral naevus; (**d**) furrow pattern with some lattice

Nail Unit Melanoma

Nail unit melanoma (NUM) is localised either under (subungual) or around (periungual) the nail. NUM is considered a variant of acral lentiginous melanoma. Acral melanomas represent a minority subgroup in Caucasians (1% to 2.5%) and is much more common in Asian races (50% to 58% of melanomas) [30–33]. In a review Haenssle et al. [34] describe a framework for assessment (not validated) of the nail. The first step in this process involves a decision as to whether there is a continuous melanocytic lesion present or a noncontinuous, non-melanocytic lesion. If it is noncontinuous non-melanocytic lesion, an attempt is made to identify what the lesion is. If it is classified as continuous melano-

Table 4.6 Classification of nail lesions

Examples of noncontinuous non-melanocytic lesions	Examples of continuous melanocytic lesions
Haemorrhage	Melanocytic naevus
Onychomycosis	Lentigo
Onychopapilloma	Racial/ethnic melanonychia
Subungual wart	Drug-induced hyperpigmentation
Neoplasms (glomus tumour, IEC/SCC)	Malignant melanoma

Adapted from Haenssle et al. [34]

cytic, then a decision needs to be made regarding further management (Table 4.6).

Ethnic nail pigmentation presents usually with homogenous brown to grey pigmentation. In benign naevi the width of the band is usually <5 mm in size varying in colour from light brown

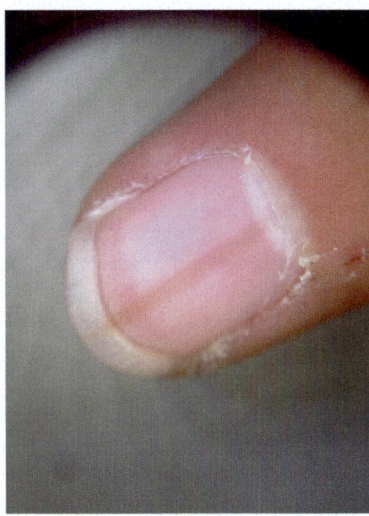

Fig. 4.17 Pigmented nail lesion in benign melanocytic naevus

to dark brown to black [35]. The bands are usually homogenous, or the individual lines within a band are evenly distributed and are a similar colour. In contrast melanoma is usually >5 mm with lines of variable thickness, spacing and colour.

An example of pigmented nail lesion can be seen in Fig. 4.17.

Hutchinson's sign is periungual (hyponychium) pigmentation accompanied by melanonychia, and it has an association with melanoma; however it has also been shown as a feature of benign melanocytic naevi [36].

Dermoscopy is a useful tool in evaluating the pigmented hyponychium; if the pattern is ridge pattern, then melanoma should be suspected, and if the pattern is parallel furrow or regular fibrillar, this suggests a benign naevus [35].

References

1. Soyer HP, Argenziano G, Chimenti S, Ruocco V. Dermoscopy of pigmented skin lesions. Eur J Dermatol. 2001;11(3):270–6.
2. Australian Cancer Network Melanoma Guidelines Revision Working Party. Clinical practice guidelines for the Management of Melanoma in Australia and New Zealand. Wellington: Cancer Council Australia and Australian Cancer Network, Sydney and New Zealand Guidelines Group; 2008.
3. Piliouras P, Buettner P, Soyer HP. Dermoscopy use in the next generation: a survey of Australian dermatology trainees. Australas J Dermatol. 2014;55:49–52. https://doi.org/10.1111/ajd.12061.
4. Anderson RR, Parrish JA. The optics of human skin. J Invest Dermatol. 1981;77:13–9.
5. Kittler H, Marghoob A, Argenziano G, Carrera C, Curiel-Lewandrowski C, Hofmann-Wellenhof R, et al. Standardization of terminology in dermoscopy/dermatoscopy: results of the third consensus conference of the International Society of Dermoscopy. J Am Acad Dermatol. 2016;74:1093–106.
6. Kittler H, Rosendahl C, Cameron A, Tschandl P. Dermatoscopy: an algorithmic method based on pattern analysis. 2011 Vienna Austria : Facultas.wuv Chapter 5 page 131.
7. Argenziano G, Soyer HP. Dermoscopy of pigmented skin lesions – a valuable tool for early diagnosis of melanoma. Lancet Oncol. 2001;2:443–9.
8. Argenziano G, Soyer HP, Chimenti S, Talamini R, Corona R, Sera F, et al. Dermoscopy of pigmented skin lesions: results of a consensus meeting via the internet. J Am Acad Dermatol. 2003;48:679–93.
9. Malvehy J, Puig S, Argenziano G, Ashfaq A, Marghoob A, Soyer HP. Dermoscopy report: proposal for standardization. Results of a consensus meeting of the International Dermoscopy Society J Am Acad Dermatol. J Am Acad Dermatol. 2007;57:84–95.
10. Marghoob A, Braun R. Proposal for a revised 2-step algorithm for the classification of lesions of the skin using dermoscopy. Arch Dermatol. 2010;146(4):426–8. https://doi.org/10.1001/archdermatol.2010.41.
11. Carrera C, Marchetti M, Dusza S, Argenziano G, Braun R, Halpern A, et al. Validity and reliability of Dermoscopic criteria used to differentiate nevi from melanoma a web-based international Dermoscopy society study. JAMA Dermatol. 2016;152(7):798–806. https://doi.org/10.1001/jamadermatol.2016.0624.
12. Carli P, Quercioli E, Sestini S, Stante M, Ricci L, Brunasso G, et al. Pattern analysis, not simplified algorithms, is the most reliable method for teaching dermoscopy for melanoma diagnosis to residents in dermatology. Br J Dermatol. 2003;148:981–4.
13. Argenziano G, Puig S, Zalaudek I, et al. Dermoscopy improves accuracy of primary care physicians to triage lesions suggestive of skin cancer. J Clin Oncol. 2006;24(12):1877–82.
14. Dolianitis C, Kelly J, Wolfe R, Simpson P. Comparative performance of 4 dermoscopic algorithms by nonexperts for the diagnosis of melanocytic lesions. Arch Dermatol. 2005;141(8):1008–14.
15. Chen L, Dusza S, Jaimes N, Marghoob A. Performance of the first step of the 2-step Dermoscopy algorithm. JAMA Dermatol. 2015;151(7):715–21. https://doi.org/10.1001/jamadermatol.2014.4642.
16. Tschandl P, Rosendahl C, Kittler H. Accuracy of the first step of the dermatoscopic 2-step algorithm for

pigmented skin lesions. Dermatol Pract Concept. 2012;2(3):a08. https://doi.org/10.5826/dpc.0203a08.

17. Pehamberger H, Steiner A, Wolff K. *In vivo* epiluminescence microscopy of pigmented skin lesions. I. Pattern analysis of pigmented skin lesions. J Am Acad Dermatol. 1987;17:571–83.

18. Steiner A, Pehamberger H, Wolff K. In vivo epiluminescence microscopy of pigmented skin lesions. II. Diagnosis of small pigmented skin lesions and early detection of malignant melanoma. J Am Acad Dermatol. 1987;17:584–91.

19. Rosendahl C, Cameron A, McColl I, Wilkinson D. Dermatoscopy in routine practice 'chaos and clues'. Aust Fam Physician. 41(7):482–7.

20. Rosendahl C, Tschandl P, Cameron A, Kittler H. Diagnostic accuracy of dermatoscopy for melanocytic and nonmelanocytic pigmented lesions. J Am Acad Dermatol. 2011;64:1068–73.

21. Rosendahl C, Cameron A, McColl I, Wilkinson D. Dermatoscopy in routine practice 'chaos and clues'. Aust Fam Physician. 2012;41(7):482–7.

22. Lallas A, Argenziano G, Moscarella E, et al. Diagnosis and management of facial pigmented macules. Clin Dermatol. 2014;32:94–100.

23. Stolz W, Schiffner R, Burgdorf WHC. Dermatoscopy for facial pigmented skin lesions. Clin Dermatol. 2002;20:276–8.

24. Lallas A, Tschandl P, Kyrgidis A, Stolz W, Rabinovitz H, Cameron A, et al. Dermoscopic clues to differentiate facial lentigo maligna from pigmented actinic keratosis. Br J Dermatol. 2016;174:1079–85.

25. Saida T, Miyazaki A, Oguchi S, et al. Significance of dermoscopic patterns in detecting malignant melanoma on acral volar skin: results of a multicenter study in Japan. Arch Dermatol. 2004;140:1233–8.

26. Braun RP, Thomas L, Kolm I, French LE, Marghoob AA. The furrow ink test: a clue for the dermoscopic diagnosis of acral melanoma vs nevus. Arch Dermatol. 2008;144:1618–20.

27. Uhara H, Koga H, Takata M, Saida T. The whiteboard marker as a useful tool for the dermoscopic "furrow ink test. Arch Dermatol. 2009;145:1331–2.

28. Saida T, Koga H, Uhara H. Key points in dermoscopic differentiation between early acral melanoma and acral nevus. J Dermatol. 2011;38(1):25–34. https://doi.org/10.1111/j.1346-8138.2010.01174.x.

29. Koga H, Saida T. Revised 3-step dermoscopic algorithm for the management of acral melanocytic lesions. Arch Dermatol. 2011;147(6):741–3. https://doi.org/10.1001/archdermatol.2011.136.

30. Duarte AF, Correia O, Barros AM, Azevedo R, et al. Nail matrix melanoma in situ: conservative surgical management. Dermatology. 2010;220:173–5.

31. Haneke E. Ungual melanoma—controversies in diagnosis and treatment. Dermatol Ther. 2012;25:510–24.

32. Chang JW. Acral melanoma: a unique disease in Asia. JAMA Dermatol. 2013;149:1272–3.

33. Jung HJ, Kweon SS, Lee JB, Lee SC, et al. A clinicopathologic analysis of 177 acral melanomas in koreans: relevance of spreading pattern and physical stress. JAMA Dermatol. 2013;149:1281–8.

34. Haenssle HA, Blum A, Hofmann-Wellenhof R, Kreusch J, Stolz W, Argenziano G, Zalaudek I, Brehmer F. When all you have is a dermatoscope start looking at the nails. Dermatol Pract Concept. 2014;4(4):11–20. https://doi.org/10.5826/dpc.0404a02.eCollection2014.

35. Hiroshi K, Toshiaki S, Hisashi U. Key point in dermoscopic differentiation between early nail apparatus melanoma and benign longitudinal melanonychia. J Dermatol. 2011;38:45–52. https://doi.org/10.1111/j.1346-8138.2010.01175.x.

36. Kawabata Y, Ohara K, Hino H, Tamaki K. Two kinds of Hutchinson's sign, benign and malignant. J Am Acad Dermatol. 2001;44(2):305–7.

Advances in Dermoscopy of Pigmented Lesions

5

Uday S. Khopkar and Ankit M. Bharti

Dermoscopy is a widely used noninvasive, diagnostic tool which magnifies the subtle clinical surface features of pigmented skin lesion as well as unveils certain subsurface structures which are not normally visible to the naked eye or even a magnifying lens. Although dermoscopy was earlier used mainly to diagnose neoplastic disorders of the skin (please see Chap. 4 on Dermoscopy of Melanoma), its use in pigmentary disorders and inflammatory disorders of the skin, as well as hair and nail disorders, has expanded the horizons of its applications immensely. This increase in the number of applications of dermoscopy has also increased the vocabulary of the dermoscopic descriptions, creating a multitude of terms to identify the colors and patterns which are sometimes specific to certain disorders and sometimes common to a number of disorders. UV light dermoscopy has added a new dimension to the application of polarized light dermoscopy in pigmentary disorders of the skin [1].

Disorders of Pigmentation

The disorders of pigmentation can be broadly divided into disorders of hyperpigmentation and hypopigmentation. The disorders of hyperpigmentation result from either increased melanin production or increased number of active melanocytes. Discoloration of the skin may also occur due to deposition of exogenous substances such as drugs and heavy metals which form complexes with the melanin [2]. The dermoscopic patterns of disorders of hyperpigmentation with well-documented data are melasma, exogenous ochronosis, pigmented purpuric dermatosis, lichen planus pigmentosus, erythema dyschromicum perstans, acanthosis nigricans, Dowling-Degos disease, reticulate acropigmentation of Kitamura, post-inflammatory hyperpigmentation, fixed drug eruption, and confluent and reticulated papillomatosis.

The disorders of hypopigmentation can result either from reduction or loss of epidermal or follicular melanocytes, due to decrease or loss of melanin synthesis or due to failure of melanin transfer to adjacent keratinocytes [2]. The disorders associated with hypopigmentation, with known dermoscopic features, are vitiligo, idiopathic guttate hypomelanosis, hypopigmented mycosis fungoides, hypomelanosis from bacterial infections (like leprosy) and parasitic infection or infestations (like leishmaniasis), and halo nevus.

U. S. Khopkar (✉) · A. M. Bharti
Department of Dermatology, Seth GS Medical
College & KEM Hospital, Mumbai,
Maharashtra, India
e-mail: drkhopkar@gmail.com

© Springer International Publishing AG, part of Springer Nature 2018
P. Kumarasinghe (ed.), *Pigmentary Skin Disorders*, Updates in Clinical Dermatology,
https://doi.org/10.1007/978-3-319-70419-7_5

Dermoscopic Findings

In the standard algorithm used to diagnose pigmented skin lesions by dermoscopy, a normal pigment network is used to differentiate between melanocytic and non-melanocytic skin lesions. The pigment network forms a honeycomb pattern which corresponds histologically to the presence of melanin in the basal keratinocytes of the epidermis along the rete ridges; the hypopigmented islands in between the network correspond to the tips of the dermal papillae and the overlying suprapapillary epidermis (Fig. 5.1) [3]. The anatomic location of the skin determines the width of network and size of the islands along with the texture of the epidermis and presence of blood vessels. The rete ridge pattern varies according to the anatomic location as on the lips, palms, soles, knees, elbows, and face and differs from that of non-glabrous skin elsewhere. Thus, there exists a variation in the pigment network which is usually absent in these locations and is replaced by a thinner and lighter pseudo-network pattern over the face and a parallel pigment pattern over the palms and soles. The pigment network may not be visible during dermoscopy of the non-glabrous skin if the rete ridge pattern is truncated or if it contains lesser melanin pigment.

Melanin pigment at its normal location in the epidermis displays brown color. However, dermoscopy of melanin in a pigmented skin lesion shows an array of colors depending on the position of melanin in the skin [3]. The melanin pigment when located in the stratum corneum appears black; in the remainder of the epidermis and upper dermis, it appears brown; in the papillary dermis, it appears gray; and in the lower papillary and reticular dermis, it appears blue. When melanin is present in large quantity in several layers, the color is black. The other colors seen on dermoscopy include red (due to vascularity and/or inflammation), white (due to depigmentation and/or scarring), yellow (due to sebaceous material and/or hyperkeratosis), orange (due to serum resulting from erosion or superficial ulceration), and jet black (due to coagulated blood).

Some of the common findings (Table 5.1) and patterns (Table 5.2) observed during dermoscopy of pigmented disorders are tabulated along with clinicopathologic correlations thereof below.

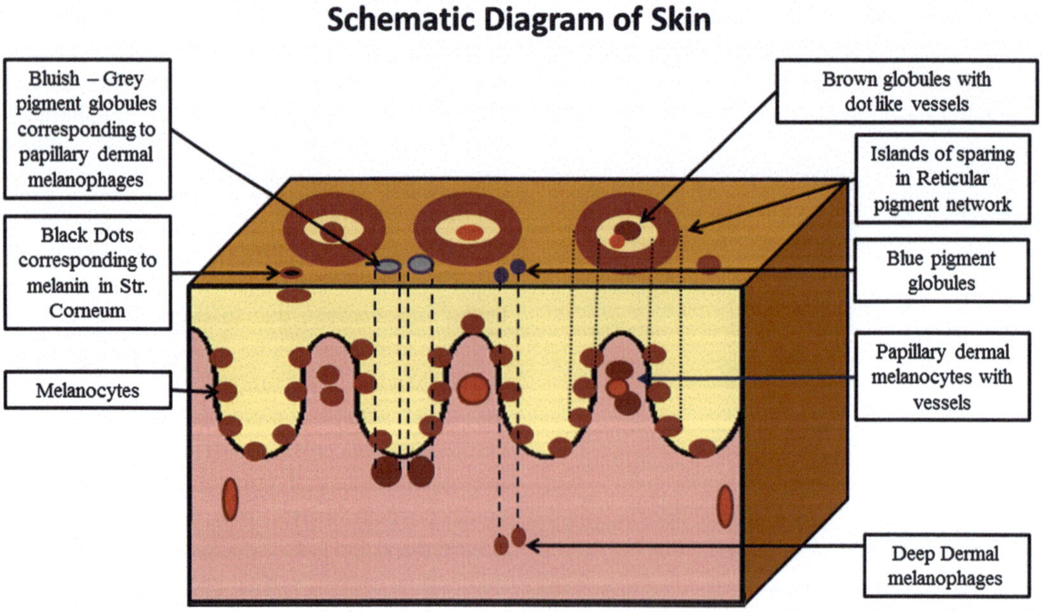

Schematic Diagram of Skin

Fig. 5.1 Schematic diagram of normal pigment network with color of melanin depending of its depth

Table 5.1 Common findings in dermoscopy of pigmentary disorders

Basic feature	Dermoscopic findings	Clinical significance
Pigment networks		
Normal pigment network	A netlike pattern of pigmentation that is seen over the normal skin, consists of homogenously pigmented lines with pale areas in between the pigment pattern, can vary slightly according to the pattern of rete ridges in different areas	Normal skin
Pseudoreticular network	The reticular pattern is incompletely irregular and blunted with large hypomelanotic areas	Normally over face
Accentuated pigment network	Darker pigment network with thick lines observed over affected skin as compared to normal	Normal dark skin, Addisonian pigmentation, café au lait macules, lichen planus pigmentosus, melasma
Granular pigment network	The network is formed by granular dark lines instead of normal homogenous pigment lines	Lichen planus pigmentosus, ashy dermatosis, post-inflammatory hyperpigmentation
Reverse pigment network	Serpiginous interconnecting broadened hypopigmented lines that surround elongated and curvilinear globules	Nevus depigmentosus, vitiligo
Reticulo-globular pattern	Patchy accentuation of pseudoreticular network surrounding globular pigmented areas	Normal face, melasma
Annular or arcuate pattern	Annular or arcuate pattern of pigment around whitish globules	Melasma
Acriform structures	Crescent-shaped dark brown pigment	Exogenous ochronosis
Hem-like pattern	Hyperpigmented dots and specks arranged in a "hem-like" pattern	Lichen planus pigmentosus
Rippled pattern	Corrugated appearance of the surface	Acanthosis nigricans, macular amyloidosis
Dots and globules		
Regular dots	Pigmented structures less than 0.1 mm	Regular, evenly distributed dots
Irregular dots	Pigmented structures less than 0.1 mm	Exogenous ochronosis
Blue-gray dots	Melanin pigment in papillary dermis	Lichen planus pigmentosus, melasma

Disorders of Hyperpigmentation

Melasma

The normal pigment network typically seen at other sites is absent on the face [4]. The pseudo-network on the face is made up of regularly arranged brown dots interrupted by follicular orifices and sebaceous glands. Early melasma shows scattered islands of reticular network of light brown or tan color with dark fine granules scattered on the surface. It shows a brown reticular pattern of pigmentation present around the opening of sweat gland and follicles producing an exaggerated pseudo-network pattern with concave borders

which is referred to as "jelly sign" (Fig. 5.2b). The epidermal reticular pattern seen in progressive lesion resembles the pseudo-network but has more diffuse blotchy large brownish pigmented globules and multiple granules superimposed on the reticular pattern. Larger patches of melasma, dark brown in color, show diffuse reticular pigmentation or irregularly shaped blotches or blackish pigmentation of various size (Fig. 5.2a). The surface of this pigmentation shows varying morphologies like arcuate, starlike, annular, and honeycomb. Granules and globules of dark brown color are also seen especially in the perifollicular region (Fig. 5.2b). The dermal component of melasma is seen as bluish streaks in reticulated pattern. The late lesions appear as

Table 5.2 Patterns in dermoscopy of pigmentary disorders

Basic feature	Dermoscopic findings	Clinical correlation
Normal pigmentation	Diffuse, well-defined hyperpigmented macule/patch	Regular – nevus whereas irregular – malignant lesion
Hypopigmentation	Areas of decreased pigmentation occurring within a pigmented structure	Pre-vitiligo, leishmaniasis, hypopigmented mycosis fungoides
Pseudo-network	A structureless pigment area interrupted by nonpigmented adnexal openings	Melasma, lichen planus pigmentosus, erythema dyschromicum perstans
Starburst pattern	Peripheral globules, pseudopods, or streaks(or a combination of all) located around the entire perimeter of the lesion	Lichen planus, idiopathic guttate hypomelanosis
Nebuloid pattern	A depigmented macule with smudged borders	Usually with unstable guttate vitiligo, occasionally with idiopathic guttate hypomelanosis
Feathery pattern	Moderately defined with feathery margins and irregular pigmentation	Usually with unstable guttate vitiligo, occasionally with idiopathic guttate hypomelanosis
Central white scar-like patch	Well-defined hypopigmented area in a pigmented lesion	Melasma, ochronosis
Regression structures	White area/blue area or combination of both	Lichen planus-like keratosis

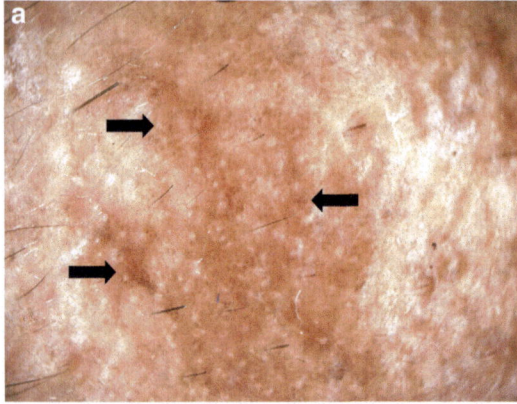 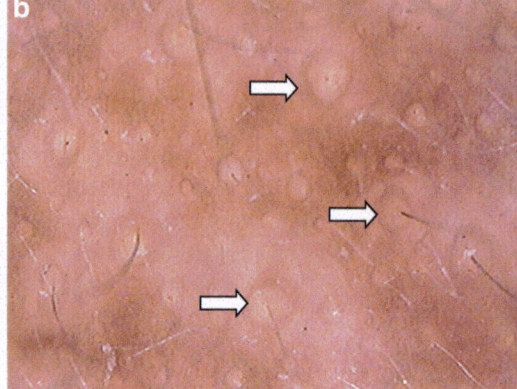

Fig. 5.2 (**a**) Low-power (40X) view of melasma with diffuse patchy reticular pigmentation with blotches (black arrow). (**b**) High-power (120X) view of melasma with exaggerated pseudo-reticular pattern with globules and jelly sign (white arrow)

grayish brown granules or arcuate or annular pigment network sparing the follicles.

Thus, dermoscopy can help in differentiating epidermal from dermal melasma, especially in later stages from lichen planus pigmentosus, seborrheic keratosis, nevus of Ota, ochronosis, lentigines, freckles, etc.

Dermoscopic evaluation also assists equivocally in identifying complications like atrophy, depigmentation, telangiectasia, exogenous ochronosis, and steroid dermatitis which have been on the rise in certain regions of the world

due to irrational use of currently available treatment option like steroids and hydroquinone [5].

Exogenous Ochronosis

Exogenous ochronosis (EO) is a disorder characterized by the deposition of microscopic, brownish-yellow or ochre-colored pigment in the dermis, giving rise to a blue-black hue in the skin [6]. Depending on origin it can be exogenous or endogenous. It is often associated with the prolonged application of various topical depigmenting agents particularly hydroquinone (HQ) leading to deposition of polymerized form of homogentisic acid in collagen in the dermis [13]. Three stages have been defined by Dogliotte in evolution of a lesion of EO: (i) initial erythema and mild pigmentary changes; (ii) hyperpigmentation, with *caviar* like hyperpigmented papules and atrophy; and (iii) papulo-nodules. Histopathologically, it is characterized by yellow-brown banana-shaped ochronotic fibres. In advanced stages, there is degeneration of the ochronotic fibres and formation of caviar-like hyperchromatic papules [7].

The dermoscopy of a melasma patch with ochronosis displays an accentuation of the pseudo-reticular pattern in areas with melasma, whereas in areas with ochronosis, it displays grayish-brown amorphous structures in the perifollicular region with few obliterating the follicular openings. There is also presence of short, thin, arciform structures along with few curvilinear or "wormlike" structures in some areas (Fig. 5.3) which histopathologically correspond to the "banana bodies" seen on histopathology [8]. It is to be noted that although the differences between "melasma" and EO Stage II and III are easily recognizable on dermoscopy, the greatest difficulty comes in differentiating melasma from Stage I EO [9].

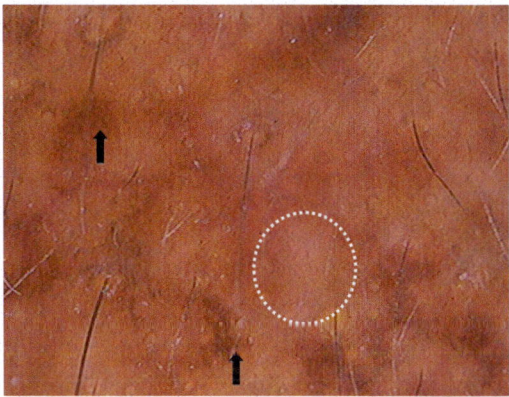

Fig. 5.3 High-power view (120X) shows macular depigmentation (Fitzpatrick's macule marked by white circle) and speckling (black arrow)

Thus the clinical significance and diagnostic utility of the arciform structures, speckling, can prove to be a useful tool to differentiate melasma from exogenous ochronosis.

Pigmented Purpuric Dermatosis

Pigmented purpuric dermatosis (PPD) is a chronic disorder of unknown etiology characterized by symmetrical hyperpigmented macules and petechiae, confined to the lower legs [10]. It is characterized by intradermal extravasation of erythrocytes or hemosiderin deposition. It can be divided into five clinical types on the basis of their clinical appearances. They are Schamberg's disease (SD) or progressive pigmented purpuric dermatosis, Majocchi's disease (MD) or purpura annularis telangiectodes, lichen aureus (LA), pigmented purpuric lichenoid dermatosis, and eczematoid purpura of Doucas and Kapetanakis. Some cases of pigmented purpuric dermatosis may clinically resemble stasis pigmentation, post-inflammatory hyperpigmentation, purpuric clothing dermatitis (khaki), leukocytoclastic vasculitis, and senile or steroid-induced purpura. Their differentiation may require dermoscopy or biopsy [17].

Common dermoscopic findings include coppery red pigment network (hemosiderin), round to oval dark brown globules (melanocytes and/or melanophages at the dermoepidermal junction), red dots (extravasated of red blood cells), and patches. Later stages show brownish or coppery-red, diffuse, homogenous background and interconnected network of gray dots. The increased number of blood vessels, some of which are dilated and swollen, appear as dotted vessels and glomerular vessels similar to those observed in psoriasis and verruca; linear vessels similar to lichen planus are also observed.

The dermoscopic patterns observed in lichen aureus, by Portela et al. and Zaballoz et al., and in Schamberg's disease by Ozkaya et al. were similar to those of PPD and not precise [10, 11].

Lichen Planus Pigmentosus

Lichen planus pigmentosus (LPP) is characterized by asymptomatic slate-gray pigmentation,
predominantly on the face and persistent in
nature. Classically, it follows an "actinic" distribution with symmetrical and diffuse pigmentation in sun-exposed areas, commonly in
dark-skinned individuals [12]. The pigmentation
is dermal and occurs without any preceding clinical evidence of inflammation.

LPP and erythema dyschromicum perstans
pose a common diagnostic dilemma due to similar appearance [13]. LPP is usually accompanied by pruritus at its onset along with frequent
relapses and remissions. The current modality
of confirming diagnosis is clinico-pathological
correlation. Dermoscopic examination of LPP
(Fig. 5.4) has revealed irregularly accentuated
reticular pigment pattern, with coarse granular
pigment at certain places. The normal reticular
pattern of pigment and the pigment surrounding
the acrosyringeal openings are blunted. There
are rounded, linear, granular discrete bluish-
gray pigment deposits evenly spaced and at
places tending to form a curvilinear pattern.
Over the extremities, a "hem-like" regular distribution of clusters of pigment is seen. There is
a tendency of the pigment to be deposited

around the acrosyringeal openings and around
follicular openings [12].

Erythema Dyschromicum Perstans and Ashy Dermatosis

Ashy dermatosis or EDP was recognized as a
separate entity when first described by Ramirez
in 1957 [13]. As against LPP, EDP cases show
more truncal affection with larger, rounded
patches of grayish pigmentation often surrounded
by a rim of faint erythema and scaling. Chapter
13 describes these conditions (acquired macular
pigmentation of uncertain aetiology) in more
detail. EDP, which is usually asymptomatic, over
the face shows uniformly accentuated reticular
pattern of pigment network on dermoscopic evaluation. The pigmented lines which form the reticular pattern are more thickened than usual, and
the lines are more granular than linear. Sometimes
the granules appear to be superimposed on lines.
The granules probably correlate with clusters of
melanophages commonly found in the papillary
dermis. The reticular pattern is complete at
places, and occasionally it disintegrated into
more discrete speckled, granular, linear, angulated, bluish-gray deposits. Over the extremities
the reticular pigment pattern around the acrosy-

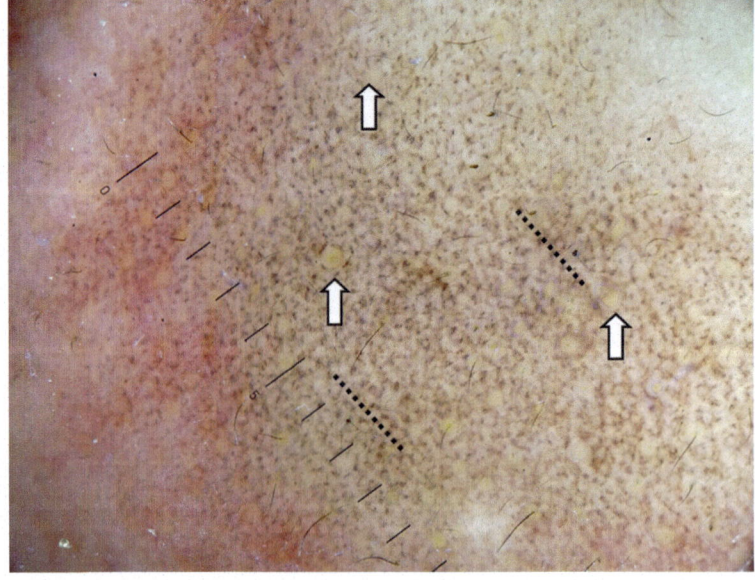

Fig. 5.4 Low-power (40X) view showing discrete bluish-gray pigment deposits with occasional curvilinear distribution sparing the acrosyringium (white arrow) and "hem-like" pattern (beside the black dotted line)

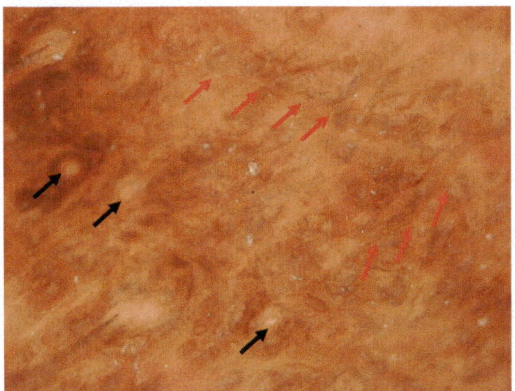

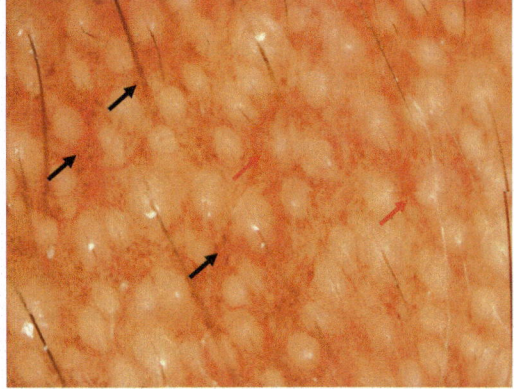

Fig. 5.5 Low-power view (40X) shows crista cutis (along red lines) and sulcus cutis with follicular plugging (black arrow)

Fig. 5.6 High-power view (120X) shows accentuated pseudo-network pattern with dark brown specks (black arrows) of pigment and telangiectasia (red arrows)

ringium is blunted. There are rounded, linear, granular discrete bluish-gray pigment deposits evenly spaced and at places tending to form a curvilinear pattern. The pigment clusters are limited by skin surface markings and do not cross them. Pigment deposits do not encircle the follicular openings.

Acanthosis Nigricans

Dermoscopy of the plaque of acanthosis nigricans over the neck shows linear crista cutis and sulcus cutis (Fig. 5.5); crista cutis displays multiple focal hyperpigmented globules which indicate follicular plugging along with white globules which represent follicular openings and eccrine ducts [14].

Periorbital Hyperpigmentation

Periorbital melanosis develops with respect to four major components: hemodynamic congestion, reduced thickness of the epidermis, dermal melanin deposition, and genetic factors [15]. It is believed to have three main etiologies: vascular, pigmented, and mixed.

The three most common dermoscopic pigmentation patterns observed are pseudo-network pattern (Fig. 5.6), blotchy pigmentation pattern,

and multicomponent pigmentation pattern. Dermoscopic evaluation of periorbital darkening/melanosis appears valuable, particularly in the determination of the degree and pattern of pigmentation as well as the extent of vascular involvement, which in turn would reflect on the choice of therapy. We have observed patchy accentuated pseudo-network pattern with speckling, white dots, and telangiectasia. In the vascular type, diffuse erythema pattern or multiple thin blood vessels or diffuse vascular network is observed [16].

Dowling-Degos Disease and Reticulate Acropigmentation of Kitamura

Dowling-Degos disease (DDD) is an autosomal dominant (with variable penetrance) genodermatosis characterized by reticular pigmentation of the flexures due to loss-of-function mutation in the keratin 5 gene (17). It is characterized by slowly progressing hyperpigmented macules involving the flexures, which begins in adult life. It shows multiple reticular pigmented macules over the flexors, neck, and occasionally on the dorsa of the hands, along with follicular keratotic papules and pitted perioral scars.

Dermoscopy of the hyperpigmented macules shows fine reticulated pigment network with some of the lesions showing annular pigmented pattern (hyperplasia and hyperpigmentation of rete ridges) with hypopigmentation in the center (follicular infundibulum). Dermoscopy of hyperpigmented lesion shows polyangulated zone with accentuation of pigment markings (Fig. 5.7a) which are usually perifollicular and shows follicular plugging. These polyangulated networks form a pseudo-reticular pattern which histopathologically corresponds to the branching epidermal hyperplasia ("antler-like") seen in this condition (Fig. 5.7b). The follicular pits on polarized light dermoscopy display irregular brownish projections representing the elongated rete ridges around the hypopigmented center with pigmentation at the tips, while the hypopigmented center corresponds to the follicular infundibulum. Palmar pits on polarized light revealed plugging with keratinous material along with breaks in the dermatoglyphic pattern by linear pigmented furrows [18].

The lesions on the palmar pits appear as depression with pigmentation at the margins. Reticular pigmentation similar to the skin is also seen on the palms. Early lesions begin as short depressed lines that interrupt the dermatoglyphic lines and eventually join to form annular pattern [19].

Similarly increasing evidence over the last few years suggests that reticulate acropigmentation of Kitamura (RAK) and Galli-Galli disease represent different phenotypic expressions of DDD [20].

RAK cases present with reticulate hyperpigmented macules and papules on the dorsum of the hands and feet, facial pits, breaks in dermatoglyphics, and epidermoid cysts. The dermoscopic examination of the hyperpigmented macules reveals a fine reticular pigment network similar to that of DDD. The patchy brown pigmented spots that are coinciding with the punctate depressions on the palms and soles seem to be specific of RAK. These spots become apparent on dermoscopy and are heterogeneous; they lack pigment networks or patterns that are previously established.

In the first reported instance of RAK, Kitamura et al. had described minute depressions in the skin surface corresponding to pigmentation which might be difficult to detect by macroscopic examination [21]. However, dermoscopy proves to be instrumental in locating them and thus promises to be useful in differentiating RAK from other pigmented disorders such as dyschromatosis symmetrica hereditaria.

Post-inflammatory Hyperpigmentation

In post -inflammatory hyperpigmentation there is irregular accentuation of normal pigment network pattern or at places partial loss of normal pigment network on the face, pseudo-reticular

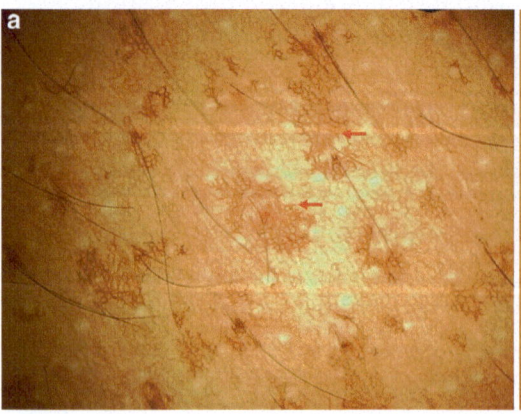
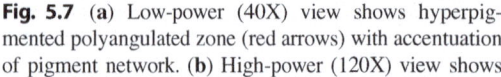
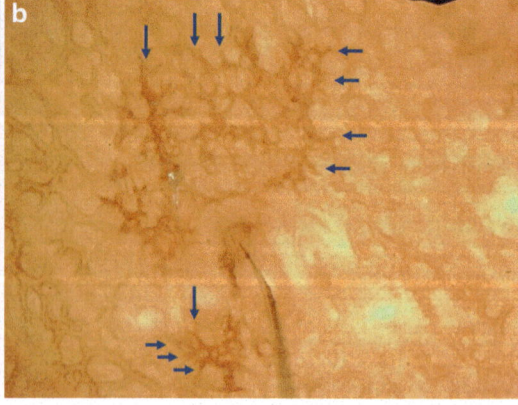

Fig. 5.7 (**a**) Low-power (40X) view shows hyperpigmented polyangulated zone (red arrows) with accentuation of pigment network. (**b**) High-power (120X) view shows polyangulated accentuation of pigment network with pseudopod-like extensions which correlate with "antler-like appearance" epidermal hyperplasia seen on histology

honeycomb-like pattern, with or without whitish irregular blotches (Fig. 5.8). The brown blotches of variable intensity may coexist depending on the underlying condition and depth of melanophages. The dermoscopy also shows granular pigment dots which represent dermal melanophages. The perifollicular sparing of pigment gives it a targetoid appearance and multiple islands of sparing which histologically represent the dermal papillae [22]. Blotchy erythema or microscaling may be present in the background.

Fixed Drug Eruption (FDE)

The dermoscopy of FDE reveals black dots, light- to dark-brown dots, and steel-blue dots. Dermoscopy of FDE displays multiple colored dots ranging from black to blue-gray corresponding to the melanin pigment deposition at different levels of the epidermis and dermis; this confirms the findings of pigment incontinence and damage at the dermoepidermal junction caused by lymphocytic infiltrate and interface damage taking place [23]. The use of dermoscopy in fixed drug eruption is not well described or documented; thus it can be considered a valid tool to a dermatologist which gives information about the depth of melanin to know the prognosis of FDE.

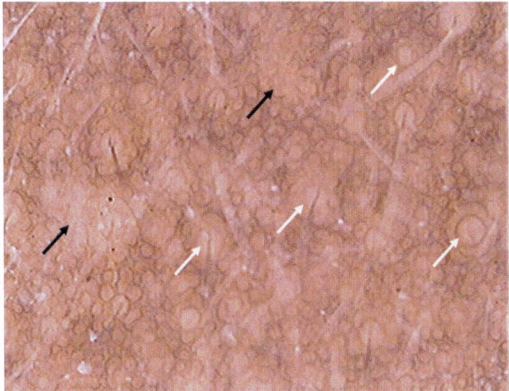

Fig. 5.8 Low-power (40X) view shows irregular accentuation of pseudo-reticular network with hypopigmented islands and acrosyringeal sparing (white arrows) and white blotches (black arrows)

Confluent and Reticulated Papillomatosis (CRP)

Confluent and reticulated papillomatosis (CRP) of Gougerot-Carteaud is a chronic disorder characterized by brown, spotted, warty papules that coalesce in the center with a peripheral reticulate pattern, leading to formation of desquamative plaques with imprecise limits [24].

Dermoscopy of CRP demonstrates bridges and furrows arranged in "crocodile skin-like" pattern which develops due to the confluent and reticulated nature of plaques and papules [14]. The furrows are brown in color and arranged in rhomboid pattern which correspond to rete ridges in the histology. The ridges demonstrate whitish structures which represent hyperkeratosis and acanthosis of follicular epidermis which indicates a possible pathology of integument. The brownish lines observed at the periphery of grayish globules give a wavy or curvilinear appearance. Thus pattern of pigmentary lines in dermoscopy gives clue to the diagnosis of CRP and can prove to be an essential tool for confirming its diagnosis.

Urticaria Pigmentosa (Cutaneous Mastocytosis)

The dermoscopy of urticaria pigmentosa has been well described by Vano-Galvan et al. He describes four major dermoscopic patterns in a study of 127 patients with cutaneous mastocytosis which include light brown blots, accentuated pigment network, reticular vascular pattern (consisting of thin reticular telangiectasias), and yellow-orange blotches [25]. An emphasis is made on the predominant pattern of accentuated pigment network and light brownish blotches which were observed more frequently in a study by Miller et al. [26]. Vano-Galvan also described that the reticular vessels which were mostly seen in patients with telangiectasia macularis eruptive perstans, and the yellow-orange blotches were more prevalent in mastocytoma help differentiate urticaria pigmentosa.

It is believed that the pigment network seen with dermoscopy is due to a high concentration of mast cell growth factor that stimulates melanocyte proliferation and melanogenesis which leads to hyperpigmentation of basal keratinocytes [26, 27].

Disorders of Hypopigmentation

Vitiligo

Dermoscopy can serve as an invaluable tool to assess the diagnosis and status of vitiligo, its stability, and repigmentation, which can be difficult to comment only on clinical examination [28]. Some of the commonly used terminologies associated with dermoscopy of vitiligo are polka-dot or salt-and-pepper appearance (perifollicular pigmentation), comet-tail appearance (micro-Koebner phenomenon), starburst appearance (nebulous pattern or galaxy sign), trichrome pattern (peripheral repigmentation), marginal and perifollicular hyperpigmentation, reticular pigmentation, and marginal reticular pigmentation. We noticed reduced pigmentary network, absent pigmentary network, reversed pigmentary network, perifollicular hyperpigmentation (see Fig. 5.11b), and perilesional hyperpigmentation in association with the evolving lesions of vitiligo [29]. Early small macules of vitiligo (guttate vitiligo) display the following four patterns:

1. Nebulous (starburst) pattern – oval or round cloudy dense white pattern with indistinct margins merging into the surrounding skin
2. Feathery pattern – slightly well-defined with feathery margins and irregular pigmentation
3. Petaloid pattern – well-defined petal-like pattern with irregular pigmented margin
4. Amoeboid pattern – hypopigmented macule with pseudopod-like extensions and hyperpigmented margins

The above patterns are similar to those seen with idiopathic guttate hypomelanosis (IGH), the only difference being that the amoeboid and petaloid patterns are much more common in IGH

than in guttate vitiligo in which the nebuloid and feathery patterns are more common [30]. Hypopigmented macules of vitiligo can be distinguished from other hypopigmented macules by UV light dermoscopy as they get accentuated with UV exposure [30]. The loss of epidermal melanin in vitiligo lesions produces a window through which the light-induced autofluorescence of dermal collagen can be seen resulting in the bright blue-white glow.

The evolving lesions of vitiligo show multiple blotches of depigmentation with loss of pigment network (Fig. 5.9) over patches forming islands of depigmentation; early lesion may also reveal perifollicular depigmentation along with unmasking of subtle unrecognizable leukotrichia (see Fig. 5.11a, b). Absence of microscaling distinguishes untreated early vitiligo from a macule which is observed in leprosy [31, 32].

The reversed pigmentary network (Fig. 5.9) described by Thatte et al. is white or depigmented netlike pattern with globules of normal pigmentation in the center and has been well documented in dermoscopy of melanoma and melanocytic nevus, yet this finding has not earlier been mentioned in vitiligo [29]. In conclusion, dermoscopy scores over routine histopathology in the diagnosis of evolving lesions of vitiligo and can obviate the need for a skin biopsy in many doubtful cases.

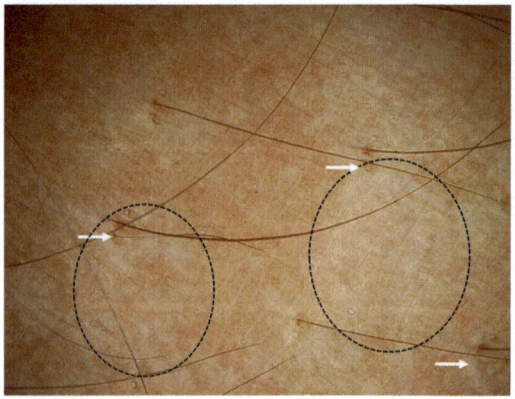

Fig. 5.9 Low-power (40X) view of evolving lesion of vitiligo shows patchy loss of pigment network with nebulous (cloudy) appearance with reversed pigmentary network (black circles) and leukotrichia (white arrow)

Idiopathic Guttate Hypomelanosis

Four dermoscopic patterns seen in guttate vitiligo or evolving lesions of vitiligo have also been described by Bambroo et al. in IGH, namely, nebuloid, petaloid, feathery, and amoeboid [30]. The nebuloid pattern of IGH is observed usually in early lesions as well as among older patients. The feathery (Fig. 5.10), amoeboid, and petaloid patterns are more commonly seen in older lesions of IGH. Ankad et al. have described the histopathology features of IGH in a study and observed the whitish areas (yellow diamond) in the center

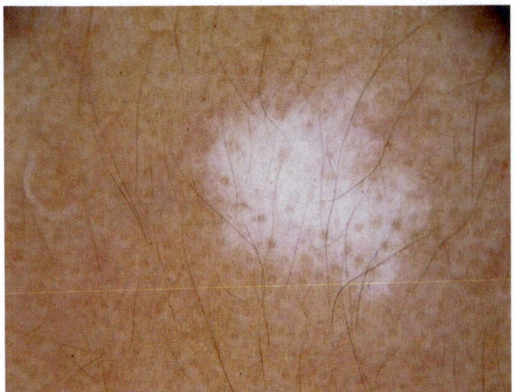

Fig. 5.10 Low-power (40X) view of IGH showing feathery pattern with loss of pigment network

of feathery patterned lesions to correlate with epidermal hyperkeratosis and denote long-standing disease [33].

Hypopigmented Mycosis Fungoides

Mycosis fungoides (MF), the most common primary cutaneous T-cell lymphoma, is a neoplastic disease characterized by classical non-infiltrated lesions (patches), plaques, tumors, and erythrodermic stages. Dermoscopic evaluation displays (i) dotted vessels, (ii) fine short linear vessels, (iii) spermatozoa-like vascular structures, (iv) orange-yellowish patchy areas, (v) white scales, and (vi) yellow scales [34]. The dermoscopic pattern can be variable in the patterns of vessels observed with dotted morphologic appearance irrespective of the diameter of the dots; similarly variable "linear vessels" are characterized by vessels with linear morphology which may or may not be curved. The term "spermatozoa-like structures" is applied to a characteristic vascular pattern observed as a dotted and a short, curved linear vessel (overall shaped as a spermatozoon). The feature "orange-yellowish patchy areas" had also been observed by Xu et al. [35].

We observed regular loss of pigment network with accentuated pseudo-reticular pigment network in certain areas with acrosyringeal

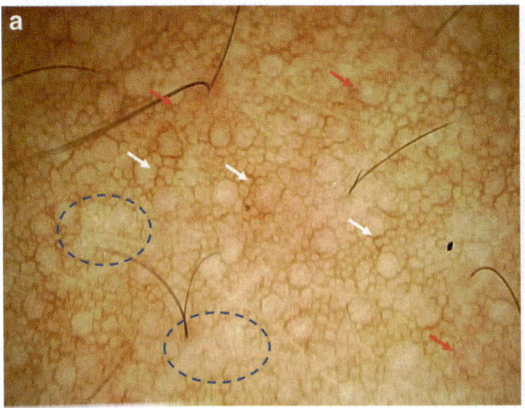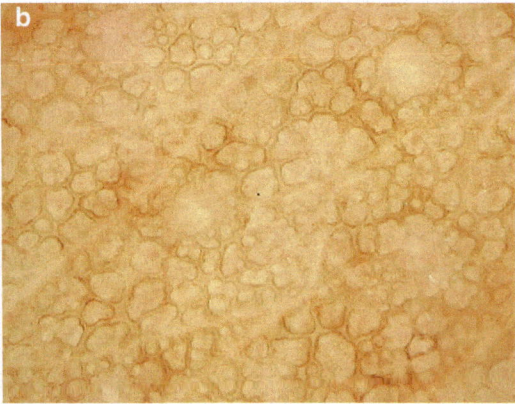

Fig. 5.11 (a) Low-power (40X) view shows skipped areas of hypopigmentation with patchy loss of normal reticular network pattern (blue circles) along with accentuated pseudo-reticular pattern (white arrows) and telangiectasia (red arrows). (b) High-power (120X) view shows patchy accentuation of pseudo-reticular pattern with hypopigmented blotches and telangiectasia

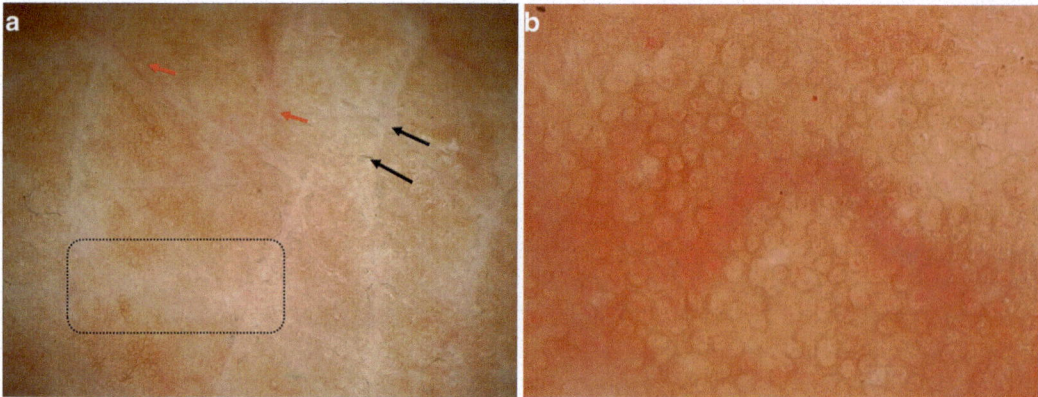

Fig. 5.12 (**a**) Low-power view (40X) shows patchy loss of pigment network (black box) with telangiectasia (red arrows), microscaling (black arrows), and loss of append- ages. (**b**) High-power view (120X) shows reduced pigment network with telangiectasia and loss of appendages

hypopigmentation and telangiectasia (Fig. 5.11a, b). Adding to it are the dotted vessels, short fine linear vessels, and spermatozoa-like vascular structures which are important to diagnose MF in pigmented skin.

Hypopigmented Patches of Leprosy

Vitiligo and leprosy are the two diseases associated with hypopigmented lesions [31]. Dermoscopy can serve as an essential supplement for aiding clinical diagnosis. Polarized light examination, of the hypopigmented patches of leprosy, shows partially obliterated pigment network without hypopigmented/depigmented islands, nor is there any perifollicular hypopigmentation, whereas the hypopigmented patches of vitiligo show multiple areas of depigmentation with loss of pigment network, forming variably sized islands of depigmentation, and loss of appendages with patchy telangiectasia and microscaling (Fig. 5.12a, b).

On UV light dermoscopy the hypopigmented patches of leprosy do not show accentuation, but scaling becomes more apparent. Hypopigmented patches of vitiligo show accentuation of patches with diffuse whitish glow and nebula-like appearance. The presence of scaling indicates xerosis associated with leprosy due to nerve damage.

Thus perifollicular pigmentation, UV accentuation, scaling, and leukotrichia can serve as important indicators to distinguish leprosy from vitiligo.

Leishmaniasis

Cutaneous leishmaniasis (CL) is a common parasitic infection caused by various species of the genus *Leishmania*, which are transmitted by the arthropod vector sand fly. Some of the most common dermoscopic features of hypopigmented patches of CL include "yellow tear-like" structures and "white starburst-like" patterns [36].

The lesions of CL show erosion, thrombotic vessel, yellow tears, white starburst-like pattern, hyperkeratosis, and both erosion and hyperkeratosis together. In advanced lesions, the vascular structures were linear irregular vessels, hairpin vessels, comma-shaped vessels, dotted vessels, arborizing telangiectasia, and glomerular vessels but no corkscrew vessels [37].

Post-kala-azar dermal leishmaniasis (PKDL) is a complication of visceral leishmaniasis (VL) which is mainly found in Sudan, Bangladesh, and India [38]. Differentiating early lesions of PKDL from lepromatous leprosy is difficult, and so dermoscopy can be instrumental in diagnosing PKDL. We observed an orange-pink appearance of the epidermis (Fig. 5.13a, b) with reticular white streaks, milia-like cysts, white starburst-

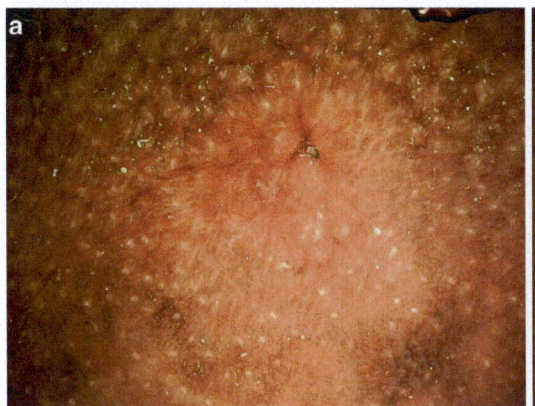 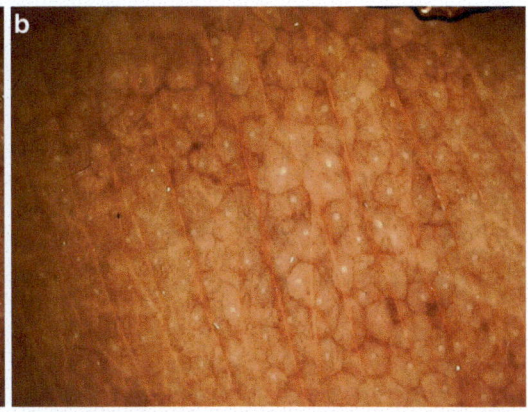

Fig. 5.13 (40X) (**a**) shows white starburst-like pattern with orange hue in the background and white dots of acrosyringeal openings. (**b**) shows polygonal globular pattern with orange hue in the background and white dots for acrosyringeal opening and peripheral reticulate hyperpigmentation

like pattern (Fig. 5.13a), scaling, and central erosions in advanced lesions of PKDL. Some lesions showed raisin-like appearance (Fig. 5.13b) with loss of eccrine duct and follicular openings and increased peripheral pigmentation, polygonal globular pattern with central white dots (eccrine ducts), and peripheral reticulate hyperpigmentation. The papular lesions gave an inflated balloon-like appearance with telangiectasias.

References

1. Nischal KC, Khopkar U. Focus dermoscope. Indian J Dermatol Venereol Leprol. 2005;71(4):300–4.
2. Ortonne JP, Passeron T. Vitiligo and other disorders of hypopigmentation. In: Bolognia JL, Jorrizzo JHSJ, editors. Dermatology, vol. 1. 3rd ed . London: Elsevier Saunders; 2012. p. 947–73.
3. Braun RP, Scope A, Marghoob AA, Kerl K, Rabinovitz HR, Malvehy J. Atlas of dermoscopy. In: Marghoob AA, Malvehy JBP, Braun RP, editors 2nd ed: Informa Healthcare (CRC Press)), Boca Raton. 2012. p. 10–33.
4. Haldar S, Khopkar U. Dermoscopy: applications and patterns in diseases of the Brown skin. In: Khopkar U, editor. Dermoscopy and trichoscopy in diseases of the brown skin: atlas and short text. New Delhi: Jaypee Bros; 2012. p. 10–37.
5. Saraswat A, Lahiri K, Chatterjee M, Barua S, Coondoo A, Mittal A, et al. Topical corticosteroid abuse on the face : a prospective , multicenter study of dermatology outpatients. Indian J Dermatol Venereol Leprol. 2011;77(2):160–6.
6. Mishra SDR. Importance of Dermatoscopy in diagnosing exogenous Ochronosis. In: Khopkar U, editor. Dermoscopy and Trichoscopy in diseases of the Brown skin: atlas and short text. New Delhi: Jaypee Bros; 2012. p. 63–9.
7. Kulandaisamy S, Thappa DM, Gupta D. Exogenous ochronosis in melasma: a study from South India. Pigment Int. 2014;1(1):17.
8. Khunger NKR. Dermoscopic criteria for differentiating exogenous ochronosis from melasma. Indian J Dermatol Venereol Leprol. 2013;79(6):819–21.
9. Tan SK. Exogenous ochronosis in ethnic Chinese Asians: a clinicopathological study, diagnosis and treatment. J Eur Acad Dermatology Venereol. 2011;25(7):842–50.
10. Ozkaya DB, Emiroglu N, Su O, Cengiz FP, Bahali AG, Yildiz P, Demirkesen C, Onsun N. Dermatoscopic findings of pigmented purpuric dermatosis. An Bras Dermatol. 2016;91(5):584–7.
11. Portela PS, Melo DF, Ormiga P, Oliveira FJ, de Freitas NC, Bastos Júnior CS. Dermoscopy of lichen aureus. An Bras Dermatol. 2013;88(2):253–5.
12. Rieder E, Kaplan J, Kamino H, Sanchez M, Pomeranz MK. Lichen planus pigmentosus. Dermatol Online J. 2013;16:19(12).
13. Haldar SS, Khopkar U. Lichen planus pigmentosus vs ashy dermatosis-through a dermoscope. In: Khopkar U, editor. Dermoscopy and trichoscopy in diseases of the brown skin: atlas and short text. New Delhi: Jaypee Bros; 2012. p. 137–56.
14. Ankad BS, Dombale V, Sujana L. Dermoscopic patterns in confluent and reticulated papillomatosis: a case report. Our Dermatology Online. 2016;7(3):323–6.
15. Ga NQ, Romero W. Dermoscopy in periorbital hyperpigmentation : an aid in the clinical type diagnosis diagnostic imaging. Surg Cosmet Dermatol. 2014;6(2):171–2.
16. Mostafa WZ, Kadry DM, Mohamed EF. Clinical and dermoscopic evaluation of patients with peri-

orbital darkening. J Egypt Women's Dermatol Soc. 2014;11(3):191–6.

17. Irvine AD, Mellerio JE. Genetics and genodermatoses. In: Burns DA, Breathnach SM, Cox N, Griffith CS, editors. Rook's textbook of dermatology. 8th ed. Oxford: Wiley Blackwell; 2010. p. 15.94–5.

18. Nirmal B, Dongre AM, Khopkar US. Dermatoscopic features of hyper and hypopigmented lesions of Dowling-Degos disease. Indian J Dermatol. 2016;61(1):125.

19. Dongre A, Khopkar U. Genodermatoses. In: Khopkar U, editor. Dermoscopy and trichoscopy in diseases of the brown skin: atlas and short text. New Delhi: Jaypee Bros; 2012. p. 257–63.

20. Braun-Falco M, Volgger W, Borelli S, Ring J, Disch R. Galli-Galli disease: an unrecognized entity or an acantholytic variant of Dowling-Degos disease? J Am Acad Dermatol. 2001;45(5):760–3.

21. Kitamura K, Akamatsu S, Hirokawa K. A special form of. Acropigmentation: acropigmentatio reticularis(in. German). Hautarzt. 1953;4:152–6.

22. Mahajan S. Melasma. In: Khopkar U, editor. Dermoscopy and trichoscopy in diseases of the brown skin: atlas and short text. New Delhi: Jaypee Bros; 2012. p. 50–62.

23. Valdebran M, Salinas RI, Ramirez N, Rodriguez A, Guzman L, Marte S, Suazo M. Esmirna Rosado: fixed drug eruption of the eyelids. A dermoscopic evaluation. Our Dermatol Online. 2013;4(3):344–6.

24. Bernardes Filho F, Quaresma MV, Rezende FC, Kac BK, da Costa Nery JA, Azulay-Abulafia L. Confluent and reticulate papillomatosis of Gougerot-Carteaud and obesity: Dermoscopic findings. An Bras Dermatol. 2014;89(3):507–9.

25. Vano-Galvan S, Alvarez-Twose I, De las Heras E, Morgado JM, Matito A, Sánchez-Muñoz L, et al. Dermoscopic features of skin lesions in patients with mastocytosis. Arch Dermatol. 2011;147:932–40.

26. Miller MD, Nery NS, Gripp AC, Maceira JP, Nascimento GM. Dermatoscopic findings of urticaria pigmentosa. An Bras Dermatol. 2013;88(6):986–8.

27. Wolff K, Komar M, Petzelbauer P. Clinical and histopathological aspects of cutaneous mastocytosis. Leuk Res. 2001;25(7):519–28.

28. Chandrashekhar L. Dermoscopy: a tool to assess stability in vitiligo. In: Khopkar U, editor. Dermoscopy and trichoscopy in diseases of the brown skin: atlas and short text. New Delhi: Jaypee Bros; 2012. p. 91–6.

29. Thatte S, Dongre A, Khopkar U. "Reversed pigmentary network pattern" in evolving lesions of vitiligo. Indian Dermatol Online J. 2015;6(3):222.

30. Bambroo M, Pande S, Khopkar U. Dermoscopy in the differentiation of idiopathic Guttate Hypomelanosis (IGH) and Guttate vitiligo. In: Khopkar U, editor. Dermoscopy and trichoscopy in diseases of the brown skin: atlas and short text. New Delhi: Jaypee Bros; 2012. p. 97–103.

31. Gutte R, Khopkar U. Dermoscopy: differentiating evolving vitiligo from a Hypopigmented patch of leprosy. In: Khopkar U, editor. Dermoscopy and trichoscopy in diseases of the brown skin: atlas and short text. New Delhi: Jaypee Bros; 2012. p. 104–13.

32. Thatte S, Khopkar U. The utility of dermoscopy in the diagnosis of evolving lesions of vitiligo. Indian J Dermatol Venereol Leprol. 2014;80(6):505.

33. Ankad BS, Beergouder SL. Dermoscopic evaluation of idiopathic guttate hypomelanosis: a preliminary observation. Indian Dermatol Online J. 2015;6(3):164–7.

34. Lallas A, Apalla Z, Lefaki I, Tzellos T, Karatolias A, Sotiriou E, et al. Dermoscopy of early stage mycosis fungoides. J Eur Acad Dermatology Venereol. 2013;27(5):617–21.

35. Xu P, Tan C. Dermoscopy of poikilodermatous mycosis fungoides (MF). J Am Dermatology. 2016;74(3):e45–7.

36. Salman A, Yucelten A, Seckin D, Ergun T, Demircay Z. Cutaneous leishmaniasis mimicking verrucous carcinoma: a case with an unusual clinical course. Indian J Dermatol Venereol Leprol. 2015;81(4):392.

37. Taheri AR, Pishgooei N, Maleki M, Goyonlo VM, Kiafar B, Banihashemi M, et al. Dermoscopic features of cutaneous leishmaniasis. Int J Dermatol. 2013;52(11):1361–6.

38. Zijlstra EE, Musa AM, Khalil EAG, El Hassan IM, El Hassan AM. Post-KalaAzar 4Dermal Leishmaniasis. Lancet Infect Dis. 2003;3:87–98.

Reflectance Confocal Microscopy in Pigmentary Disorders

Nesrine Brahimi and Pascale Guitera

Introduction to In Vivo Reflectance Confocal Microscopy

In the last decade, in vivo reflectance confocal microscopy (RCM) has started to extend into public hospitals and even private practices. The RCM provides real-time images with cellular resolution, in some ways resembling histopathological images. It has become useful technique for non-invasive analysis of the epidermis and the upper dermis up to the papillary dermis. Due to its technical improvements, multiple studies have shown an increase in accuracy of skin cancer diagnosis [1–3].

Basic and Technical Principles

In the vivo confocal microscope, near-infrared light (830 nm) from a diode laser is focused to the depth of the skin. The depth of penetration into

N. Brahimi (✉)
Melanoma Diagnostic Centre, Royal Prince Alfred Hospital, Sydney, NSW, Australia
e-mail: dr.nesrine.brahimi@gmail.com

P. Guitera
Department of Dermatology, Melanoma Diagnostic Centre, Royal Prince Alfred Hospital and Melanoma Institute Australia, University of Sydney, Sydney, NSW, Australia
e-mail: pascale.guitera@melanoma.org.au

the skin is around 200 μm. This light passes between cellular structures having different refraction indices. It is naturally reflected and then captured through a pinhole in front of the detector, allowing a narrow lateral resolution (1.0 μm). The images are recomposed with computer software into a two-dimensional greyscale image. The highly reflective skin components, essentially melanin, but also collagen, haemoglobin and keratin, appear white and bright. Immersion oil (Crodamol® STS; Croda Inc., Edison, NJ, USA) is applied to the skin to match the refractive index of the stratum corneum, improving penetration depth of light. An automated stepper function 'VivaStack' permits collection of a stack of images at progressive depths from the stratum corneum to upper dermis.

Up to now, there are two types of reflectance confocal scanning microscopes appropriate for in vivo skin examination. The first was the VivaScope 1500®, Caliber Inc., Henrietta, New York, USA. Each image corresponds to a horizontal section at a selected depth, with approximately 500 x 500 μm field of view (FOV). A structure of mosaic images can be captured in a total area of 8x8 mm horizontal FOV. The VivaScope 1500® is also combined with a VivaCam, which is a handheld dermatoscope with high-resolution images that allow dermatologists to plan subsequent imaging with the microscope, targeting dermoscopy features of interest, and to orientate the lesion.

© Springer International Publishing AG, part of Springer Nature 2018
P. Kumarasinghe (ed.), *Pigmentary Skin Disorders*, Updates in Clinical Dermatology,
https://doi.org/10.1007/978-3-319-70419-7_6

The imaging requires that the skin is fixed with a disposable adhesive window to the head of the microscope, and for larger lesions, not completely comprised within the FOV, the operator needs to displace the probe to different areas so it is time-consuming, but the device can be centred on the lesion or on the portion with the most interesting dermoscopic features.

Recently, in 2011, the VivaScope 3000® (Fig. 6.1) was introduced. It is a small, movable handheld device applied directly to the skin (without contention of an adhesive window) for imaging lesions. Thus, it is easier to collect images on curved facial contours such around the eyes, nose and ears and also for widespread lesions as the operator can move freely between lesional and perilesional skin or between the areas of interest. But there is no micro–/macro correlation or any possibility of dermoscopic images corresponding exactly to the confocal field of focus. It can be difficult to know whether the 1 mm orifice is correctly positioned on the lesion or the area of concern.

The imaging with this device is faster, and imaging of several sites is easier especially when there are several foci within a large lesion or for investigation of tumour/lesion margins.

The image captured by the handheld RCM microscope is a frame of 1 mm × 1 mm FOV. There is no possibility of obtaining large mosaics but only individual and the 'stacks' of images.

Melanin is one of the main targets of RCM [4], so this technique appears to be an interesting method for the evaluation of pigmentary disorders. Patients and clinicians prefer RCM as a non-invasive method compared to biopsy for the evaluation of pigmentary changes especially when lesions are localised on the face. Both hyperpigmentary and hypopigmentary disorders are caused by abnormal amounts of melanin in the skin and could be suitable for exploration by in vivo RCM. As in histopathology, the interpretation of the images must be done according to the clinical history and symptoms.

Pathology and Confocal Correlations

Firstly, the morphology and size of the main cells of the skin are described, then the features of the different layers are described, so the reader has a basic understanding of the specific vocabulary of RCM [5–7].

Skin Layers

Epidermal Layer
Stratum Corneum
This corresponds to a very bright layer highly refractile and granular that can be first seen when entering horizontally in the epidermis [8].

Fig. 6.1 Handheld VivaScope 3000 (Courtesy of Caliber Imaging & Diagnostics, Inc.)

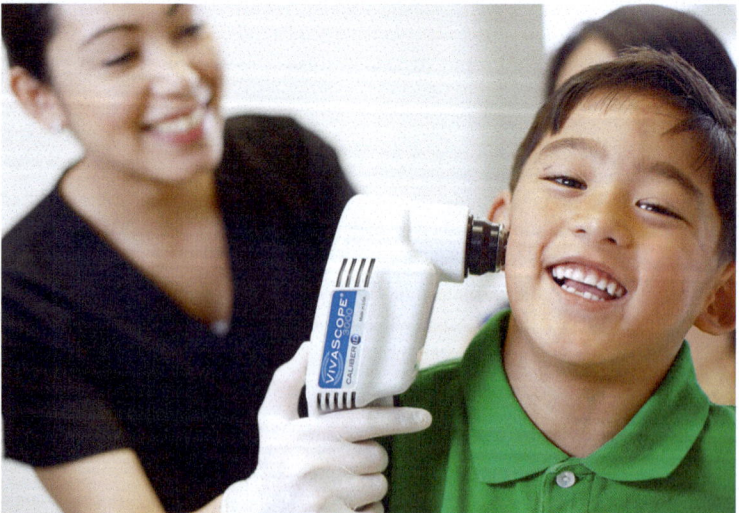

Stratum Granulosum

The stratum granulosum is formed by polygonal cells with moderately refractile granular cytoplasm and dark central nuclei arranged in a regular honeycomb.

Stratum Spinosum

The stratum spinosum is formed by smaller polygonal cells with moderately refractile cytoplasm and dark central nuclei arranged in a regular honeycomb pattern as well.

Basal Layer and Dermo-Epidermal Junction

Edged and Non-edged Papillae

The dermal papillae delineated by a rim of bright cells made of pigmented basal keratinocytes and melanocytes. In contrast, non-edged papillae are seen in melanoma where the atypical cells have distorted the normal delineation. On the face the papillae are often non-visible with a direct transition to the dermal layer. In lighter skin phototypes, the pigmented basal cells are difficult to distinguish from surrounding cells.

Clusters and Nests

These correspond to small or big aggregates of dense cells located in the dermis with no connection with the basal layer of the epidermis. The clusters can be described as dense, sparse-cell or even cerebriform (very specific of nodular melanoma) [9].

Dermal Layer

The papillary dermis composed of laced collagen network shows moderately refractile fibrillar structures giving a weblike pattern, but sometimes it can show a bundle-like appearance. The blood vessels are weakly refractile but can be identified by the movement of blood cells' flow [8].

The *reticular dermis* 150 μm below the surface is difficult to see due to backscatter of light from the structures of the epidermis.

The Cells and Patterns

Keratinocytes are cohesive polygonal-shaped cells, displaying a honeycomb pattern with variably bright granular cytoplasm. They can appear very bright when they are densely pigmented [5].

Melanocytes are highly refractive and they appear as round or oval cells, sometimes fusiform with dendritic prolongations. They have a diffuse bright cytoplasm; they are visualised either solitarily or in nests in the epidermis or the dermis [5].

Melanophages are *usually* smaller than melanocytes. The melanophages are oval or stellate and can be solitary cells or aggregates of cells in dermal papillae. They are rich in melanin. Melanophages can appear irregularly shaped, plump bright cells with ill-defined borders and no visible nucleus [5].

Pagetoid cells are considered when large nucleated cells are twice the size of basal keratinocytes with a dark nucleus and bright cytoplasm, particularly within superficial layers. They correspond to atypical melanocytes in melanoma and Paget cells in extra-mammary Paget's disease [10, 11].

Dendritic cells are Langerhans cells that are highly refractile on RCM. Sometimes they are difficult to differentiate from dendritic melanocytes, reactive or neoplastic. Dendritic cells increase in inflammatory conditions [12].

Honeycomb pattern is a normal pattern of the spinous-granular layers formed by bright polygonal outlines of keratinocytes.

Cobblestone pattern corresponds to the honeycomb pattern but when keratinocytes are pigmented appearing like closely cohesive bright cobblestone, separated by a less refractive polygonal outline.

Disarranged pattern is characterised by disarray of the normal architecture of the superficial layers with unevenly distributed bright granular particles and cells.

Pigmentary Disorders

We describe the main pigmentary disorders in two separate sections, the acquired pigmentary skin disorders (melasma and vitiligo) and melanocytic lesions (naevi and melanoma).

Acquired Pigmentary Skin Disorders

Melasma

Melasma is characterised by an increased number of bright keratinocytes arranged in a bright cobblestone pattern that can be visible sometimes focally.

At the dermo-epidermal junction, melasma displays an increased rimming around the dermal papillae or around adnexal epithelium that substitutes the junctional rimming visible in other anatomical sites (but not on the face normally). An increased density of small and uniform pigmented keratinocytes and melanocytes due to the large amount of melanin at basal cell layer is obvious [7], and it is more pronounced in lesional areas (Fig. 6.2c) compared to perilesional normal skin (Fig. 6.2d). Dendritic cells are also found at basal cell layer with bright cytoplasm corresponding to activated melanocytes. Melanophages (plump irregularly shaped bright cells with ill-defined borders) are found mostly around the vessels of the dermis [13]. They are small but larger than inflammatory cells.

These images display a sudden transition from the stratum spinosum to the papillary dermis that is less refractile as solar elastosis corresponds to moderately refractile lacelike structures and suggests the existence of chronic solar damage in melasma.

The dermal papillary rings are usually invisible in lesional and perilesional normal skin because of the nature of the facial skin organisation and the chronic sun damage corresponding to flattened rete ridges enhancing this abrupt transition from the stratum spinosum to papillary dermis, in most RCM images [14].

These findings suggested the possibility of future clinical applications of RCM for melasma diagnosis and evaluation of treatment efficacy.

Vitiligo

RCM has been recently used to examine, monitor and follow vitiligo patients during the treatments [15].

In the Active Stage of Vitiligo

The most typical confocal feature is that the bright dermal papillary rings present at the dermo-epidermal junction level in normal skin lose their integrity (Fig. 6.3c) or totally disappear and look like shadows of pre-existing papillary rings. Additionally, the absence of bright keratinocytes is usually seen beyond these rings in healthy and phototypes > II subjects in vitiligo lesions. At the junction, few melanocytes and pigmented keratinocytes can be seen organised in ring structures.

The border between vitiligo lesions and normal skin can be indistinct, and highly refractile cells which correspond to infiltrated inflammatory cells could be seen within the papillary dermis at the edge of the lesions [15]. On non-vitiligo areas, a bright ringed pattern of the junction is observed (Fig. 6.3d), but it is different from the normal skin of healthy persons where the bright ring around dermal papillae is clearly visible. Half ring structures and sometimes undulated borders can be seen particularly when the half rings are linked together. Some dendritic melanocytes are seen at the junction level [15].

In the Stable Stage of Vitiligo

The RCM in stable vitiligo shows a complete loss of melanin in lesional skin but a clear border between lesional and normal skin. The inflammatory cells are not found at the edge of lesional skin [16].

Lai et al. showed in their study three kinds of *re-pigmentation patterns*:

- Marginal-dendritic and highly refractile melanocytes, which can be seen moving from the adjacent normal-appearing area to the lesional area
- Perifollicular melanocytes that can be seen surrounding the hair follicle
- Diffuse melanocytes that were evenly distributed in the lesional area

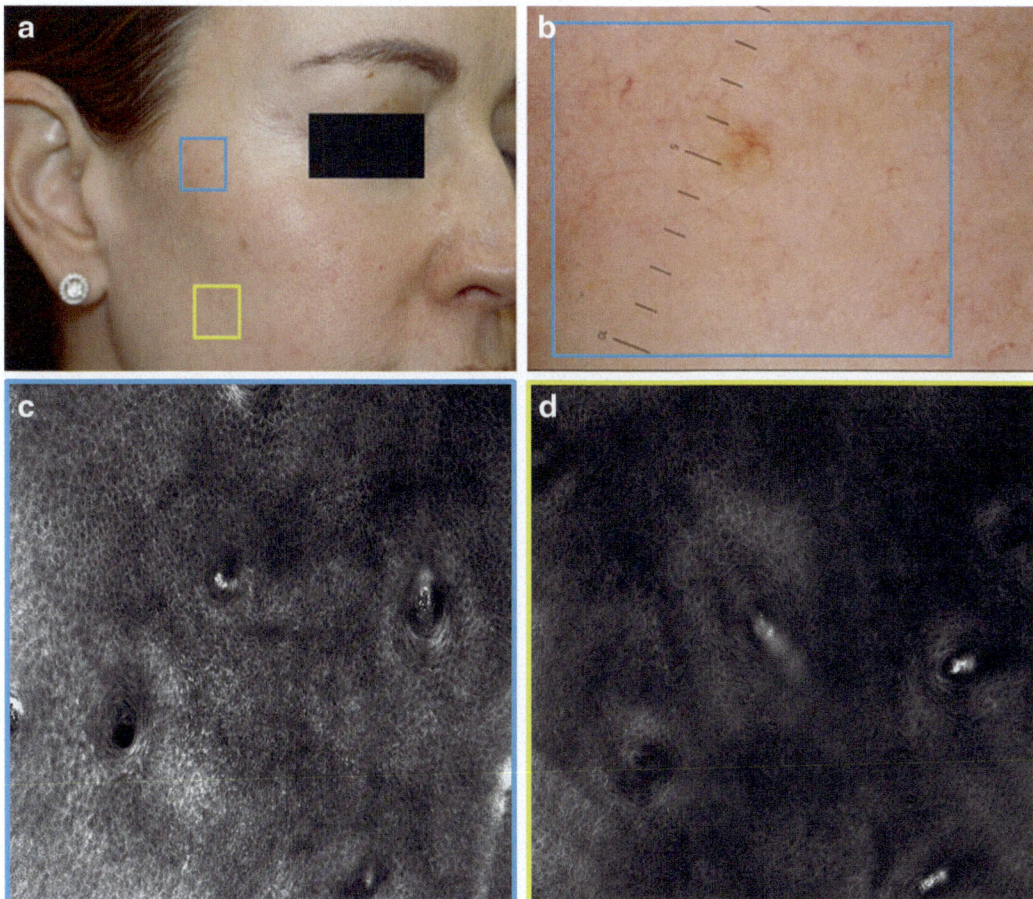

Fig. 6.2 (**a**) Clinical photograph showing a woman in her thirties with a melasma on her right cheek. (**b**) Dermoscopy showing a homogenous network. Image showing at the epidermis level a brighter honeycomb pattern lesional skin (**c**) compared to normal skin (**d**)

In recent RCM studies [17], Xiang W et al. reported that in the re-pigmented skin areas after several months of UVB narrowband therapy, the presence of activated melanocytes can be seen.

RCM appears to be an interesting tool for assessing repigmentation in patients with vitiligo.

Melanocytic Lesions

Naevi
Naevus Depigmentosus
Naevus depigmentosus (ND) is a congenital disorder characterised by a nonprogressive hypopigmented lesion, which may not be apparent at birth.

A histopathological study [18] showed that both the amount of melanin and the number of melanocytes were decreased compared with those in the perilesional normal skin, without any change in the number of melanocytes in patients with ND.

Confocal features show that the content of melanin is obviously decreased in lesional skin, but the dermal papillary rings stay intact. The dermal papillary rings in adjacent normal-appearing skin retained integrity and their brightness [16]. Small bright cells are generally homogeneously distributed and keep their brightness but still with low density compared with non-lesional skin. The borders between lesional and normal skin are well defined [15, 17].

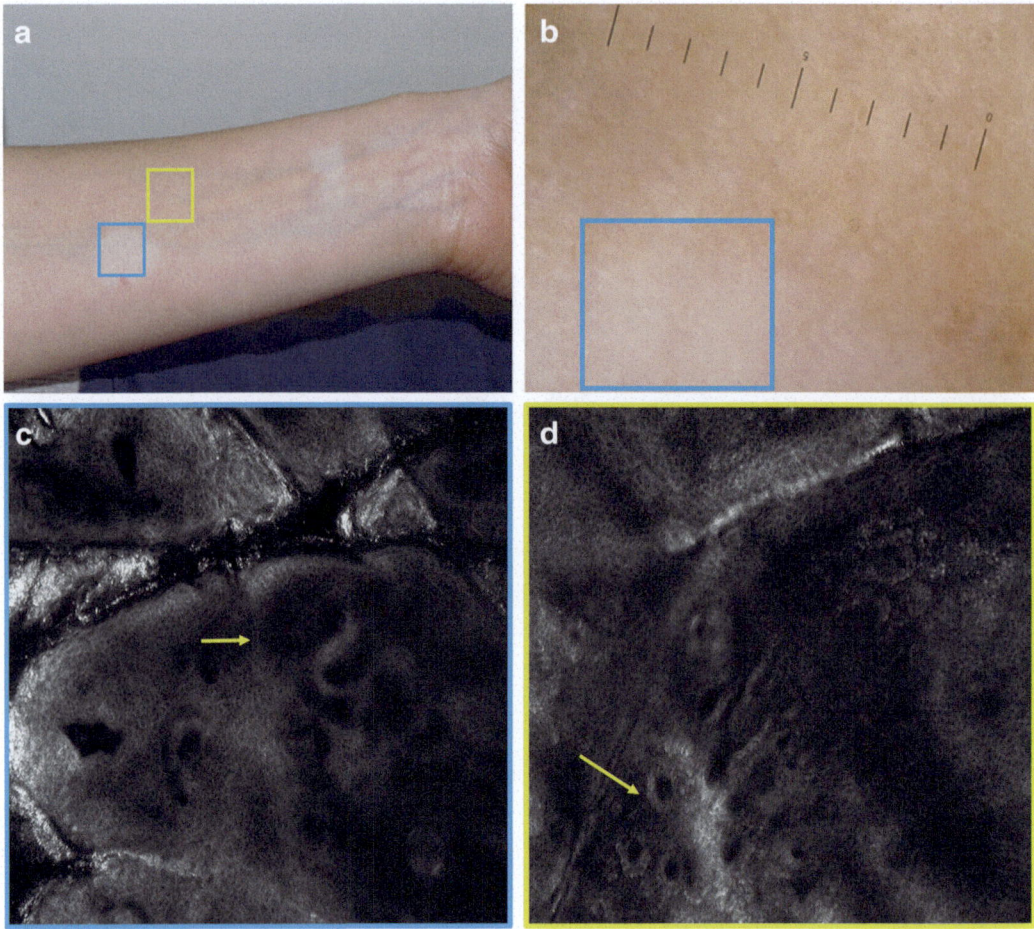

Fig. 6.3 (**a**) Clinical photograph showing a woman in her thirties with an active vitiligo on her inner left. (**b**) Dermoscopy showing an absent pigmentary network. (**c**) Image showing shadows of pre-existing papillary rings (→) on lesional skin. (**d**) Image showing at the junction level normal dermal papillae rim (→) on normal skin

Naevus Anaemicus

Naevus anaemicus (NA) is a congenital nonfamilial localised naevus characterised by a well-defined, hypopigmented, irregularly hypopigmented patch formed from the confluent macules (Fig. 6.6a, b), usually located on the trunk [19]. On RCM, the dermal papillary rings show no abnormalities in the lesional skin of NA (Fig. 6.4c, d). It is consistent with the normality of melanocytes in the epidermis of NA as shown in histopathology. There are no differences in dermal papillary rings between the lesional skin and the adjacent normal-appearing skin of NA [16, 17].

Thus, combining RCM with the clinical history, it is easy to discriminate NA from vitiligo or naevus depigmentosus [10–12].

Spitz Naevus and Reed Naevus

Spitz naevus was first described by Sophie Spitz [20]. It is an acquired melanocytic tumour later reclassified as benign and considered likely to occur also in older patients. Clinical presentation varies, but it usually presents as a pink-red raised papule occurring in young patients, mostly on the face or lower extremities, while Reed naevi are seen in older people on the legs (Fig. 6.5a, b). Pigmented naevi can sometimes mimic a melanoma

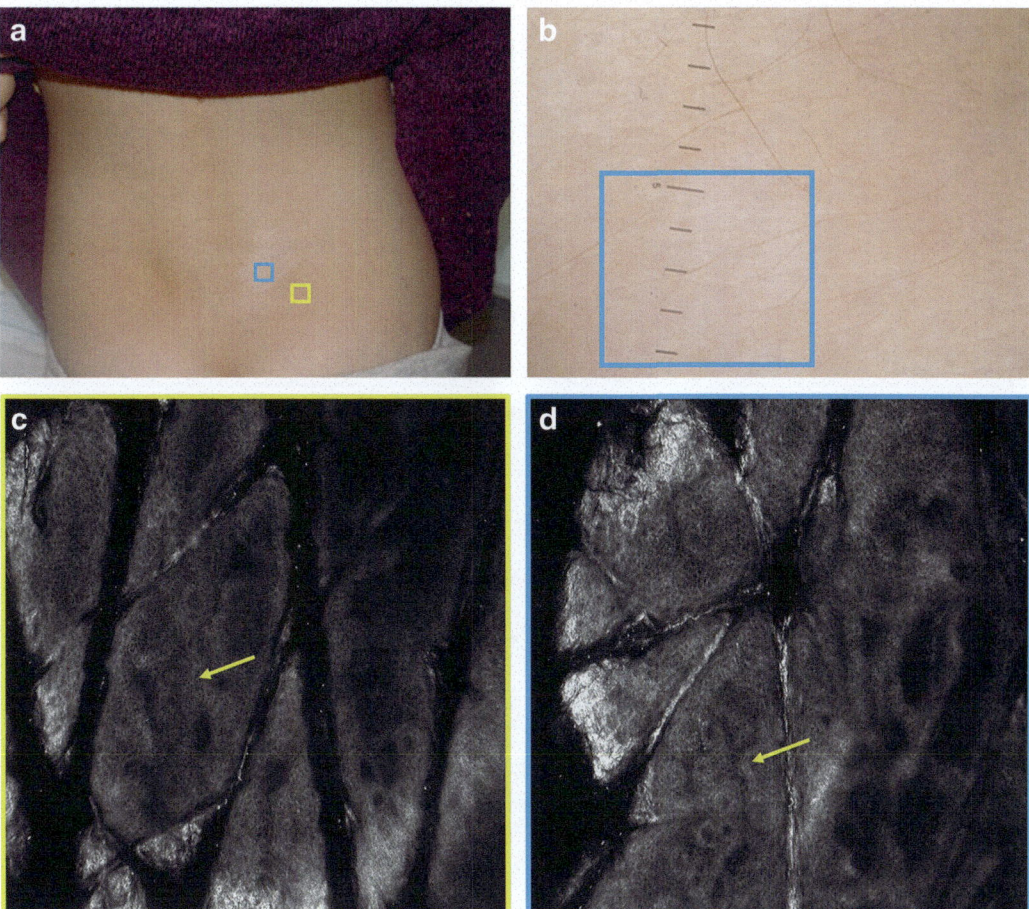

Fig. 6.4 (**a**) Clinical photograph showing girl in her early childhood with a naevus anaemicus on lower back noticed at birth. (**b**) Dermoscopy showing an absent pigmentary network. Images showing at the junction level some honeycomb pattern (→) on both normal (**c**) and pigmented areas (**d**)

and differentiating them can be difficult. As Spitz and Reed naevi share some similar histological findings, we describe their most common RCM features together.

The specific RCM features correlate with histology [1]. In the superficial layers of the epidermis, pagetoid cells are present (Fig. 6.5c) throughout the lesion, particularly constituted by small dendritic cells while dense cell clusters seen at the periphery. At the junction, the papillae are non edged, and atypical cells are present in the basal layer and dermo-epidermal junction.

In the dermis, a large confluent irregular dermal cluster of reflective polygonal cells can be found. There is also an increased vascularity [21].

Naevus Spilus

Naevus spilus (NS) is seen in approximately 2–3% of the population [22]; it is a naevoid disorder characterised by several brown shade small, pigmented macules over a large macule of cafe-au-lait macule (Fig. 6.6a, b) or a tan pigmentation. NS is considered as a subtype of congenital melanocytic naevus [23]. The darker pigmented speckles of NS slowly increase in number and size over time. Melanoma can rarely occur on NS particularly on areas that may change during life [24].

On RCM [25], a typical honeycomb pattern at epidermal layers is observed, but a normal regular cobblestone pattern can also be found. At the dermo-epidermal junction, a regular ringed

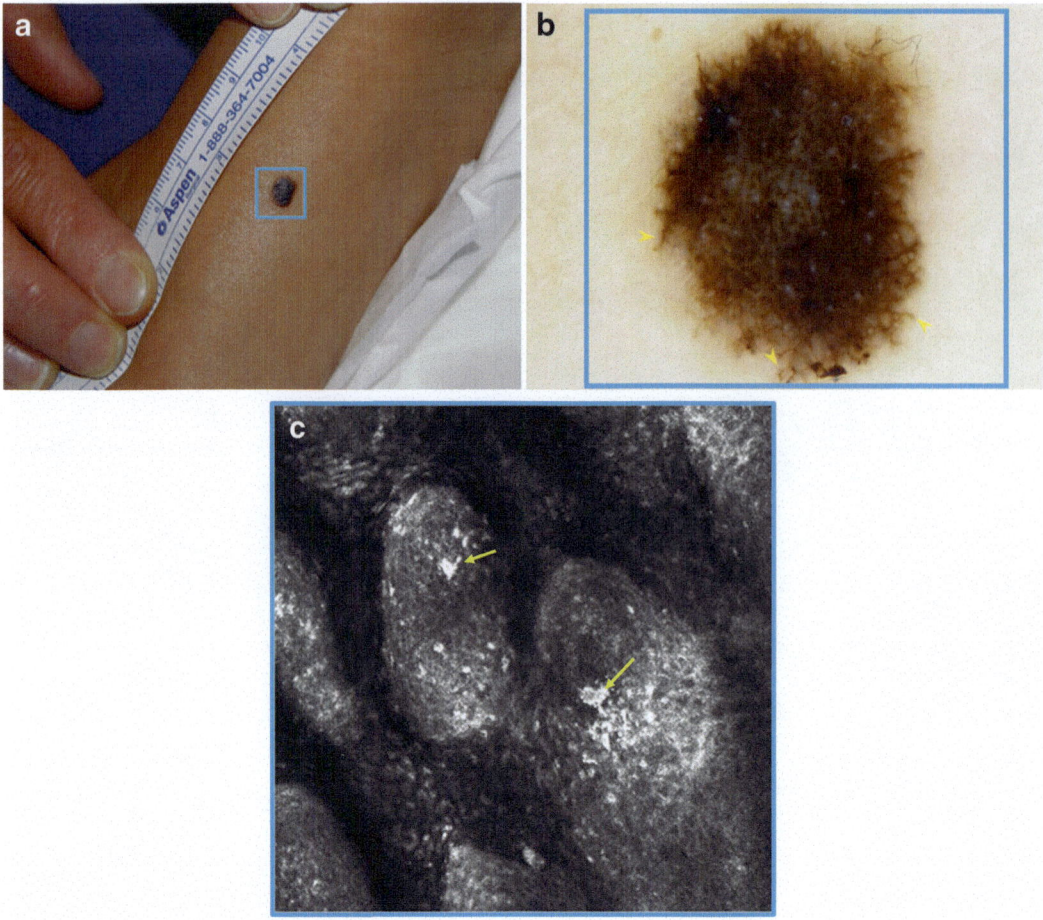

Fig. 6.5 (**a**) Clinical photograph showing a teenaged girl with a Reed naevus on the right sole. (**b**) Dermoscopy showing a multifocal pigment distribution characterised by small areas revealing dark and light brown and grey colour with non-regular peripheral streaks (➤). (**c**) Image showing at the epidermal layer some big oval bright cells (→) correlating to pagetoid cells

pattern is uniformly distributed with well-defined dermal papillae surrounded by a rim of bright monomorphous cells, correlating to pigmented keratinocytes and melanocytes (Fig. 6.6c). Additionally, small junctional aggregates of melanocytes bulging into the dermal papillae are found. At the upper dermis, focal gathered plump bright cells correlating to melanophages can be found. Rarely transition to melanoma has been described in NS and is easy to be diagnosed with RCM. It may show as a sudden disarray of the normal architecture of the superficial layers with the presence of non-edged and distorted papillae due to numerous, scattered, large, irregular, round, junctional and pagetoid cells with a dark nucleus and bright cytoplasm [26].

Dysplastic or Atypical Naevus

Dysplastic naevus (DN) is still a controversial entity clinically or histologically. In fact, DN is an interesting concept not only as simulants but also as possible precursors to melanoma. They can be described as being on a continuum between common acquired naevi and melanoma because they are intermediate between these two entities [27, 28].

In 1992, the National Institutes of Health recommended that the term 'dysplastic naevus' be abandoned and replaced with 'nevus with architectural disorder, accompanied by a statement describing the presence and degree of melanocyte atypia' (mild, moderate or severe) [29]. However, the term 'dysplastic naevus' is still widely used by clinicians and pathologists.

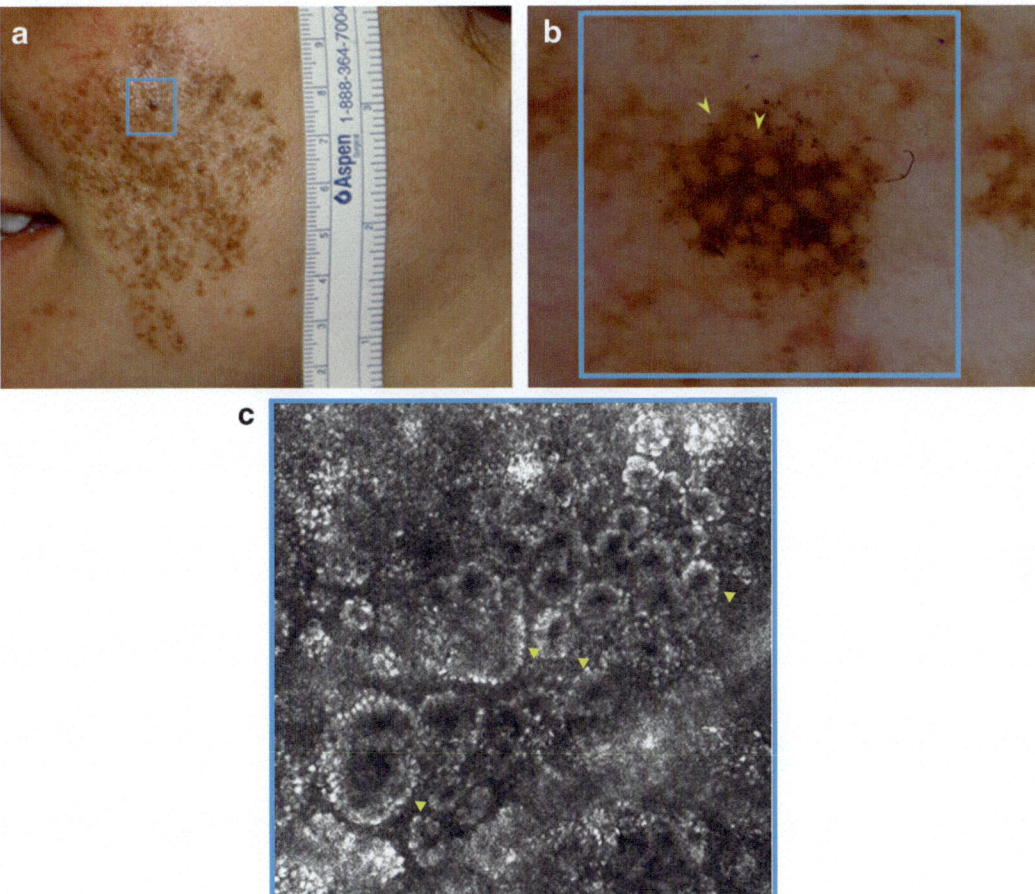

Fig. 6.6 (a) Clinical photograph showing a woman in her thirties with a Spilus naevus on the left cheek with dark brown speckles that changed recently. (b) Dermoscopy showing a reticular, homogenous, dot/globular (►) at the periphery. (c) Image showing a well-defined edged papillae (►) surrounded by a rim of monomorphous cells, correlating to pigmented keratinocytes

In RCM, two separate groups can be recognised [30].

Mild Atypia
The global symmetry of the architecture is preserved. An extensive lentiginous proliferation of bright cells correlating to melanocytes, spread through the lesion, is found but sometimes limited only to the periphery. The pagetoid cells are rare within a mild irregular epidermal architecture (Fig. 6.7c). The papillae are edged. At the junction, nests are present surrounded by inflammatory infiltrates (formed by bright very small particles) with small bright cells and thick collagen fibres.

Moderate to Severe Atypia
In contrast to the mild atypia, there is a disorganisation of the global architecture. In the epidermis, the normal organisation of the keratinocytes in a honeycombed or cobblestone (when pigmented) architecture is noted but within an irregular pattern. Large roundish nucleated pagetoid cells can be observed but are rare. At the junction, edged papillae are clearly detectable but sometimes distorted, elongated due to the fusion of rete ridges. They are normally well outlined, but atypical roundish junctional cells can be observed.

In severe DN, round and dendritic cells are usually more obvious.

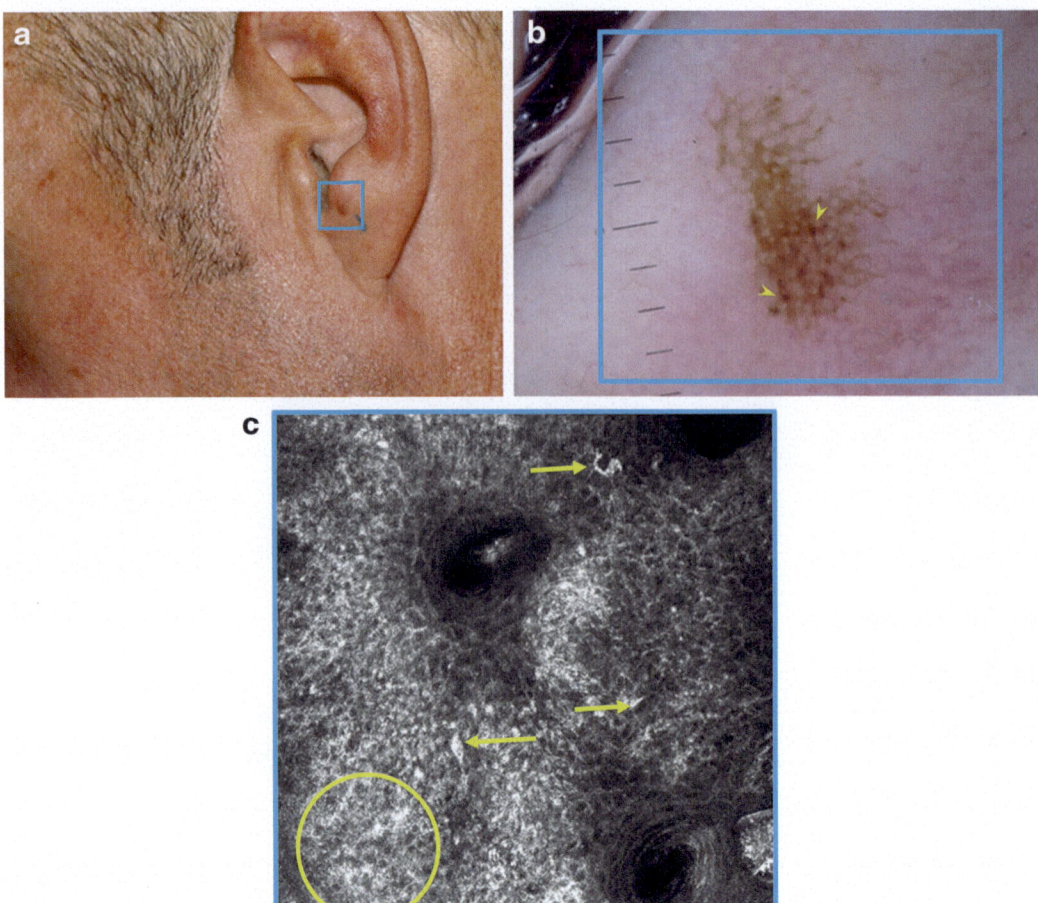

Fig. 6.7 (a) Clinical photograph showing a man in his fifties with a pigmented lesion on the left ear lobe recently appeared. (b) Dermoscopy showing a reticular pattern with dots/globules (➤). (c) Image showing at the lower layers of the epidermis a distorted pattern (◯) with mild atypia (→)

Studies demonstrate that combinations of the above cited features have high sensitivity and specificity for differentiating melanoma from naevi, including DN [1].

Melanoma

Malignant melanoma (MM) is a common and severe form of skin cancer. Its incidence has increased worldwide during the last decades [31]. Early screening of melanoma is crucial for the management of patients leading to a better long-term prognosis. Melanoma is a multifactorial disease modulated by genetic susceptibility and interacting with environmental factors [32]. These factors include the Caucasian phenotype, benign pigmented naevi [33], clinically and histologically atypical naevi and a family history of melanoma [34]. These factors may also determine subtypes and anatomic localisation of melanoma [31]. Even dermoscopy, which is a non-invasive tool that permits the visualisation of subsurface structures, improves diagnostic accuracy to as high as 85% for clinicians who are trained in its use [35]; its accuracy level remains low for a potentially life-threatening disease. The diagnosis of melanoma needs to be done at early stage to get a better prognosis. The diagnosis of malignant melanoma by RCM relies on specific cytological and architectural features [36, 37].

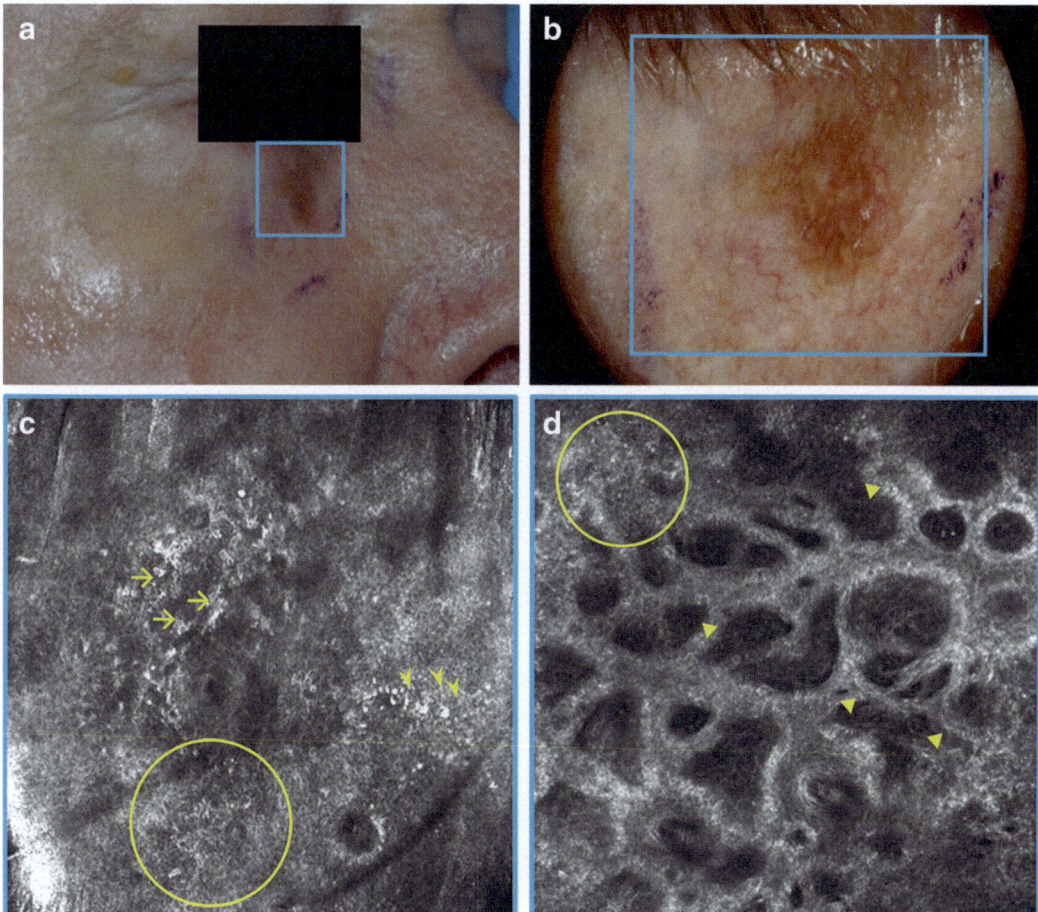

Fig. 6.8 (**a**) Clinical photograph showing a man in his sixties with pigmented macule on his lower eyelid appeared since 3 months. (**b**) Dermoscopy showing a reticular pattern. (**c**) Image showing at the epidermal layers a distorted pattern (○) with big oval bright cells correlating to a pagetoid proliferation (→) and some monomorphous cells, correlating to pigmented keratinocytes (▸) in an early stage of lentigo maligna. (**d**) Image showing at junction level a disorganisation with a distorted pattern (○) with non-edged papillae (▸)

We describe only the superficial spreading melanoma in situ and the lentigo maligna type in this chapter as they can be in the differential diagnosis of pigmentary disorders.

Superficial Spreading Melanoma In Situ

On RCM images [32], a disarray of the normal architecture of the superficial layers of the epidermis with a disarranged pattern among nonspecific architecture (loss of the honeycomb and cobblestone pattern) is generally found with the presence of bright round or dendritic pagetoid cells in the spinous or granular cell layer (Fig. 6.8c).

At the junction level, there are increased numbers of large atypical bright cells (with dendritic or roundish morphology) and loose cell clusters with junctional thickenings.

At dermal papillae there are non-edged papillae without a demarcated, but a distorted border of atypical bright cells (Fig. 6.8d). In the dermis, melanophages can be scattered in the papillary dermis defined as plump bright cells.

Lentigo Maligna

The lentigo maligna type shows a disruption of the normal epidermal and junctional architecture, prominent harsh branching dendrites and atypical bright nucleated cells. The epidermis shows a complete disarrangement with an atypical honeycombed pattern or disarray and presence of heterogeneously shaped large round pagetoid cell infiltration [32].

RCM in melanoma is not only useful to establish a diagnosis but also to delineate the extent of the lesion [38] which is a major challenge to avoid recurrence [39]. In a very bad sun-damaged skin, it can be subtle and difficult to establish a diagnosis. But still, in melanoma RCM helps to target a biopsy, to draw margins and to follow up different kinds of treatments such as radiotherapy and topical treatments (imiquimod) and also allows to monitor when there are narrow surgical margins due to the anatomic localisation [40].

Limitations and Future

The limitations of the confocal microscopy include the limited depth penetration that allows imaging of only the epidermis and the superficial dermis up to 300 μm and obviously less in hyperkeratotic or ulcerated lesions, and RCM does not permit a definite differentiation from different kinds of neoplasms.

The bulky size of the RCM microscopes is to be taken in consideration for the clinical practice and time taken in preparing the patient (about 10 min) and more when mapping.

Although RCM gives relatively comparable resolution that provides cellular and subcellular details, it is in black and white with no possibility of staining, so it is less reliable than conventional histology. The interpretation of the images is difficult for beginners and even challenging for the experts with the same pitfalls as is pathology (uncertain malignancy of atypical Spitz naevi, transition of lentigo maligna in sun-damaged skin, etc.). Finally, the high cost of the current microscopes is also an obstacle (about 100 K AUD).

Training and technical limitations may improve in the near future. In fact, several technological developments are promising to potentially reducing the time, size and cost of imaging. In the future RCM may play a major role in teledermatology, and it may make confocal microscopy applications more practical for obtaining a rapid expert diagnosis.

Summary

Acquired pigmentary skin disorders
Melasma
Epidermis
Increase of highly refractile keratinocytes
Dendritic cells
Dermo-epidermal junction
Papillary rings strongly visible around the dermal papillae
Dermis
Melanophages
Collagen bundles
Vitiligo (active)
Epidermis
Absence of bright keratinocytes
Dermo-epidermal junction
Shadow of papillary rings
Few melanocytes
Dermis
Inflammatory cell infiltration
Melanocytic lesions
Naevus depigmentosus
Epidermis
Normal honeycomb pattern
Dermo-epidermal junction
Normal dermal papillae but less bright than non-lesional skin
Dermis
Small bright cells
Naevus anaemicus
Epidermis
Normal honeycomb pattern
Dermo-epidermal junction
Normal dermal papillae and melanocyte in lesional skin
Dermis
Normal architecture
Spitz/reed naevus
Epidermis
Normal honeycomb or cobblestone pattern
Dermo-epidermal junction
Alteration papillae not well defined
Nests of atypical cells
Melanophages
Dermis
Melanophages and dense nests

Melanocytic lesions

Spilus naevus
Epidermis
Typical honeycomb or cobblestone pattern
Dermo-epidermal junction
Well-defined dermal papillae
Small junctional aggregates of melanocytes
Dermis
Focal melanophages gathered focally in the
papillary dermis

Dysplastic naevi
Epidermis
Atypical honeycomb and cobblestone patterns
Dermo-epidermal junction
Atypia from mild to severe in size and shape
Disorganised nests
Dermis
Nests in the papillary dermis

Superficial spreading melanoma
Epidermis
Atypical honeycomb or cobblestone pattern
Pagetoid cells
Dermo-epidermal junction
Disorganisation
Ill-defined and non-edged papillae
Atypical cells in the basal layer
Dermis
Dense or scarce nests
Increased reticulation of the collagen

Melanoma
Epidermis
Disarranged pattern with atypical honeycomb or
cobblestone pattern
Pagetoid and dendritic cells
Dermo-epidermal junction
Disorganisation
Ill-defined and non-edged papillae
Atypical cells in the basal layer
Dermis
Clusters
Plump bright cells

References

1. Pellacani G, Guitera P, Longo C, Avramidis M, Seidenari S, Menzies S. The impact of in vivo reflectance confocal microscopy for the diagnostic accuracy of melanoma and equivocal melanocytic lesions. J Invest Dermatol. 2007;127(12):2759–65.
2. Xiong YD, Ma S, Li X, Zhong X, Duan C, Chen Q. A meta-analysis of reflectance confocal microscopy for the diagnosis of malignant skin tumours. J Eur Acad Dermatol Venereol. 2016;30(8):1295–302.
3. Guida S, Pellacani G, Cesinaro AM, Moscarella E, Argenziano G, Farnetani F, et al. Spitz naevi and

melanomas with similar dermoscopic patterns: can confocal microscopy differentiate? Br J Dermatol. 2016;174(3):610–6.
4. Rajadhyaksha M, Grossman M, Esterowitz D, Webb RH, Anderson RR. In vivo confocal scanning laser microscopy of human skin: melanin provides strong contrast. J Invest Dermatol. 1995;104(6):946–52.
5. Busam KJ, Charles C, Lee G, Halpern AC. Morphologic features of melanocytes, pigmented keratinocytes, and melanophages by in vivo confocal scanning laser microscopy. Mod Pathol. 2001;14(9):862–8.
6. Scope A, Benvenuto-Andrade C, Agero AL, Malvehy J, Puig S, Rajadhyaksha M, et al. In vivo reflectance confocal microscopy imaging of melanocytic skin lesions: consensus terminology glossary and illustrative images. J Am Acad Dermatol. 2007;57(4):644–58.
7. Xiang W, Peng J, Song X, Xu A, Zhang D, Liu J, et al. In vivo visualization of honeycomb pattern, cobblestone pattern, ringed pattern, and dermal papillae by confocal laser scanning microscopy. Skin Res Technol. 2016;22(1):32–9.
8. Rajadhyaksha M, Gonzalez S, Zavislan JM, Anderson RR, Webb RH. In vivo confocal scanning laser microscopy of human skin II: advances in instrumentation and comparison with histology. J Invest Dermatol. 1999;113(3):293–303.
9. Segura S, Pellacani G, Puig S, Longo C, Bassoli S, Guitera P, et al. In vivo microscopic features of nodular melanomas: dermoscopy, confocal microscopy, and histopathologic correlates. Arch Dermatol. 2008;144(10):1311–20.
10. Pan ZY, Liang J, Zhang QA, Lin JR, Zheng ZZ. In vivo reflectance confocal microscopy of extramammary Paget disease: diagnostic evaluation and surgical management. J Am Acad Dermatol. 2012;66(2):e47–53.
11. Pellacani G, Cesinaro AM, Seidenari S. Reflectance-mode confocal microscopy for the in vivo characterization of pagetoid melanocytosis in melanomas and nevi. J Invest Dermatol. 2005;125(3):532–7.
12. Hoogedoorn L, Peppelman M, van de Kerkhof PC, van Erp PE, Gerritsen MJ. The value of in vivo reflectance confocal microscopy in the diagnosis and monitoring of inflammatory and infectious skin diseases: a systematic review. Br J Dermatol. 2015;172(5):1222–48.
13. Ardigo M, Cameli N, Berardesca E, Gonzalez S. Characterization and evaluation of pigment distribution and response to therapy in melasma using in vivo reflectance confocal microscopy: a preliminary study. J Eur Acad Dermatol Venereol. 2010;24(11):1296–303.
14. Kang HY, Bahadoran P, Suzuki I, Zugaj D, Khemis A, Passeron T, et al. In vivo reflectance confocal microscopy detects pigmentary changes in melasma at a cellular level resolution. Exp Dermatol. 2010;19(8):e228–33.

15. Pan ZY, Yan F, Zhang ZH, Zhang QA, Xiang LH, Zheng ZZ. In vivo reflectance confocal microscopy for the differential diagnosis between vitiligo and nevus depigmentosus. Int J Dermatol. 2011;50(6):740–5.
16. Lai LG, Xu AE. In vivo reflectance confocal microscopy imaging of vitiligo, nevus depigmentosus and nevus anemicus. Skin Res Technol. 2011;17(4):404–10.
17. Xiang W, Xu A, Xu J, Bi Z, Shang Y, Ren Q. In vivo confocal laser scanning microscopy of hypopigmented macules: a preliminary comparison of confocal images in vitiligo, nevus depigmentosus and postinflammatory hypopigmentation. Lasers Med Sci. 2010;25(4):551–8.
18. Sehgal VN, Srivastava G. Hereditary hypo/depigmented dermatoses: an overview. Int J Dermatol. 2008;47(10):1041–50.
19. Ahkami RN, Schwartz RA. Nevus anemicus. Dermatology. 1999;198(4):327–9.
20. Spitz S. Melanomas of childhood. Am J Pathol. 1948;24(3):591–609.
21. Pellacani G, Longo C, Ferrara G, Cesinaro AM, Bassoli S, Guitera P, et al. Spitz nevi: in vivo confocal microscopic features, dermatoscopic aspects, histopathologic correlates, and diagnostic significance. J Am Acad Dermatol. 2009;60(2):236–47.
22. Vaidya DC, Schwartz RA, Janniger CK. Nevus spilus. Cutis. 2007;80(6):465–8.
23. Schaffer JV, Orlow SJ, Lazova R, Bolognia JL. Speckled lentiginous nevus--classic congenital melanocytic nevus hybrid not the result of "collision". Arch Dermatol. 2001;137(12):1655.
24. Haenssle HA, Kaune KM, Buhl T, Thoms KM, Padeken M, Emmert S, et al. Melanoma arising in segmental nevus spilus: detection by sequential digital dermatoscopy. J Am Acad Dermatol. 2009;61(2):337–41.
25. Prodinger C, Tatarski R, Laimer M, Ahlgrimm-Siess V. Large congenital nevus spilus-improved follow-up through the use of in vivo reflectance confocal microscopy. Dermatol Pract Concept. 2013;3(2):55–8.
26. Laing ME, Coates E, Jopp-McKay A, Scolyer RA, Guitera P. Atypical naevus spilus: detection by in vivo confocal microscopy. Clin Exp Dermatol. 2014;39(5):616–9.
27. Goldstein AM, Tucker MA. Dysplastic nevi and melanoma. Cancer Epidemiol Biomark Prev. 2013;22(4):528–32.
28. Rosendahl CO, Grant-Kels JM, Que SK. Dysplastic nevus: fact and fiction. J Am Acad Dermatol. 2015;73(3):507–12.
29. NIH consensus conference. Diagnosis and treatment of early melanoma. JAMA. 1992;268(10):1314–9.
30. Pellacani G, Farnetani F, Gonzalez S, Longo C, Cesinaro AM, Casari A, et al. In vivo confocal microscopy for detection and grading of dysplastic nevi: a pilot study. J Am Acad Dermatol. 2012;66(3):e109–21.
31. Nikolaou V, Stratigos AJ. Emerging trends in the epidemiology of melanoma. Br J Dermatol. 2014;170(1):11–9.
32. Usher-Smith JA, Emery J, Kassianos AP, Walter FM. Risk prediction models for melanoma: a systematic review. Cancer Epidemiol Biomark Prev. 2014;23(8):1450–63.
33. Scheibner A, Milton GW, McCarthy WH, Norlund JJ, Pearson LJ. Multiple primary melanoma - a review of 90 cases. Australas J Dermatol. 1982;23(1):1–8.
34. Gupta BK, Piedmonte MR, Karakousis CP. Attributes and survival patterns of multiple primary cutaneous malignant melanoma. Cancer. 1991;67(7):1984–9.
35. Braun RP, Saurat JH, French LE. Dermoscopy of pigmented lesions: a valuable tool in the diagnosis of melanoma. Swiss Med Wkly. 2004;134(7–8):83–90.
36. Guitera P, Menzies SW. State of the art of diagnostic technology for early-stage melanoma. Expert Rev Anticancer Ther. 2011;11(5):715–23.
37. Guitera P, Menzies SW, Longo C, Cesinaro AM, Scolyer RA, Pellacani G. In vivo confocal microscopy for diagnosis of melanoma and basal cell carcinoma using a two-step method: analysis of 710 consecutive clinically equivocal cases. J Invest Dermatol. 2012;132(10):2386–94.
38. Guitera P, Moloney FJ, Menzies SW, Stretch JR, Quinn MJ, Hong A, et al. Improving management and patient care in lentigo maligna by mapping with in vivo confocal microscopy. JAMA Dermatol. 2013;149(6):692–8.
39. Guitera P, Haydu LE, Menzies SW, Scolyer RA, Hong A, Fogarty GB, et al. Surveillance for treatment failure of lentigo maligna with dermoscopy and in vivo confocal microscopy: new descriptors. Br J Dermatol. 2014;170(6):1305–12.
40. Guitera P, Pellacani G, Crotty KA, Scolyer RA, Li LX, Bassoli S, et al. The impact of in vivo reflectance confocal microscopy on the diagnostic accuracy of lentigo maligna and equivocal pigmented and non-pigmented macules of the face. J Invest Dermatol. 2010;130(8):2080–91.

Update on Albinism

7

Masahiro Hayashi and Tamio Suzuki

Introduction

Albinism is a generic clinical term that describes conditions characterized by hypopigmentation of skin, hair, and eyes or eyes alone of affected individuals. It is caused by pathologic variants of genes that are associated with melanin synthesis, melanocyte differentiation/migration, or membrane trafficking.

Albinism contains two subtypes, non-syndromic albinism, with symptoms restricted to impaired melanin biosynthesis, and syndromic albinism, which displays various non-pigmentary symptoms including bleeding diathesis, lung fibrosis, and immunodeficiency. Recent advances in genetic analysis enable us to detect additional types of albinism and the genes responsible for these disorders. Here we update and review the clinical features and pathophysiology of albinism.

Non-syndromic Albinism

Oculocutaneous Albinism (OCA)

Definition

Oculocutaneous albinism (OCA) is a rare, autosomal recessive condition characterized by hypopigmentation of skin, hair, and eyes. Visual disturbances such as nystagmus, impaired visual acuity, and stereoscopic vision are seen to various degrees because of the lack of L-DOPA, an intermediate metabolite of melanin biosynthesis, in retinal and visual development. Systemic manifestations of OCA are restricted to hypopigmentation (non-syndromic OCA). Currently seven types of OCA have been identified (Table 7.1), and all of the genes responsible, with the exception of OCA5 (for which the gene responsible has not yet been identified), are associated with melanin biosynthesis or migration of melanocyte/melanocyte precursor cells. Recently, a Japanese family with OCA4 in autosomal dominant inheritance was reported [10].

Epidemiology

The overall prevalence of OCA is estimated at around 1:10,000–20,000; however, the ratio of each type varies depending on geographic region and ethnicity. OCA1 is the most common type of OCA in the general population. OCA2 is much more common among the Igbo (previously referred to as Ibo) population in Nigeria, with a

M. Hayashi (✉) · T. Suzuki
Department of Dermatology, Yamagata University
Faculty of Medicine, Yamagata, Japan
e-mail: czk11223@nifty.ne.jp

© Springer International Publishing AG, part of Springer Nature 2018
P. Kumarasinghe (ed.), *Pigmentary Skin Disorders*, Updates in Clinical Dermatology,
https://doi.org/10.1007/978-3-319-70419-7_7

Table 7.1 Ocular albinism and oculocutaneous albinism (non-syndromic albinism)

Disease name	Inheritance	Genes	Chromosomal location	MIM
OCA1	AR	*TYR*	11q14.3	203,100
OCA2	AR	*OCA2*	15q12-q13.1	203,200
OCA3	AR	*TYRP-1*	9p23	203,290
OCA4	AR	*SLC45A2*	5p13.2	696,574
OCA5	AR	Unknown	4q24	615,312
OCA6	AR	*SLC24A5*	15q21.1	609,802
OCA7	AR	*C10orf11*	10q22.2-q22.3	615,179
OA1	X-linked	*GPR143*	Xp22.3	300,500

OCA oculocutaneous albinism, *OA* ocular albinism

prevalence of around 1:1100 [2], while this type is much less common in the Caucasian population. OCA3, previously known as rufous OCA in Africa, is rare among other regions and ethnicities. OCA4 is relatively rare in the general population, found in around 3% of albino individuals; however, it accounts for 27% of Japanese albinos and is one of the major types of OCA in Japan [11]. OCA5 has been reported in one consanguineous Pakistani family [4]. OCA6 was initially identified in a Chinese family [5], although this type has subsequently been reported in several families and sporadic individuals of Chinese, European, French Guinean, and Middle Eastern origin [12]. OCA7 was initially reported from a consanguineous Danish albino family in the Faroe Islands [6]. Recently an additional case with OCA7 harboring novel *C10orf11* mutation has been reported from Iran [13].

Responsible Genes and Pathophysiology

The scheme of melanin synthesis in melanosomes and genes responsible for types of OCA is shown in Fig. 7.1 (modified from a reference figure [14]). OCA1 is caused by the pathologic mutation of the tyrosinase gene (*TYR*), which encodes a rate-limiting enzyme in melanin synthesis. OCA1 is divided into four subtypes, OCA1A, OCA1B, OCA1 temperature sensitive (TS), and OCA1 minimal pigment (MP). OCA1A completely lacks TYR activity; the rest of them retain slight TYR activity and may show unique clinical manifestation, depending on the impact of the mutation. Regarding OCA1TS, certain

specific mutations in *TYR* cause a conformational change of the TYR protein, leading to the production of a thermolabile variant. TYR activity is decreased around 37 °C and retained to at least approximately 31 °C. Pigmentation is found on extremities with relatively low body temperature [15]. OCA1MP has no eumelanogenesis but limited just pheomelanogenesis, the individuals with OCA1MP show white skin and hair and severe visual impairment, resembling OCA1A, but they develop some freckles [16]. King et al. reported that an individual with OCA1MP showed the accumulation of pigment only in the irises that increases with age [17]. *OCA2* encodes the melanosomal transporter OCA2 (also known as P protein), which plays an important role in pH control inside melanosomes. Since eumelanin synthesis is tightly controlled by pH within melanosomes, aberrant function of OCA2 would affect and impair melanin synthesis. The impact on melanin biosynthesis varies among the mutations, which may explain the clinical variations in hypopigmentation. OCA2 is also suggested to involve membrane trafficking of melanosome-related proteins such as TYR [18]. OCA3 is caused by mutation of *tyrosinase-related protein-1* (*TYRP-1*), which encodes an important protein in the stabilization of TYR in melanosomes. Since there is a collateral eumelanin synthesis pathway, the impact of *TYRP-1* mutation on eumelanin synthesis is not so large, which seems reasonable in view of the relatively mild albinism phenotype of OCA3. Many cases of OCA3 have been reported in Africa [19], and OCA3 seems to be rare in other regions; however, it may be overlooked in

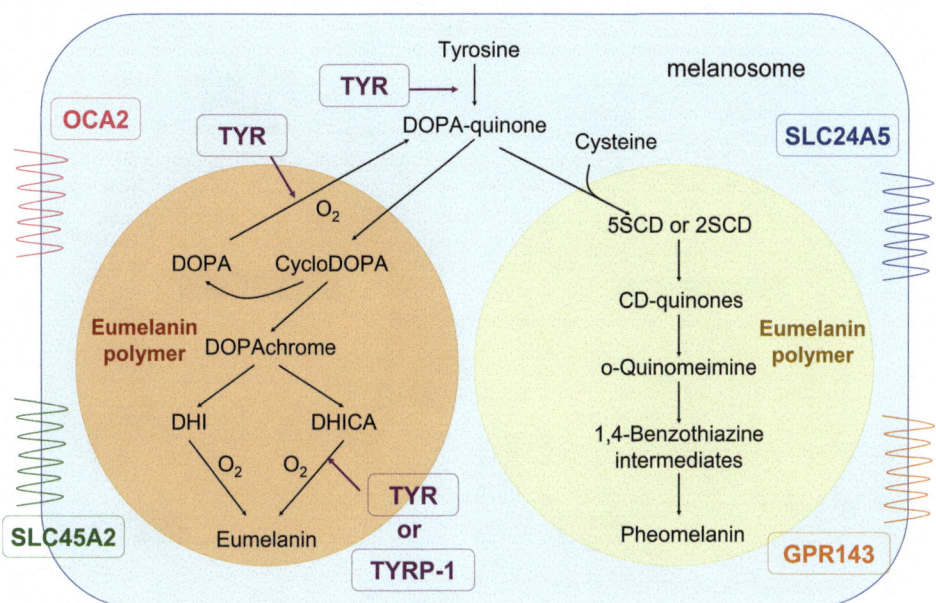

Fig. 7.1 Scheme of melanin production pathway in melanosomes (Modified from reference figure, with permission [14])

individuals of non-African ethnicity because the effect of diluted pigmentation in OCA3 is mild. SLC45A2, a melanosomal transporter protein, is responsible for OCA4. SLC45A2 is considered to be involved in pH control inside the melanosome along with OCA2; thus, mutation of *SLC45A2* would impair melanin biosynthesis with wide clinical variation [20]. OCA5 was reported in a consanguineous Pakistani albino family [4]. Individuals with OCA5 display hypopigmentation of skin, golden hair, and ocular symptoms. Linkage analysis mapped the responsible locus to 4q24; however, subsequent sequence analysis of candidate genes failed to detect the pathological mutation. OCA6 is caused by the mutation of *SLC24A5* [5]. SLC24A5 acts as an ion transporter on melanosomal membranes along with OCA2 and SLC45A2 [21]. The eumelanin content of hair in individuals with OCA6 is significantly lower than that of unaffected family members (heterozygous carriers). Electron microscopy of skin from individuals with OCA6 revealed fewer mature melanosomes (stage IV) but more immature melanosomes (stages II and III) in both the cell body and dendrites of melanocytes compared with unaffected

individuals. This finding suggests that SLC24A5 protein is required for the maturation of melanosomes or for the production of pigment in mature melanosomes [5]. *C10orf11*, which is considered a melanocyte differentiation gene, is responsible for OCA7. Immunohistochemistry of skin from human fetuses showed C10orf11-positive cells (melanoblasts) on the dermis, which migrates from the neural crest, while no positive cells for C10orf11 were observed in either fetal or adult retinal pigment epithelium. This finding suggests that C10orf11 is also associated with melanocyte migration [6].

Clinical Features

These types of OCA principally demonstrate hypopigmentation of skin and hair and ocular changes; the degree of hypopigmentation varies among the types of OCA and affected individuals (Figs. 7.2, 7.3, 7.4, and 7.5). Ocular changes include hypopigmentation in retinal pigment epithelium and in the iris, infantile nystagmus, photophobia, impaired visual acuity, foveal hypoplasia, and misrouting of the optic nerve at the chiasm. Individuals with OCA1A do not have melanin pigment at all, leading to non-tanning white skin,

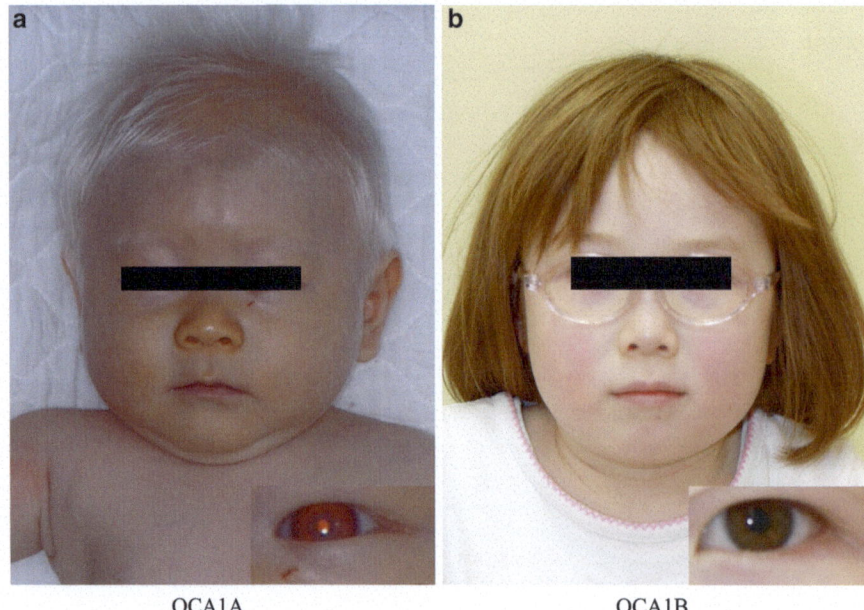

OCA1A   OCA1B

Fig. 7.2 Clinical findings of OCA1. (**a**) OCA1A, 2-month-old boy. He demonstrates complete lack of melanin. Iris is translucent and reddish. (**b**) OCA1B, 5-year-old girl. She retains some amount of melanin synthesis. Iris is brownish

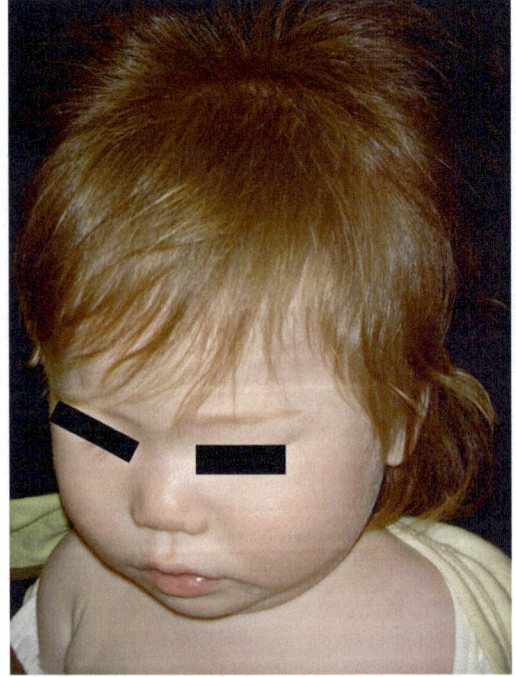

OCA2

Fig. 7.3 Clinical findings of OCA2. 6-month-old boy. His hair is brown; skin is not as pale as OCA1A

white hair, and reddish irises, while those with OCA1B retain slight melanin biosynthesis. In OCA3, melanin biosynthesis is relatively retained compared to other type of OCA, and visual alteration tends to be mild. The hypopigmentation of OCA2 and OCA4 varies among individuals, and pigmentation tends to recover as individuals mature. The symptoms of OCA6 are similar to those of OCA2 and OCA4, presumably because the responsible genes are found in the same functional entity, ion transporters on melanosomes. Visual impairment in OCA7 is severe in contrast to the mild hypopigmentation of skin and hair.

Differential Diagnosis

Since the symptoms of the different types of OCA show significant overlap, genetic analysis is necessary for definitive diagnosis. The coexistence of systemic symptoms such as bleeding diathesis, interstitial pneumonia, immunodeficiency, and/or neurological defects is useful in suggesting syndromic OCA. Prader-Willi syndrome and Angelman syndrome, which are characterized by mental retardation, are sometimes accompanied by the symptoms of OCA2 because both conditions are caused by the deletion of

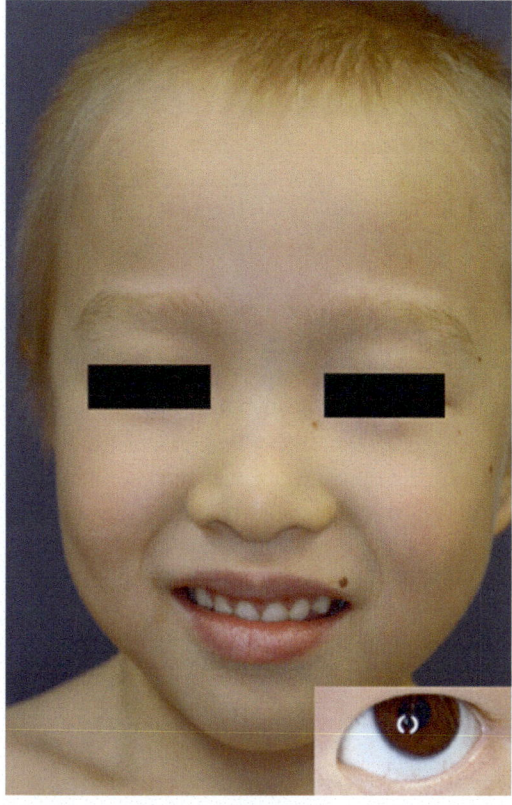

OCA3

Fig. 7.4 Clinical findings of OCA3. 5-year-old boy. His hair is light brown; iris is dark brown, and the eyes do not show nystagmus [66]

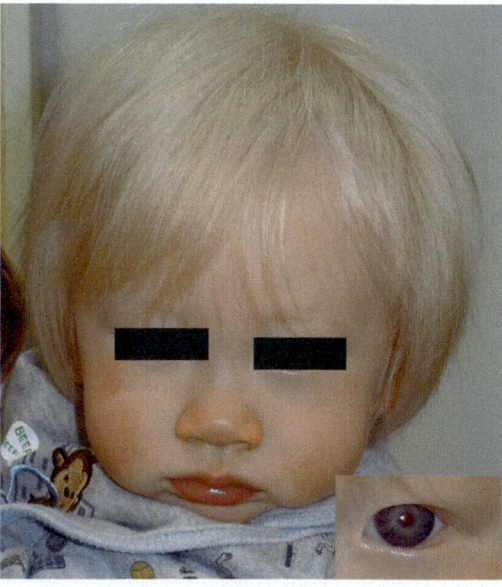

OCA4

Fig. 7.5 Clinical findings of OCA4. 11-month-old girl. Her melanin synthesis is slight; iris is translucent and reddish blue

chromosome 15q, which contains the *OCA2* gene. Other congenital or nutritional disorders including phenylketonuria, histidinemia, homocystinuria, selenium deficiency, copper deficiency, and kwashiorkor may show hypopigmentation of skin and hair (albinism). These can also be distinguished by the accompanying symptoms.

Intervention and Treatment

No curative treatment has been found for OCA to date. Early diagnosis is important to allow initiation of appropriate interventions for skin and eye symptoms. For skin, sun protection through the wearing of protective clothing and the regular application of sunscreen are essential to prevent sunburn and secondary skin changes and to decrease the risk of skin cancer in later life.

Regular skin checkups for skin cancer are recommended for adult individuals with OCA, especially in cases of severe hypopigmentation. Early referral to ophthalmologists is mandatory to introduce proper ophthalmologic interventions such as corrective glasses or surgical correction of strabismus and nystagmus. Dark sunglasses may alleviate photophobia. Once pathologic mutations are detected in an affected family member, prenatal diagnosis would be scientifically possible and may be an option for parents and other family members.

Prognosis

The lifespan of individuals with OCA may be similar to that of unaffected individuals. However, several epidemiological studies showed that a relatively large number of albino people constitute in the younger age groups in Africa [22]. In addition, retrospective survey of African albinos with skin cancers described that late presentation mainly due to lack of fund and poor access to healthcare facilities lead to more advanced disease status [23]. Lack of preventive resources including sunscreens could give albino people a chance to have more ultraviolet exposure, which is a major risk factor of skin carcinogenesis [22]. These data might imply that the mortality of people with albinism at younger age might be higher than people without albinism, though more specific data are required to accurately speculate this issue. In terms of public health issue of albino people particularly in African countries, they have been reported to face social stigma and discrimination because of lack of accurate knowledge and education about albinism, leading to have albino people live in lower economic status [22].

With the exception of OCA1A, hypopigmentation of skin and hair tends to be alleviated as individuals mature. Although there is no case-control data regarding whether early ophthalmologic intervention can prevent the progression of visual impairment, generally speaking, this impairment is not progressive and may gradually improve with age. An increased risk for skin cancers, particularly squamous cell carcinoma (SCC) [24] and basal cell carcinoma (BCC) [24, 25], has been reported. The incidence rate of melanoma in individuals with OCA is controversial [26] because of the lack of large population studies; however, it is generally considered that the risk of melanoma is increased in individuals with OCA compared to unaffected individuals [27]. Melanin is a kind of scavenger that removes free radicals from tissue [28]; thus decrease or lack of melanin will lead to increases in risk of melanoma [24, 25, 29–31], SCC, and BCC.

Ocular Albinism (OA)

Definition
OA is a genetic disorder characterized by decreased pigmentation of eyes and visual disturbance. The most common and recognized form is X-linked OA (also called as OA1); however, OA comprises heterogeneous conditions accompanied by extraocular symptoms such as sensorineural deafness [32], sensorineural deafness with autosomal recessive inheritance [33], or congenital malformation of the maxillary bone [34]. Although hypopigmentation of skin and hair can be seen in some individuals, these manifestations are usually mild and not as visible as those of OCA.

Epidemiology
The prevalence of OA has been reported as 1 out of 60,000 and 1 out of 50,000 in a Danish cohort and a US cohort, respectively [3, 35].

Responsible Genes and Pathophysiology
OA1 is caused by a defective G protein-coupled receptor 143 gene (GPR143) located on chromosome Xp.22.2. GPR143 is a melanosome-associated G-protein-coupled receptor involved in melanosome biogenesis during melanocyte differentiation. Electron microscopy showed that the number of melanosomes decreased but their size increased in skin melanocytes and retinal pigment epithelium from OA1 patients [36]. GPR143 regulates melanosome size and number via activation of the microphthalmia-associated transcription factor (MITF), which is a key regulator of melanocyte differentiation [37].

Clinical Features
OA1 is characterized by hypopigmentation in retinal pigment epithelium and iris, nystagmus, photophobia, impaired visual acuity, and foveal hypoplasia. Misrouting of the optic nerve in the chiasm is also observed in visual evoked potential (VEP) testing. These ophthalmologic findings greatly overlap with those of types of OCA. Theoretically, hypopigmentation of skin is not seen in individuals with OA; however, some individuals show mild dilution of the pigmentation in skin and hair compared to unaffected male siblings.

Differential Diagnosis
OCA can be excluded by the absence of hypopigmentation of skin and hair. In Caucasian individuals with pale skin and blond hair, it may be impossible to determine whether the individuals have hypopigmentation of their skin and hair. In such case, genetic analysis of GRP143 and OCA genes may be needed to obtain a definitive diagnosis.

There are rare genetic disorders that demonstrate congenital nystagmus, and this can also be distinguished by the absence of hypopigmentation of the iris and retinal pigment epithelium.

Intervention and Treatment

As with the ocular symptoms of OCA, no curative treatment for OA1 exists to date. Early referral to ophthalmologists is mandatory to initiate appropriate interventions. For visual impairment, wearing corrective glasses is necessary, and dark sunglasses may alleviate photophobia. Surgical correction may be preferred for strabismus and nystagmus in some individuals. Regular ophthalmologic examination should be introduced.

Prognosis

OA1 is likely to be a nonprogressive disorder; visual acuity is usually stable throughout the lifespan of an individual and sometimes improves gradually until adulthood. Nystagmus also tends to improve as individuals mature, but is unlikely to disappear [3].

Syndromic Albinism

Hermansky-Pudlak Syndrome (HPS)

Definition

Hermansky-Pudlak syndrome (HPS) is an autosomal recessive disorder characterized by OCA and other non-pigmentary symptoms such as bleeding diathesis, due to platelet storage pool deficiency and accumulation of ceroid in tissues [38]. It is genetically and clinically heterozygous, with ten types of HPS and their responsible genes reported to date (Table 7.2). On electron microscopy, platelets from individuals with HPS do not contain dense granules, which is a gold standard diagnostic finding.

Epidemiology

HPS is a rare disorder, with an estimated prevalence in the general population of 1:500,000–1:1,000,000 [39]. The region with the highest known prevalence of HPS is Puerto Rico, where approximately one in 1800 persons is affected and approximately one in 1800 persons is affected, and approximately one in 22 is a carrier [40]. Almost all of these individuals are type1 or type3. Regarding the non-Puerto Rican population, HPS1 is a relatively common type of albinism in Japan and China [1, 41, 42].

Responsible Genes and Pathophysiology

HPS is caused by the disruption of lysosomal-related organelles (LROs), which play important roles in membrane trafficking in many types of cells and organs. The symptoms, including OCA, bleeding diathesis, and deposition of ceroid bodies, are due to the disruption of membrane trafficking of melanosome-related protein, platelet dense granules, and lysosomes. LROs are synthesized by several protein complexes including biogenesis of lysosome-related organelles complex (BLOC)-1, BLOC-2, and BLOC-3 and the adaptor protein (AP)-3 complex, which consist of several HPS proteins (Fig. 7.6). Thus, disruption of HPS proteins causes pigmentary and various non-pigmentary symptoms.

BLOC-3 is composed of two subunits, HPS1 and HPS4 [43]. Analysis of fibroblasts derived from BLOC-3-deficient mice showed altered distribution of late endosomes/lysosomes, suggesting that BLOC-3 may play a role in the proper distribution and motility of organelles, although its pathophysiology in the development of HPS1 and HPS4 remains to be clarified. Depending on where it is expressed, the AP-3 complex has two forms, the ubiquitous form and the neuron-specific form [44]. The ubiquitous form plays a role in the efficient trafficking of TYR and OCA2 in melanocytes [45, 46]. The neuron-specific form is necessary for synaptic vesicle formation from endosomes, which allows the release of neurotransmitters along developing axons [47]. Although both forms share three subunits, AD-3α, AD-3δ, and AP-3 μ, the difference between the two forms is the presence of AP-3β3A in the ubiquitous form and the presence of AP-3β3B in the neuron-specific form (Fig. 7.6). The gene for HPS2 (*AP3B1*) encodes the β3A subunit. Recently, *AP3D1* encoding AP-3δ has been reported to be the gene

Table 7.2 Syndromic oculocutaneous albinism

Disease name	Inheritance	Genes	Chromosomal location	MIM
HPS1	AR	*HPS1*	10q24.2	203,300
HPS2	AR	*HPS2/AP3B1*	5q14.1	608,233
HPS3	AR	*HPS3*	3q24	614,072
HPS4	AR	*HPS4*	22q12.1	614,073
HPS5	AR	*HPS5*	11p15.1	614,074
HPS6	AR	*HPS6*	10q24.32	614,075
HPS7	AR	*HPS7/DTNBP1*	6p22.3	614,076
HPS8	AR	*HPS8/BLOC1S3*	19q13.32	614,077
HPS9	AR	*HPS9/PLDN*	15q21.1	614,171
HPS10	AR	*HPS10/AP3D1*	19p13.3	617,050
GS1	AR	*MYO5A*	15q21.2	214,450
GS2	AR	*RAB27A*	15q21.3	607,624
GS3	AR	*MLPH* and *MYO5A*	2q37.3	609,227
CHS	AR	*LYST*	1q42.3	214,500
Cross syndrome	AR	Unknown	Unknown	257,800
Albinism-deafness syndrome	X-linked	Unknown	Xq26.3-q27.1	300,700
Tietz syndrome	AD	*MITF*	3q14.1-q12.3	103,500
ABCD syndrome	AR	*EDNRB*	13q22	600,501

HPS Hermansky-Pudlak syndrome, *GS* Griscelli syndrome, *CHS* Chediak-Higashi syndrome, *ABCD* albinism, black lock, cell migration disorder of the neurocytes of the gut, and deafness

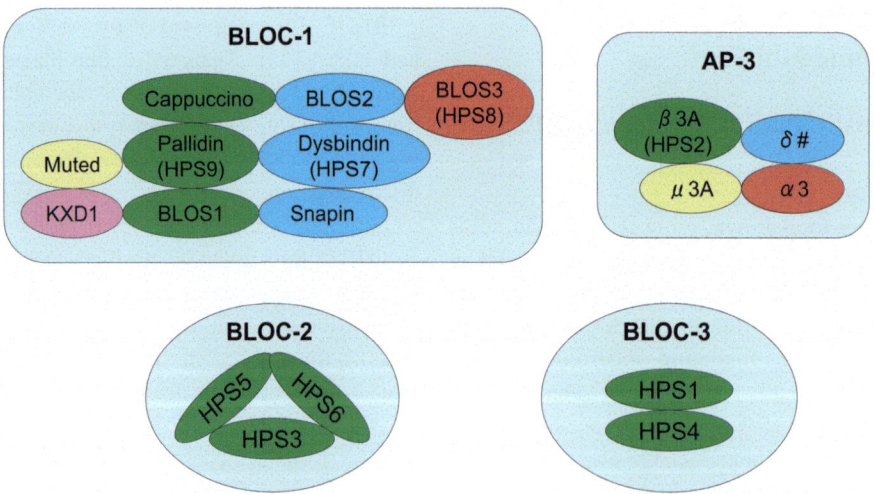

Fig. 7.6 Scheme of representative lysosomal-related organelles (LROs) which are related to HPS proteins. BLOC: Biogenesis of lysosome-related organelles com- plex. AP-3: Adaptor protein complex-3 (Modified from reference figure, with permission [38])

responsible for HPS10 [44]. Clinical symptoms of HPS2 and HPS10 are consistent with these molecular findings, since defective β3A subunit (HPS2), which is a component of the ubiquitous form, but not the neuron-specific form, does not cause neurological abnormalities, while defective AP-3δ subunit (HPS10) is associated with neurological symptoms [44]. BLOC-2 is composed of three subunits, which are responsible for HPS3, HPS5, and HPS6, respectively. Melanocytes from individuals with HPS with deficient BLOC-2 showed mislocalization of TYR and TYRP-1 and accumulation of TYR-containing vesicular structures in the cytoplasm. These findings suggest that BLOC-2 is located downstream of BLOC-1 and might play a role in fusion of BLOC-1-dependent transport intermediates with maturing melanosomes [46]. BLOC-1 is a large complex consisting of at least nine subunits, including HPS7, HPS8, and HPS9. BLOC-1 may play a role in the trafficking of TYR and TYRP-1 cooperating with AP-1 and AP-3, although the details remain to be clarified. BLOC-1-deficient mice show prominent hypopigmentation [48].

Clinical Features

Patients with HPS show various degrees of hypopigmentation, impaired visual acuity, and bleeding tendency (Fig. 7.7). It is noteworthy that patients with HPS1 or HPS4 frequently demonstrate life-threatening symptoms such as interstitial pneumonia, granulomatous colitis mimicking Crohn's disease, and, rarely, cardiomyopathy after middle age. HPS2 and HPS10 are associated with immunodeficiency and uncontrolled lymphocyte and macrophage activation, leading to subsequent hemophagocytic syndrome. HPS3, HPS5, and HPS6 show relatively mild phenotypes lacking pneumonia and colitis.

Differential Diagnosis

The definitive diagnosis of HPS is confirmed by the lack of platelet dense granules on electron microscopy. The differential diagnosis of HPS includes non-syndromic OCA and CHS. The symptoms of non-syndromic OCA are restricted to hypopigmentation and visual impairment. CHS is characterized by silvery hair, recurrent pyogenic infection, and subsequent fatal hemophagocytic syndrome, considered the "accelerated phase." Large granules are seen in polymorphonuclear cells from individuals with CHS, which is diagnostic. Immunodeficiency is observed in HPS2 and HPS10.

Fig. 7.7 Clinical findings of HPS1. 1-year-old boy. He has blonde hair and pale skin. Multiple purpuras due to bleeding diathesis are seen on his leg

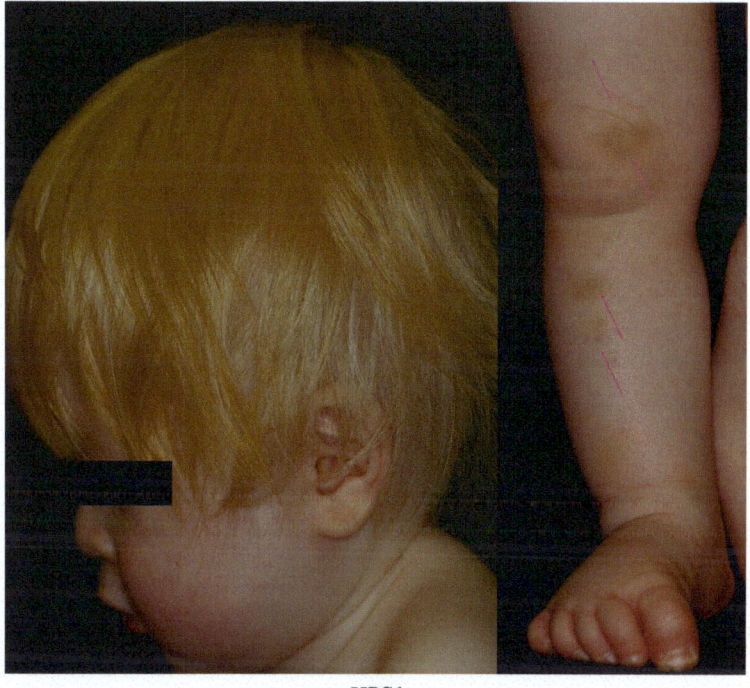

HPS1

Intervention and Treatment

For hypopigmentation of skin and visual impairment, early intervention should be introduced (see "Intervention and Treatment" in the non-syndromic OCA and OA sections). No curative treatment has been found to date for hypopigmentation. Pirfenidone, corticosteroid, and immunosuppressants have been used to treat pulmonary fibrosis, although the efficacy of these therapies remains controversial [49]. Infliximab [50] and granulocyte colony-stimulating factor (G-CSF) [51] are suggested to be effective for colitis and neutropenia/immune deficiency, respectively. Colectomy may be necessary for severe colitis. Hematopoietic stem cell transplantation (HSCT) may be required to prevent the development of hemophagocytic syndrome in individuals with HPS2 [51].

Prognosis

Hypopigmentation of skin and hair tends to be alleviated as individuals mature. Visual impairment is usually nonprogressive. The prognosis of individuals with HPS1, which is the most common subtype of HPS, can be determined by the interstitial pneumonia.

Chediak-Higashi Syndrome (CHS)

Definition and General Description

CHS is a rare genetic disease with autosomal recessive inheritance characterized by reduced pigmentation of skin and eyes, silvery or metallic colored hair, immunodeficiency, and debilitating neurologic abnormalities. Large granules in polymorphonuclear neutrophils on blood smear are diagnostic, and pigment clumping on the hair shaft is also seen. To date, fewer than 500 cases have been reported. Around 90% of individuals with CHS develop lymphoproliferative syndrome, which is known as the "accelerated phase" of the disease and tends to be fatal.

Responsible Genes and Pathophysiology

The gene responsible for CHS is *LYST*, located on 1q42.3, which encodes lysosomal trafficking regulator (LYST), also known as CHS1. Although the biological function of CHS1 is yet to be determined, electron microscopy of epidermal melanocytes from an individual with CHS shows the accumulation on the periphery of the cytoplasm of large melanosomes, which are not transferred to neighboring keratinocytes. Peroxidase-positive large inclusion bodies are seen in polymorphonuclear neutrophils and occasionally in lymphocytes, which is a characteristic finding in CHS. Neurological abnormalities may be caused by lysosome dysfunction in neurons and glial cells [52]. Considering these findings, LYST may play roles in vesicle trafficking in various cell types.

Clinical Features

Individuals with CHS show various degrees of hypopigmentation of skin and eyes, silvery or metallic colored hair, and immunodeficiency. Approximately 90% of individuals with CHS develop lymphoproliferative syndrome, which is called the "accelerated phase" of the disease and tends to be fatal. Neurological findings including low IQ scores, cerebellar ataxia, and peripheral neuropathy appear in childhood or adolescence and tend to progress gradually. A case report exists of two brothers with *LYST* mutation, who showed slowly progressive neurological symptoms including spastic paraplegia, cerebral ataxia, and peripheral neuropathy, but lacked hypopigmentation [53].

Differential Diagnosis

Differential diagnosis includes diseases showing hypopigmentation of skin, hair, and eyes and/or immunodeficiency. Non-syndromic OCA is restricted to hypopigmentation and ocular symptoms, with a lack of immunodeficiency or neurological abnormalities. Individuals with HPS2 and HPS10 demonstrate neutropenia and immunodeficiency in addition to albinism. Individuals with Griscelli syndrome demonstrate similar symptoms to those with CHS; however, Griscelli syndrome can be distinguished from CHS by the lack of large inclusion bodies in polymorphonuclear neutrophils. Individuals with HPS also lack dense granules in platelets. Genetic analysis of CHS1 assists in making a diagnosis of CHS.

Intervention and Treatment

HSCT is the only treatment for hematological and immunological abnormalities. For hypopigmentation of skin and visual impairment, early intervention should be introduced (see "Intervention and treatment" in the OCA and OA sections). To date, no curative treatment has been established for hypopigmentation.

Prognosis

Most individuals with CHS are required to undergo HSCT, and without this treatment, they will die within the early part of their first decade of life. Individuals with mild symptoms or those who do not develop the accelerated phase may survive for a long period of time, although debilitating neurological abnormalities such as loss of balance, difficulty with ambulation, and peripheral neuropathy may appear [52].

Griscelli Syndrome (GS)

Definition and General Description

Griscelli syndrome (GS) is a rare autosomal recessive genetic disorder characterized by hypopigmentation of skin and hair with large clumps of pigment in the hair shaft on light microscopy. Three forms of GS have been identified to date. GS1 is characterized by hypopigmentation with neurological abnormalities, GS2 features hypopigmentation accompanied by hematologic immunodeficiency and hematologic abnormalities, and GS3 is restricted to hypopigmentation.

Responsible Genes and Pathophysiology

The genes responsible for the three types of GS are *MYO5A*, *RAB27A*, and *MLPH*, respectively. They form a complex in melanocytes, connect melanosomes to the actin network, and are involved in melanosome transport at the periphery of melanocytes [54] (Fig. 7.8). MYO5A binds to actin filaments and moves along them like a wheel, MLPH connects RAB27A and MYO5A, and RAB27A connects to melanosomes. Since MYO5A is associated with neurological development and function [55], defective MYO5A can cause severe neurological deterioration. On the other hand, a transcript variant in brain tissue does not contain exon-F of *MYO5A* [56]. Individuals showing hypopigmentation of skin and hair identical to GS3 showed homozygous deletion of MYO5A exon-F [54]. RAB27A is also associated with the release of lytic granules from CD8-positive T cells [57]. Defective RAB27A causes immunodeficiency and uncontrolled T cell and macrophage activation leading to fatal hemophagocytic syndrome [54].

Clinical Features

GS is characterized by hypopigmentation of skin and silvery hair with large clumps of pigment in the hair shaft. GS1 is associated with severe developmental delay and mental retardation. GS2 is associated with recurrent pyogenic infections and uncontrolled T cell and macrophage activation leading to hemophagocytic syndrome, the so-called accelerated phage, which could be fatal without immunosuppressive treatment or stem cell bone marrow transplantation. GS3 is restricted to hypopigmentation of skin and hair.

Differential Diagnosis

The presence of large clumps of pigment in the hair shaft is diagnostic for GS. The differential diagnosis of GS includes non-syndromic OCA, CHS, and HPS. Non-syndromic OCA can be excluded based on the presence of non-pigmentary symptoms. GS3 can be distinguished from non-syndromic OCA by the presence of large clumps of pigment in the hair shaft. Similarly, these hair findings can be used to distinguish GS2 from CHS. Peripheral blood smears from individuals with CHS demonstrate giant inclusion bodies in polymorphonuclear neutrophils and some lymphocytes. HPS2 and HPS10 show hypopigmentation together with immunodeficiency, although HPS lacks platelet dense granules on electron microscopy.

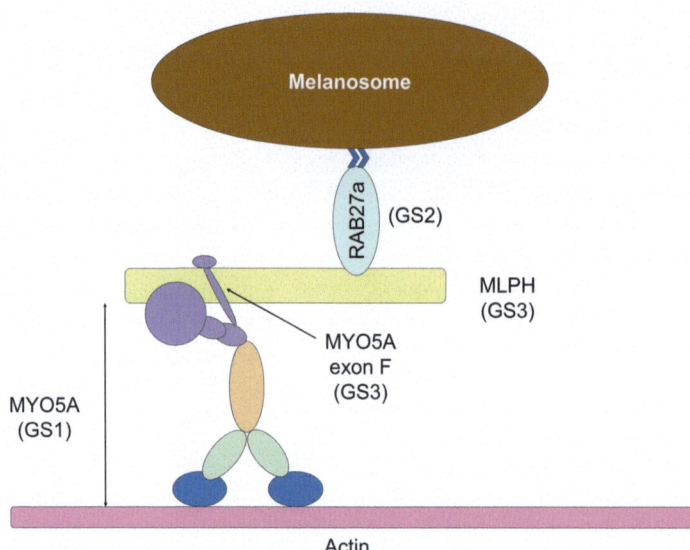

Fig. 7.8 Scheme of protein complex involved in melanosome transport and corresponding type of Griscelli syndrome (GS). Head of MYO5A binds to actin filament. Tails of MYO5A and RAB27A are attached to MLPH. RAB27A binds melanosome complex. This protein complex moves on actin filament and involved in melanosome transfer at the periphery of the cytoplasm in melanocytes. Exon-F of MYO5A is expressed only in melanocytes; its disruption causes hypopigmentation of skin and hair only (Modified from reference figure, with permission [67])

Intervention and Treatment

For hypopigmentation of skin and visual impairment, early intervention should be introduced (see "Intervention and treatment" in the OCA and OA sections). No curative treatment yet exists for the neurological symptoms. However, rehabilitation could alleviate these neurological symptoms. Stem cell bone marrow transplantation is the only method to cure the hematological and immunological abnormalities.

Prognosis

Most patients with GS1 and GS2 reported in the literature died before the age of 10. Cağdaş et al. reported healthy 21- and 24-year-old patients with GS3 with only pigmentary dilution [58].

Tietz Syndrome

Definition and General Description

Tietz syndrome is a rare genetic disorder with autosomal dominant inheritance characterized by hypopigmentation of skin and hair and congenital complete deafness [59]. Tietz reported that the affected individuals did not show hypopigmentation of eyes, but others have reported that individuals with Tietz syndrome also demonstrate albinoid fundi [60]. Tietz syndrome is caused by the mutation of *MITF*, which is also the gene responsible for Waardenburg syndrome type II. The pathogenesis of Tietz syndrome and why different phenotypes appear as a result of *MITF* mutation remain unclear.

Albinism, Black Lock, Cell Migration Disorder of the Neurocytes of the Gut, and Deafness (ABCD) Syndrome

Definition and General Description

ABCD syndrome is a rare genetic disorder with autosomal recessive inheritance characterized by hypopigmentation of skin and eyes, a black mark on the left temporal region, bilateral deafness, and agangliosis of the colon [61]. The symptoms of this syndrome overlap with those of

Waardenburg syndrome. Gross et al. reported five individuals with this syndrome in a consanguineous Kurdish family, all of whom died within the first 5 weeks of life [61]. Verheij et al. [62] identified an individual with ABCD syndrome who harbored a homozygous mutation of the endothelin B receptor gene (*EDNRB*) and whose parents had heterogeneous mutations of *EDNRB*, while neither parent showed symptoms of Waardenburg syndrome.

Cross Syndrome

Definition and General Description

Cross syndrome (also called Kramer syndrome) is a rare genetic disorder with autosomal recessive inheritance, characterized by hypopigmentation of skin, eyes, and hair and cerebral defects [63]. Neurological findings include spasticity, psychomotor retardation, ataxia, and athetoid movements. The responsible gene has not yet been identified. Although several complications such as urinary tract abnormalities [64] and Batter syndrome [65] have been reported, it remains unclear whether these complications are related symptoms or merely a coincidence.

Conclusions

Clinical and basic research about albinism enable us not only to detect their responsible genes or genetic diagnosis of affected individuals but also to expand knowledge and shed light on melanocyte biology and the mechanism of membrane trafficking, contributing to advances of molecular biology.

On the other hand, no mutations in known albinism-related genes are detected in around 20% of affected individuals [8]. A genome-wide association study has shown that a single nucleotide polymorphism (SNP) in the regulatory region upstream of the *KIT ligand* (*KITLG*) gene is involved in blond hair in Northern Europeans [9], suggesting that genetic alterations in noncoding regions near albinism-related genes can also be involved in the pathogenesis of albinism, as well as potential albinism genes yet to be identified [8]. Vigorous investigation will further clarify the pathophysiology of albinism.

References

1. Ito S, Suzuki T, Inagaki K, Suzuki N, Takamori K, Yamada T, et al. High frequency of Hermansky-Pudlak syndrome type 1 (HPS1) among Japanese albinism patients and functional analysis of HPS1 mutant protein. J Invest Dermatol. 2005;125(4):715–20.
2. Okoro AN. Albinism in Nigeria. A clinical and social study. Br J Dermatol. 1975;92(5):485–92.
3. Lewis RA. Ocular albinism, X-linked. In: Pagon RA, Adam MP, Ardinger HH, Wallace SE, Amemiya A, Bean LJH, et al., editors. GeneReviews(R). Seattle: University of Washington, Seattle, University of Washington, Seattle. All rights reserved; 1993.
4. Kausar T, Bhatti MA, Ali M, Shaikh RS, Ahmed ZM. OCA5, a novel locus for non-syndromic oculocutaneous albinism, maps to chromosome 4q24. Clin Genet. 2013;84(1):91–3.
5. Wei AH, Zang DJ, Zhang Z, Liu XZ, He X, Yang L, et al. Exome sequencing identifies SLC24A5 as a candidate gene for nonsyndromic oculocutaneous albinism. J Invest Dermatol. 2013;133(7):1834–40.
6. Gronskov K, Dooley CM, Ostergaard E, Kelsh RN, Hansen L, Levesque MP, et al. Mutations in c10orf11, a melanocyte-differentiation gene, cause autosomal-recessive albinism. Am J Hum Genet. 2013;92(3):415–21.
7. Okamura K, Abe Y, Araki Y, Wakamatsu K, Seishima M, Umetsu T, Kato A, Kawaguchi M, Hayashi M, Hozumi Y, Suzuki T. Characterization of melanosomes and melanin in Japanese patients with Hermansky-Pudlak syndrome types 1,4, 6, and 9. Pigment Cell Melanoma Res. 2017. https://doi.org/10.1111/pcmr.12662.
8. Montoliu L, Gronskov K, Wei AH, Martinez-Garcia M, Fernandez A, Arveiler B, et al. Increasing the complexity: new genes and new types of albinism. Pigment Cell Melanoma Res. 2014;27(1):11–8.
9. Sulem P, Gudbjartsson DF, Stacey SN, Helgason A, Rafnar T, Magnusson KP, et al. Genetic determinants of hair, eye and skin pigmentation in Europeans. Nat Genet. 2007;39(12):1443–52.
10. Oki R, Yamada K, Nakano S, Kimoto K, Yamamoto K, Kondo H, et al. A Japanese family with autosomal dominant oculocutaneous albinism type 4. Invest Ophthalmol Vis Sci. 2017;58(2):1008–16.
11. Inagaki K, Suzuki T, Shimizu H, Ishii N, Umezawa Y, Tada J, et al. Oculocutaneous albinism type 4 is one

of the most common types of albinism in Japan. Am J Hum Genet. 2004;74(3):466–71.

12. Morice-Picard F, Lasseaux E, Francois S, Simon D, Rooryck C, Bieth E, et al. SLC24A5 mutations are associated with non-syndromic oculocutaneous albinism. J Invest Dermatol. 2014;134(2):568–71.

13. Khordadpoor-Deilamani F, Akbari MT, Karimipoor M, Javadi GR. Homozygosity mapping in albinism patients using a novel panel of 13 STR markers inside the nonsyndromic OCA genes: introducing 5 novel mutations. J Hum Genet. 2016;61(5):373–9.

14. Hearing VJ. Determination of melanin synthetic pathways. J Invest Dermatol. 2011;131(E1):E8–e11.

15. King RA, Townsend D, Oetting W, Summers CG, Olds DP, White JG, et al. Temperature-sensitive tyrosinase associated with peripheral pigmentation in oculocutaneous albinism. J Clin Invest. 1991;87(3):1046–53.

16. Kono M, Kondo T, Ito S, Suzuki T, Wakamatsu K, Ito S, et al. Genotype analysis in a patient with oculocutaneous albinism 1 minimal pigment type. Br J Dermatol. 2012;166(4):896–8.

17. King RA, Wirtschafter JD, Olds DP, Brumbaugh J. Minimal pigment: a new type of oculocutaneous albinism. Clin Genet. 1986;29(1):42–50.

18. Kondo T, Namiki T, Coelho SG, Valencia JC. Hearing VJ. Oculocutaneous albinism: developing novel antibodies targeting the proteins associated with OCA2 and OCA4. J Dermatol Sci. 2015;77(1):21–7.

19. Manga P, Kromberg JG, Box NF, Sturm RA, Jenkins T, Ramsay M. Rufous oculocutaneous albinism in southern African blacks is caused by mutations in the TYRP1 gene. Am J Hum Genet. 1997;61(5):1095–101.

20. Inagaki K, Suzuki T, Ito S, Suzuki N, Adachi K, Okuyama T, et al. Oculocutaneous albinism type 4: six novel mutations in the membrane-associated transporter protein gene and their phenotypes. Pigment Cell Res. 2006;19(5):451–3.

21. Ito S, Wakamatsu K. Diversity of human hair pigmentation as studied by chemical analysis of eumelanin and pheomelanin. J Eur Acad Dermatol Venereol. 2011;25(12):1369–80.

22. Hong ES, Zeeb H, Repacholi MH. Albinism in Africa as a public health issue. BMC Public Health. 2006;6:212.

23. Mabula JB, Chalya PL, McHembe MD, Jaka H, Giiti G, Rambau P, et al. Skin cancers among Albinos at a University teaching hospital in Northwestern Tanzania: a retrospective review of 64 cases. BMC Dermatol. 2012;12:5.

24. Box NF, Duffy DL, Irving RE, Russell A, Chen W, Griffyths LR, et al. Melanocortin-1 receptor genotype is a risk factor for basal and squamous cell carcinoma. J Invest Dermatol. 2001;116(2):224–9.

25. Gudbjartsson DF, Sulem P, Stacey SN, Goldstein AM, Rafnar T, Sigurgeirsson B, et al. ASIP and TYR pigmentation variants associate with cutaneous melanoma and basal cell carcinoma. Nat Genet. 2008;40(7):886–91.

26. Streutker CJ, McCready D, Jimbow K, From L. Malignant melanoma in a patient with oculocutaneous albinism. J Cutan Med Surg. 2000;4(3):149–52.

27. Asuquo ME, Ngim O, Ebughe G, Bassey EE. Skin cancers amongst four Nigerian albinos. Int J Dermatol. 2009;48(6):636–8.

28. Herrling T, Jung K, Fuchs J. The role of melanin as protector against free radicals in skin and its role as free radical indicator in hair. Spectrochim Acta A Mol Biomol Spectrosc. 2008;69(5):1429–35.

29. Wenczl E, Van der Schans GP, Roza L, Kolb RM, Timmerman AJ, Smit NP, et al. (Pheo)melanin photosensitizes UVA-induced DNA damage in cultured human melanocytes. J Invest Dermatol. 1998;111(4):678–82.

30. Yoshizawa J, Abe Y, Oiso N, Fukai K, Hozumi Y, Nakamura T, et al. Variants in melanogenesis-related genes associate with skin cancer risk among Japanese populations. J Dermatol. 2014;41(4):296–302.

31. Fernandez LP, Milne RL, Pita G, Floristan U, Sendagorta E, Feito M, et al. Pigmentation-related genes and their implication in malignant melanoma susceptibility. Exp Dermatol. 2009;18(7):634–42.

32. Bassi MT, Ramesar RS, Caciotti B, Winship IM, De Grandi A, Riboni M, et al. X-linked late-onset sensorineural deafness caused by a deletion involving OA1 and a novel gene containing WD-40 repeats. Am J Hum Genet. 1999;64(6):1604–16.

33. Morell R, Spritz RA, Ho L, Pierpont J, Guo W, Friedman TB, et al. Apparent digenic inheritance of Waardenburg syndrome type 2 (WS2) and autosomal recessive ocular albinism (AROA). Hum Mol Genet. 1997;6(5):659–64.

34. Somsen D, Davis-Keppen L, Crotwell P, Flanagan J, Munson P, Stein Q. Congenital nasal pyriform aperture stenosis and ocular albinism co-occurring in a sibship with a maternally-inherited 97 kb Xp22.2 microdeletion. Am J Med Genetics A. 2014;164a(5):1268–71.

35. Rosenberg T, Schwartz M. X-linked ocular albinism: prevalence and mutations--a national study. Eur J Hum Genet. 1998;6(6):570–7.

36. Garner A, Jay BS. Macromelanosomes in X-linked ocular albinism. Histopathology. 1980;4(3):243–54.

37. Falletta P, Bagnato P, Bono M, Monticone M, Schiaffino MV, Bennett DC, et al. Melanosome-autonomous regulation of size and number: the OA1 receptor sustains PMEL expression. Pigment Cell Melanoma Res. 2014;27(4):565–79.

38. Wei AH, Li W. Hermansky-Pudlak syndrome: pigmentary and non-pigmentary defects and their pathogenesis. Pigment Cell Melanoma Res. 2013;26(2):176–92.

39. Gahl WA, Huizing M. Hermansky-Pudlak syndrome. In: Pagon RA, Adam MP, Ardinger HH, Wallace SE, Amemiya A, Bean LJH, et al., editors.

GeneReviews(R). Seattle: University of Washington, Seattle, University of Washington, Seattle. All rights reserved; 1993.

40. Witkop CJ, Nunez Babcock M, Rao GH, Gaudier F, Summers CG, Shanahan F, et al. Albinism and Hermansky-Pudlak syndrome in Puerto Rico. Boletin de la Asociacion Medica de Puerto Rico. 1990;82(8):333–9.

41. Wei A, Lian S, Wang L, Li W. The first case report of a Chinese Hermansky-Pudlak syndrome patient with a novel mutation on HPS1 gene. J Dermatol Sci. 2009;56(2):130–2.

42. Wei A, Wang Y, Long Y, Wang Y, Guo X, Zhou Z, et al. A comprehensive analysis reveals mutational spectra and common alleles in Chinese patients with oculocutaneous albinism. J Invest Dermatol. 2010;130(3):716–24.

43. Suzuki T, Li W, Zhang Q, Karim A, Novak EK, Sviderskaya EV, et al. Hermansky-Pudlak syndrome is caused by mutations in HPS4, the human homolog of the mouse light-ear gene. Nat Genet. 2002;30(3):321–4.

44. Ammann S, Schulz A, Krageloh-Mann I, Dieckmann NM, Niethammer K, Fuchs S, et al. Mutations in AP3D1 associated with immunodeficiency and seizures define a new type of Hermansky-Pudlak syndrome. Blood. 2016;127(8):997–1006.

45. Falcon-Perez JM, Nazarian R, Sabatti C, Dell'Angelica EC. Distribution and dynamics of Lamp1-containing endocytic organelles in fibroblasts deficient in BLOC-3. J Cell Sci. 2005;118(Pt 22):5243–55.

46. Sitaram A, Marks MS. Mechanisms of protein delivery to melanosomes in pigment cells. Physiology (Bethesda). 2012;27(2):85–99.

47. Blumstein J, Faundez V, Nakatsu F, Saito T, Ohno H, Kelly RB. The neuronal form of adaptor protein-3 is required for synaptic vesicle formation from endosomes. J Neurosci Off J Soc Neurosci. 2001;21(20):8034–42.

48. Dell'Angelica EC. The building BLOC(k)s of lysosomes and related organelles. Curr Opin Cell Biol. 2004;16(4):458–64.

49. Kanazu M, Arai T, Sugimoto C, Kitaichi M, Akira M, Abe Y, et al. An intractable case of Hermansky-Pudlak syndrome. Internal Med (Tokyo, Japan). 2014;53(22):2629–34.

50. Felipez LM, Gokhale R, Guandalini S. Hermansky-Pudlak syndrome: severe colitis and good response to infliximab. J Pediatr Gastroenterol Nutr. 2010;51(5):665–7.

51. Enders A, Zieger B, Schwarz K, Yoshimi A, Speckmann C, Knoepfle FM, et al. Lethal hemophagocytic lymphohistiocytosis in Hermansky-Pudlak syndrome type II. Blood. 2006;108(1):81–7.

52. Tardieu M, Lacroix C, Neven B, Bordigoni P, de Saint BG, Blanche S, et al. Progressive neurologic dysfunctions 20 years after allogeneic bone marrow transplantation for Chediak-Higashi syndrome. Blood. 2005;106(1):40–2.

53. Shimazaki H, Honda J, Naoi T, Namekawa M, Nakano I, Yazaki M, et al. Autosomal-recessive complicated spastic paraplegia with a novel lysosomal trafficking regulator gene mutation. J Neurol Neurosurg Psychiatry. 2014;85(9):1024–8.

54. Ménasché G, Ho CH, Sanal O, Feldmann J, Tezcan I, Ersoy F, et al. Griscelli syndrome restricted to hypopigmentation results from a melanophilin defect (GS3) or a MYO5A F-exon deletion (GS1). J Clin Investig. 2003;112(3):450–6.

55. Langford GM, Molyneaux BJ. Myosin V in the brain: mutations lead to neurological defects. Brain Res Brain Res Rev. 1998;28(1–2):1–8.

56. Lambert J, Naeyaert JM, Callens T, De Paepe A, Messiaen L. Human myosin V gene produces different transcripts in a cell type-specific manner. Biochem Biophys Res Commun. 1998;252(2):329–33.

57. Bizario JC, Feldmann J, Castro FA, Menasche G, Jacob CM, Cristofani L, et al. Griscelli syndrome: characterization of a new mutation and rescue of T-cytotoxic activity by retroviral transfer of RAB27A gene. J Clin Immunol. 2004;24(4):397–410.

58. Cagdas D, Ozgur TT, Asal GT, Tezcan I, Metin A, Lambert N, et al. Griscelli syndrome types 1 and 3: analysis of four new cases and long-term evaluation of previously diagnosed patients. Eur J Pediatr. 2012;171(10):1527–31.

59. Tietz W. A syndrome of deaf-mutism associated with albinism showing dominant autosomal inheritance. Am J Hum Genet. 1963;15:259–64.

60. Smith SD, Kelley PM, Kenyon JB, Hoover D. Tietz syndrome (hypopigmentation/deafness) caused by mutation of MITF. J Med Genet. 2000;37(6):446–8.

61. Gross A, Kunze J, Maier RF, Stoltenburg-Didinger G, Grimmer I, Obladen M. Autosomal-recessive neural crest syndrome with albinism, black lock, cell migration disorder of the neurocytes of the gut, and deafness: ABCD syndrome. Am J Med Genet. 1995;56(3):322–6.

62. Verheij JB, Kunze J, Osinga J, van Essen AJ, Hofstra RM. ABCD syndrome is caused by a homozygous mutation in the EDNRB gene. Am J Med Genet. 2002;108(3):223–5.

63. Cross HE, McKusick VA, Breen W. A new oculocerebral syndrome with hypopigmentation. J Pediatr. 1967;70(3):398–406.

64. Tezcan I, Demir E, Asan E, Kale G, Muftuoglu SF, Kotiloglu E. A new case of oculocerebral hypopigmentation syndrome (cross syndrome) with additional findings. Clin Genet. 1997;51(2):118–21.

65. White CP, Waldron M, Jan JE, Carter JE. Oculocerebral hypopigmentation syndrome associated with Bartter syndrome. Am J Med Genet. 1993;46(5):592–6.

66. Okamura K, Yoshizawa J, Abe Y, Hanaoka K, Higashi N, Togawa Y, et al. Oculocutaneous albinism (OCA) in Japanese patients: five novel mutations. J Dermatol Sci. 2014;74(2):173–4.

67. Van Gele M, Dynoodt P, Lambert J. Griscelli syndrome: a model system to study vesicular trafficking. Pigment Cell Melanoma Res. 2009;22(3):268–82.

Recent Advances in Pathogenesis and Medical Management of Vitiligo

8

Muhammed Razmi T and Davinder Parsad

Introduction

Vitiligo is an acquired disorder of melanogenesis caused by melanocyte destruction, involving a complex interaction between environmental and genetic factors, ultimately resulting in the characteristic depigmented patches [1]. The disease runs an unpredictable course but is often progressive with stable phases in between [2]. It usually begins during childhood or early adulthood. Vitiligo on the exposed body parts often leads to social embarrassment, psychological turmoil and aesthetic disfigurement [3]. An aggressive management is warranted in vitiligo because of the stigma, social isolation and psychological stress associated with the disease.

Recently, there has been an increase in the awareness activities on vitiligo by various patient support organisations. Vitiligo research has also gained much attention nowadays in pigment cell research community. This chapter deals with the updates on the classification and recent advances in pathogenesis and medical management of vitiligo.

M. Razmi T (✉) · D. Parsad
Department of Dermatology, Venereology and Leprology, Postgraduate Institute of Medical Education and Research, Chandigarh, India
e-mail: dr.razmi.t@gmail.com; parsad@me.com

Epidemiology

Worldwide prevalence of vitiligo is 0.5–2%, but up to 8.8% has been reported in India, with no sex predilection [4, 5]. In approximately 50% of cases, vitiligo appears before the age of 20 years, and 70–80% of patients develop the disease by the age of 30 years [6]. Non-segmental vitiligo can occur at any age, whereas a younger age of occurrence is seen in segmental vitiligo [7].

Classification

The Bordeaux Vitiligo Global Issues Consensus Conference (VGICC) [8] classified vitiligo in to two major forms, namely, segmental vitiligo (SV) and non-segmental vitiligo (NSV). Focal vitiligo was assigned a separate category – 'undetermined' vitiligo – until more definitive classification can be made on clinical grounds [8].

Segmental (unilateral) vitiligo It has an early onset, rapid progression, early stabilisation and unilateral or segmental distribution with no specific triggering factors [9]. Depigmentation process in SV occurs rapidly within the segment over a period of 6–24 months and then usually halts without any further progression [8]. Prevalence of SV ranges from 5% to 16% of all patients with vitiligo [9]. Autoimmune disorders are reported less frequently in patients with SV and their family members than in those with NSV [10]. However, there are recent reports of associated autoimmune diseases in SV as well [11]. Demonstration of inflammation in early stages of SV [12] and the concept of mixed vitiligo has challenged the so far considered non-immune background of SV. Segmental vitiligo most commonly affects the face (Fig. 8.1), followed by the trunk, neck, extremities and scalp in descending order. VGICC has subdivided SV into uni-, bi- or plurisegmental based on the distribution. Based on the pattern of involvement, SV over face is classified by Hann [13] and over trunk by van Geel [14]. These patterns do not strictly follow a dermatomal or blaschkolinear distribution [11]. Several hypotheses for the pathogenesis of SV have been proposed, including neuronal mechanisms, somatic mosaicism and microvascular skin homing, through or without immune destruction of melanocytes [15]. Since hair follicular melanocyte reservoir is affected early in the disease process, SV responds poorly to medical

modalities. High rate of repigmentation with surgical techniques is frequently achieved, owing to its less immunologic background.

Non-segmental (bilateral) vitiligo Although not fully satisfactory, the term 'NSV' is currently used as an umbrella term for different clinical subtypes of vitiligo that are all clearly distinct from SV including acrofacial, generalised, mucosal (more than one mucosal site), universal, mixed and rare variants [8]. Non-segmental vitiligo typically starts over acral areas and gradually involves other parts of the body. Contrary to SV, in NSV, hair follicle melanocytes are initially spared from immune-mediated attack. However, hair depigmentation may occur with disease progression when hair follicle melanocyte stem cells are exhausted following repeated melanocyte contribution to the depigmented epidermis. Acrofacial vitiligo (Fig. 8.2) involves distal digits and periorificial facial areas. Lip-tip vitiligo (Fig. 8.3) is a variety in which tips of fingers, toes, nipples, penis, and lips become depigmented. Common vitiligo (formerly referred to as vitiligo vulgaris) (Fig. 8.4) is the most common

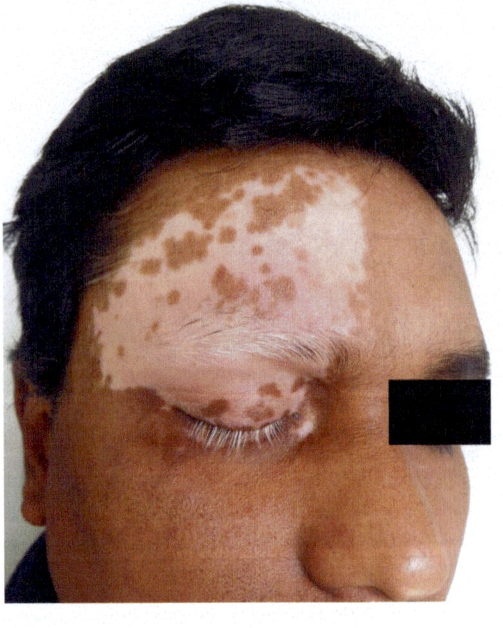

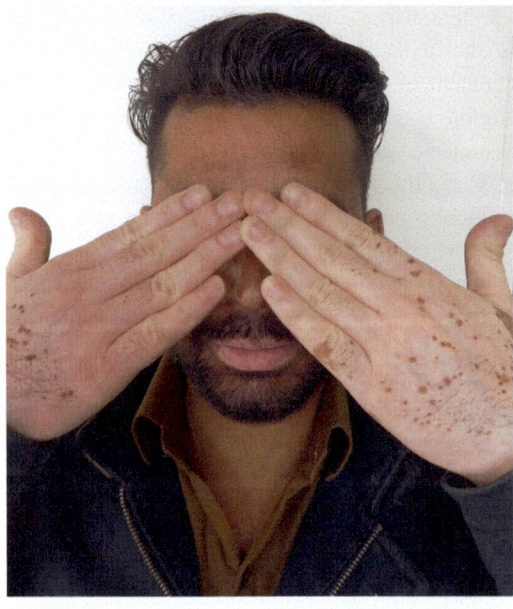

Fig. 8.1 Segmental vitiligo. Depigmented patch over the right half of the forehead extending to the right upper eyelid. Unilateral involvement (not crossing the midline of the body), irregular borders and the predominant leukotrichia are easy clinical pointers to segmental vitiligo in this patient

Fig. 8.2 Acrofacial vitiligo. Depigmented patches involving the lips and hands. Minimal perifollicular repigmentation can be seen. Lesions are refractory to the treatment in this type of vitiligo

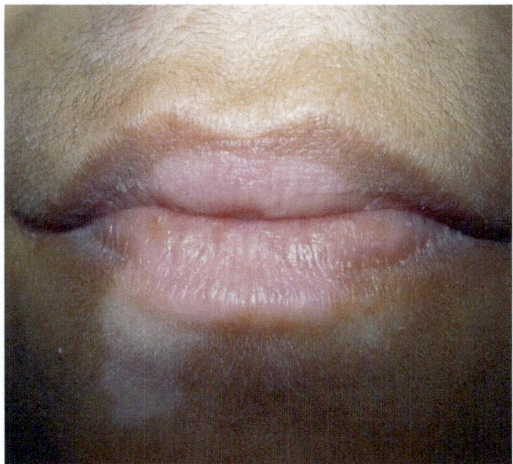

Fig. 8.3 Lip-tip vitiligo. Involvement of the upper and lower lips as a part of acrofacial vitiligo in this patient. Periorificial pattern of depigmented patches can be appreciated in the area adjoining the lower lip and the philtrum. The patient had refractory lesions over tips of fingers, toes and nipples

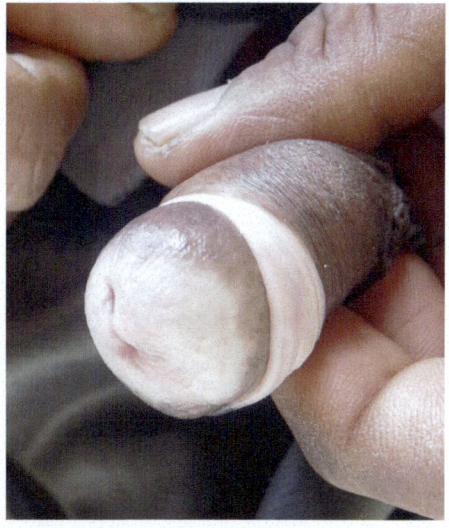

Fig. 8.5 Genital (mucosal) vitiligo. Isolated involvement of the genital mucosa for years classifies this case as focal vitiligo under 'unclassified vitiligo' as per VGICC (Vitiligo Global Issues Consensus Conference 2012). The patient had no difficulty in retracting the foreskin and hence lichen sclerosus was ruled out clinically

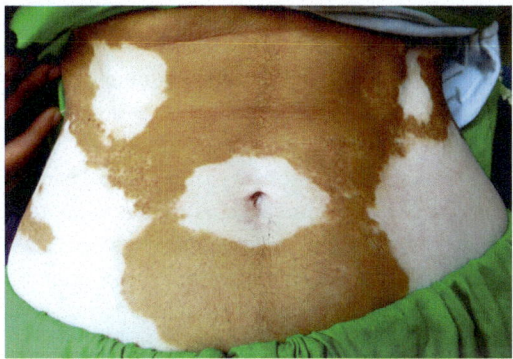

Fig. 8.4 Common vitiligo. Multiple depigmented patches distributed symmetrically on the abdomen. VGICC (Vitiligo Global Issues Consensus Conference 2012) discourages the use of 'vitiligo vulgaris', since the term 'vulgaris' conveys a negative connotation to the patients and the general public

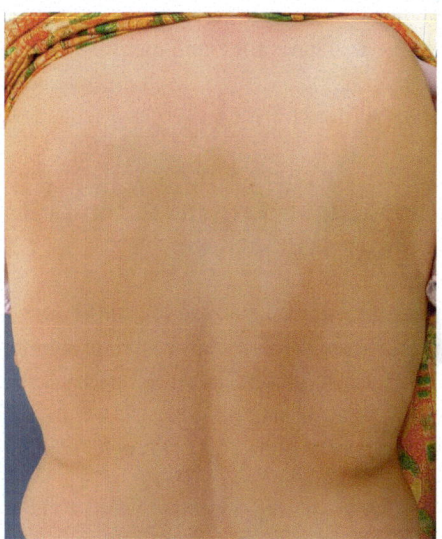

Fig. 8.6 Universal vitiligo. Nearly complete depigmentation of the body in this lady of Indian origin (Fitzpatrick skin type IV). She had got breakthrough repigmentation recently over her malar area (scapular areas in this picture), after a brief period of sun exposure for which she attended our clinic for depigmentation therapy

form of NSV and is composed of several scattered depigmented macules distributed symmetrically all over the body. Mucosal vitiligo affects mucosae of both mouth and genitalia. If it is found in isolation, i.e. affecting only one mucosa (Fig. 8.5), it is considered as focal vitiligo under 'unclassified vitiligo' as per VGICC. Universal vitiligo (Fig. 8.6) is the most severe form of NSV, where complete or nearly complete depigmentation can be noted. Mixed vitiligo has been defined as the coexistence of NSV and SV in the same patient and is classified as a subgroup of NSV [16]. This association may be viewed as an example of a superimposed segmental manifestation of a generalised polygenic disorder, in which segmental involvement precedes disease generalisation and is more resistant to therapy [8]. Vitiligo minor and follicular vitiligo are rare variants. Vitiligo minor [17], reported mainly in dark-skinned individuals, refers to incomplete pigment defects leaving pale skin, apart from coexistent depigmented patches of vitiligo. Follicular vitiligo [18] is a rare subtype of NSV where hair follicular melanocytes are preferentially destroyed compared to epidermal melanocytes, with marked generalised hair whitening in contrast to limited skin involvement.

Focal vitiligo refers to a small isolated patch (Fig. 8.5) that does not follow a typical segmental distribution and which has not evolved into SV/NSV after a period of 1–2 years [8]. This form of vitiligo may evolve into either SV or NSV. Accurate prediction of fate of focal vitiligo is still not possible [19].

In vitiligo punctata, lesions present as sharply demarcated depigmented punctate macules involving any area of the body [8]. Other forms of vitiligo that have not found mention in VGICC are inflammatory vitiligo, multichrome vitiligo and blue vitiligo [20].

Recent Insights into the Pathogenic Mechanisms in Vitiligo

Pathogenic mechanisms causing vitiligo are still elusive. Various theories have been proposed for the melanocyte defects in vitiligo, but there is a lack of consensus among scientists on the pathophysiology of vitiligo. Even though the convergence or integrated theory [21], which encompasses autoimmune hypothesis [22], self-destruct hypothesis [23], biochemical theory and genetics, fairly depicts various causative steps in melanocyte loss, the overall contribution of each step as well as triggering event in the pathogenic cascade is still debatable.

Genetic susceptibility in vitiligo is established by various studies. However, only 23% concordance has been seen in monozygotic twins, lower than that of psoriasis and atopic dermatitis [24, 25]. In an epidemiological analysis of Caucasian probands and their families, the risk of vitiligo in a patient's siblings was about 6.1%, 18 times the population frequency, suggesting a strong genetic component in disease pathogenesis [25]. It refers mostly to increased susceptibility of melanocytes to immune-mediated attacks. However, polymorphisms in non-immune genes like *TYR* (the gene encoding tyrosinase), *MC1R* (the gene encoding melanocortin 1 receptor), and *MTHFR* (the gene encoding methylene tetrahydrofolate reductase) have also been described [24, 26]. Of the 23 new risk loci of vitiligo susceptibility genes in the recent genome-wide analysis among European-ancestry subjects [27], 15 loci are associated with immune system and 6 loci regulate apoptosis. Gene expression profiling of generalised vitiligo was different from segmental vitiligo [28]. The inverse relationship of genetic susceptibility to vitiligo with melanoma, as shown by a recent genome-wide analysis study [27], is consistent with the threefold reduction in melanoma incidence among patients with vitiligo [29] and the prolonged survival of patients with melanoma who develop vitiligo during immunotherapy [30].

Autoimmune hypothesis is currently the leading hypothesis to describe vitiligo pathogenesis. The role of autoimmunity in vitiligo is supported by the presence of antibodies against melanocytes, association with polymorphisms at immune loci, presence of prominent T-cell perilesional infiltrates and cytokine expression and by the association with other autoimmune diseases [25]. Interferon (IFN)-γ/CXCL10 axis and IL-17-mediated responses are considered as the two key components of the autoimmune response that perpetuate disease activity in vitiligo [31]. In a recent genome-wide analysis, nearly all vitiligo susceptibility genes have been found to encode components of the immune system, suggesting a deregulated immune response in vitiligo [32].

Innate immunity Deregulated innate immune system plays an important role in the initiation and maintenance of melanocyte directed attack in vitiligo. In vitiligo, the disease process is likely to begin with release of stress signals by melanocytes or possibly by keratinocytes. These exosomes or damage-associated molecular patterns (DAMPs) attract natural killer cells to the stressed melanocytes and also activate nearby dendritic cells into antigen-presenting cells. S100B, a DAMP protein expressed in melanocytes, was found to be a possible biomarker for vitiligo activity and a potential target for treatment [33]. An important role of inducible heat-shock protein 70 (HSP70i) , released by stressed melanocytes, in vitiligo induction and disease progression has been suggested [34]. A recent study highlighted the role of HSP70 in promoting interferon alpha production by plasmacytic dendritic cells and subsequent induction of keratinocytes to produce CXCL9 and CXCL10 [35]. Moreover, melanocytes upon stress by phenols and other chemical agents, respond by accumulation of unfolded proteins in endoplasmic reticulum (unfolded protein response, UPR). Even though this homeostatic response is intended for cell survival, prolonged stress leads to production of IL-6 and IL-8, providing a direct link between cellular stress and immune activation [36].

Adaptive immunity Patients with vitiligo have higher numbers of cytotoxic CD8+ T cells in blood, compared with healthy controls, which correlate with disease activity; and isolated CD8+ T cells from vitiligo patients can identify and kill normal human melanocytes in vitro [37]. Functional studies in mice have confirmed the crucial role of the IFN-γ–CXCL10– CXCR3 axis in both the progression and maintenance of depigmentation [38]. Elevated levels of CXCL10 were noted in NSV patients, especially in the presence of autoimmune thyroid disorders, suggesting a common TH$_1$-mediated immune pathogenesis in both the diseases [39]. Melanocyte derived CXCL12 and CXCL5 were found to be associated with onset and progression of vitiligo through activation of melanocyte-specific immunity [40]. The role of CD4+ T cells in the pathogenesis of vitiligo is still unclear, although a possible role of deregulated regulatory T cells has been suggested [41, 42].

Oxidative stress Melanocytes in vitiligo patients are inherently susceptible to oxidative stresses

owing to the imbalance of the pro-oxidant and antioxidant systems. Oxidative stress compromises the function of cellular proteins and membrane lipids. Impairment in autophagy, a lysosome-dependent degradation pathway that protects cells from oxidative insults, is a speculated mechanism for melanocyte damage [43]. Oxidative stress-driven modification of the TRP1–calnexin complex can lead to reduced TRP1 stability with subsequent production of toxic melanin intermediates [44]. Modification and inactivation of acetylcholinesterase further promotes and maintains skin oxidative damage [45]. Oxidative stress impairs WNT-β catenin pathway which helps in melanoblast differentiation. Using a WNT agonist, Regazzetti et al. have demonstrated melanocyte differentiation from stem cells in vitiligo skin explants [46]. Oxidation end products were found to be increased in NSV compared to healthy controls and were directly correlated with extent, duration and activity of vitiligo [47]. A recent study that suggested similar immune pathogenesis in halo nevus and vitiligo has demonstrated H_2O_2-associated autoimmune phenotype in both the conditions. Moreover, elevated H_2O_2 concentration correlated well with CXCL10 levels in skin lesions [48].

Cellular metabolic alterations Unaffected epidermis in vitiligo is characterised by deregulation of the biopterin metabolism [49] that could lead to inhibition of antioxidant enzyme activities and of melanin synthesis [50, 51]. Aberrant signalling pathways have been noted even in non-lesional skin of vitiligo patients, which result in increased expression of p53, hence a pre-senescent cellular profile, which could be melanocyte specific [5]. Increased p53 expression was found to be associated with defects in stem cell reservoir in a mice study [52]. Interestingly, the p53 deregulation correlates with a protection from non-melanoma skin cancer [53]. Several lines of evidence suggest that mitochondria are key in mediating melanocyte dysfunction [5]. Keratinocytes also exhibit oxidative stress, phosphorylation of p38, overexpression of p53 and a senescent phenotype in perilesional vitiligo skin [54]. It is important to note that various melanocyte growth factors are secreted by keratinocytes. UV light triggers differentiation of melanocyte stem cells through WNT proteins derived from irradiated keratinocytes [55]. A recent immunohistochemical study in vitiligo patients has demonstrated aberrant Notch-1 signalling (required for development and maintenance of melanocyte lineage) in acral vitiligo and attributed it to be the cause of their treatment resistance [56]. Senescence of dermal fibroblasts was noted in NSV, and it can lead to decreased secretion of growth factors and cytokines for melanocyte survival resulting in vitiligo progression [57]. In summary, metabolic alterations within melanocytes and its neighbouring cells or a disruption in the 'cross talk' between them may lead to melanocyte loss in vitiligo.

Melanocytorrhagy Defective attachment within the epidermis leads to detachment of melanocytes from the basal layer, to be eliminated through superficial epidermis, where they are more prone to apoptosis [58]. Demonstration of altered expression and/ or distribution of E-cadherin or co-localised aquaporin-3 in vitiligo skin has attracted further interest in this hypothesis recently [59, 60].

Medical Management

Literature on the conventional medical modalities and light-based therapies are discussed briefly, focusing mainly on topic introduction and recent updates as an exhaustive discussion is beyond the scope of this chapter. We will discuss novel medical modalities in vitiligo and summarise the treatment protocol for vitiligo as per current evidence.

Update on Conventional Medical Treatments and Light-Based Therapy in Vitiligo

Conventional medical treatments include topical medications like corticosteroids, tacrolimus, vitamin D analogues and systemic agents like corticosteroids. Light-based therapy includes NBUVB, photochemotherapy and lasers. Recent

studies have found that a combination of light-based therapy with topical medication yields greater efficacy compared to either treatment as monotherapy [31, 61–65]. Light-based therapies are increasingly being used as adjuvants to surgical modalities.

Conventional Topical Agents

1. *Topical corticosteroids*: Topical steroids are the first-line treatment for body lesions, barring intertriginous and genital areas, and have the best response over sun-exposed sites and in newer lesions [66, 67]. Preceding laser dermabrasion and combination with NBUVB are found to increase the treatment efficacy in refractory vitiligo [68]. A recent cross-sectional study did not show an increased risk of glaucoma or cataract in vitiligo patients with periorbital topical steroid use [69].

2. *Topical calcineurin inhibitors*: Apart from inhibition of T-cell activation, the role of tacrolimus in inducing melanocyte migration and differentiation has been described recently [70]. Vitiligo European Task Force considers it as the first-line treatment for facial vitiligo, unlike its use as second-line agent in atopic dermatitis [66, 67]. Twice-daily application ensures optimal results [71]. Occlusion, preceding microdermabrasion, sunlight and adjuvant NB-UVB or 308-nm laser have all been reported to augment therapeutic response to topical calcineurin inhibitors [66]. Black-box warning by FDA of potential risk of carcinoma and lymphoma warrants avoidance of tacrolimus use in children less than the age of 2 years. However, two recent reviews on long-term usage of topical calcineurin inhibitors in atopic dermatitis have not reported an increased risk of malignancy [72, 73]. Twice-weekly application of 0.1% tacrolimus ointment was found to be successful in retaining the attained pigmentation in vitiligo that may address the local relapse (40% within the first year) [74].

3. *Topical vitamin D analogues*: Calcipotriene, calcipotriol and tacalcitol have all been used topically in vitiligo, and act by modulation of the local immune response and direct influ-

ence on melanogenesis. Recently, protective role of tacalcitol against oxidative damage in human epidermal melanocytes has also been demonstrated [75]. It is mutually beneficial when combined with topical corticosteroids; irritation of vitamin D analogues and atrophogenic effects of topical steroids are reduced [76]. Combination with light-based therapy has shown variable response [67, 77, 78]. Lack of superior results on combination with phototherapy may be due to photoprotective effect of vitamin D analogues decreasing the efficacy of phototherapy and its degradation on light exposure. Hence, they should be applied after the phototherapy session.

Conventional Systemic Agents

1. *Systemic steroids*: Though widely used in active vitiligo, literature on its use in vitiligo is sparse. Steroids are commonly used as pulse therapy – suprapharmacological doses at regular intervals – to augment the response and reduce side effects. Oral mini-pulse therapy (OMP) involves oral administration of betamethasone or dexamethasone at a single dose of 5 mg on 2 consecutive days per week. A low-dose OMP schedule with oral dexamethasone 2.5 mg per day on 2 consecutive days in a week is also found to be effective in halting progression of vitiligo with minimal side effects [79]. Oral methylprednisolone mini-pulse therapy (0.5 mg/kg on 2 consecutive days per week) combined with NBUVB has also shown similar results [80]. A recent RCT has found that NBUVB plus OMP and NBUVB alone are clinically superior over OMP alone in treating stable vitiligo patients [81].

Light-Based Therapies

1. *Photochemotherapy*: Topical or systemic photochemotherapy combines use of long-wave UVA (320–340 nm) with psoralen (PUVA) or khellin (KUVA) to stimulate melanogenesis. Prolonged therapy lasting for months with 100–200 treatment sessions given two to three times per week may be needed for optimal outcome. If no response is observed even after approximately 50 sessions or 6 months, PUVA should be discontinued [67, 82]. KUVA is less phototoxic and less mutagenic than PUVA, but hepatotoxicity limits its widespread use. Oral PUVA was found to be more efficacious than PUVA sol (UVA obtained through sunlight) in a recent prospective comparative study [83].

2. *Nontargeted phototherapy*: Narrowband UVB (NBUVB) is currently the treatment of choice in active, widespread vitiligo involving more than 10–20% body surface area. Combined use of various medical modalities and, recently, fractional CO_2 laser and platelet-rich plasma were found to enhance the efficacy of NBUVB [84, 85]. A recent systematic review of RCTs reveals equivalent efficacy of NBUVB to UVA, PUVA or 308-nm excimer laser in the treatment of vitiligo with acceptable side effect profile [86]. Carcinogenic risk of NBUVB therapy is poorly defined. However, recent studies have shown no increased risk of malignancies with long-term use of NBUVB [87]. Total body irradiation in NBUVB chambers is preferred in generalised vitiligo. Even though the vitiligo lesions are devoid of melanin to protect from UV rays, MED (minimal erythema dose) of vitiligo patients varies depending on the phototypes of the individuals. Hence a higher starting dose of NBUVB (50% of MED) is increasingly used nowadays. Treatment is normally given twice or three times weekly and is continued up to 1–2 years as long as there is ongoing repigmentation. Maintenance phototherapy is not recommended [67].

   Broadband (BB)-UVA was also found to be useful in vitiligo. A recent RCT evaluating efficacy of different doses of BB-UVA in vitiligo showed BB-UVA at a dose of 15 J/cm^2 / session had comparable efficacy to PUVA [88].

3. *Targeted phototherapy* [89]: In this modality, super-erythemogenic doses of radiation are delivered selectively to the lesions in a short

duration thereby enhancing efficacy, achieving faster response and attaining longer duration of remission. It is helpful to treat difficult areas such as scalp, nose, genitals, oral mucosa and ears. It also helps to tailor the dose according to the refractoriness of the lesions. Targeted phototherapy includes lasers (excimer laser and low-energy helium–neon (He–Ne) lasers) and non-laser devices (monochromatic Excimer Lamp or Light 308 nm, mercury arc lamps, plasma lamps and microphototherapy). Combination with topical modalities is found to enhance efficacy. Digital phototherapy device skintrek®, a novel targeted UV therapy modality, reduces carcinogenic risk, premature skin ageing and avoids tanning of healthy surrounding skin by delivering light energy only to the lesional skin. Positive results in psoriasis and mycosis fungoides make this method a promising therapeutic option for vitiligo [90, 91]. A literature review on targeted phototherapy in vitiligo showed it to have good response in localized involvement, resistant lesions and in children [92]. A recent study has demonstrated similar efficacy with once a week targeted NBUVB exposure compared to twice a week schedule, thus obviating the need of frequent hospital visits [93].

In home-based phototherapy, motivated patients are trained to use phototherapy units, either standard chambers or hand-held devices, at their homes. It is a convenient and cost-effective approach which increases treatment compliance and hence efficacy [94]. Further well-conducted studies are needed to ascertain the safety and efficacy of this approach.

Other Interventions

1. *Camouflage*: Methods to conceal depigmented patches may be permanent like cosmetic tattoos; tanning agents like dihydroxyacetone; general cosmetics like tinted cover creams, compact, liquid and stick foundations, fixing powders, and dyes for leukotrichia; and various topical camouflage agents like the newest product, Microskin™. Clinical studies on camouflaging in vitiligo are sparse. A recent literature review favours temporary methods for camouflaging [95].

2. *Depigmenting agents*: Methods of permanent depigmentation should be explored only in patients with extensive refractory vitiligo. Further depigmenting cycles may be needed sometimes for possible spontaneous repigmentation over vitiligo lesions. Patients with darker skin phototypes V and VI are ideal candidates, although those with lighter phototypes I and II may also obtain better cosmetic improvement. Motivated patients, after proper psychological evaluation and counselling, can apply 20% monobenzone ethyl ester (MBEH) cream twice or thrice a day. Sun exposure may decrease the efficacy and hence sunscreens are advised. If no satisfactory depigmentation occurs even after 4 months, treatment should be discontinued. Retinoic acid may also augment the depigmenting action of MBEH by accelerating keratinocyte turnover and, hence, melanocyte loss, or by impairing glutathione-dependent defence. But 0.025% retinoic acid plus 10% MBEH may worsen the eczematous side effects of MBEH. The Q-switched ruby laser (QSR) alone or in combination with methoxyphenol and cryotherapy has also been used for depigmentation [96, 97].

3. *Psychological interventions*: Prevalence of psychiatric morbidity in vitiligo patients ranges from 25% to 75%, depending on the extension and site of the disease, phototype, ethnicity and cultural background [67]. Being a disease that is associated with psychological morbidity, various psychological interventions may have a role in controlling the disease activity. However, there is a paucity of literature on psychological intervention in vitiligo. A recent Cochrane review couldn't retrieve any new literature on psychological interventions since the 2010 review which had commented on cognitive behavioural therapy [98]. Recently, group climatotherapy [99] and cognitive behavioural self-help [100]/therapy [101] have been found to improve quality of life and social anxiety in vitiligo patients.

Newer Medical Modalities

1. *Tofacitinib*: A case report has highlighted the usefulness of this systemic Janus kinase 1/3 inhibitor, proposed to act by blockade of interferon-gamma signalling and downstream CXCL10 expression [102]. It is considered to be the first therapy in vitiligo acting on the pathogenic pathway. Later, a case series has suggested that tofacitinib might require concomitant light exposure for the repigmentation outcome [103]. Ruxolitinib, another JAK inhibitor, was studied in a patient with alopecia areata and vitiligo and showed fairly good, yet not long-standing, repigmentation over the face [104]. An open-label study of twice-daily topical ruxolitinib 1.5% cream showed significant repigmentation in facial vitiligo with poor response at other body parts [105]. As the data on long-term safety of these drugs is not available at present, it is too early to draw a solid conclusion about the position of these drugs in the treatment of vitiligo.

2. *Simvastatin*: Simvastatin, by blocking activation of STAT1, inhibits interferon-gamma signalling and has shown to halt vitiligo and attain repigmentation in a mouse model [106]. A case report highlighted repigmentation of vitiligo lesions, while the patient was on treatment with high-dose simvastatin [107]. But a recent phase 2 clinical trial using 80 mg per day dose of simvastatin did not support its use in vitiligo, owing mainly to dosage limitations in humans compared to mice [108]. Addition of simvastatin did not have any impact on the repigmentation outcome of topical betamethasone [109].

3. *Afamelanotide*: It is an analogue of α-melanocyte-stimulating hormone that has shown to induce melanogenesis. It was licensed in Europe to reduce the photosensitivity pain in erythropoietic protoporphyria [110]. A recent randomised multicentre trial has found that the combination of afamelanotide (16 mg) implant and narrowband UVB phototherapy resulted in statistically superior and faster repigmentation, compared to narrowband UVB monotherapy [111]. Melanocortin

1 receptor (MC1R) is not present in melanocyte stem cells; thus, concomitant induction of these stem cells with phototherapy is required for the optimal repigmentation outcome of afamelanotide [112]. Adverse effects of afamelanotide include fatigue, gastrointestinal intolerance and hyperpigmentation.

4. *Minocycline*: It has been shown that minocycline can rescue melanocytes from oxidative stress in vitro [113]. The mechanism of action includes inhibition of free radical and cytokine production, interference with protein synthesis, anti-apoptotic properties and modulation of matrix metalloproteinases activity. A randomised clinical trial comparing oral minocycline (100 mg/day) to oral mini-pulse corticosteroids found that the two treatments were comparable in arresting the progression of actively spreading vitiligo with minimal side effects in each group [114]. But a prospective comparative trial showed that NB-UVB was statistically more useful than oral minocycline in unstable vitiligo in terms of efficacy and the resulting stability [115].

5. *Prostaglandin analogues*: Latanoprost, a prostaglandin F2-alpha analogue, is well known for causing, among the possible side effects, increased pigmentation of the iris and periocular hyperpigmentation [116]. Latanoprost was found to be better than placebo and comparable with NB-UVB in inducing skin repigmentation, with enhanced efficacy when combined with NB-UVB [117]. Efficacy of latanoprost and tacrolimus was found to be comparable, when used in combination with phototherapy and microneedling [118]. Any doubts regarding malignant melanoma induction due to latanoprost administration have been excluded [119]. A recent study has shown that bimatoprost as a monotherapy or in combination with mometasone is more effective than mometasone alone in the treatment of non-facial vitiligo [120]. However, more robust clinical studies comparing prostaglandin analogues with other alternatives are needed.

6. *Oral vitamins, antioxidants and other supplements*: Owing to their antioxidant properties,

silymarin [121]; pseudocatalase/superoxide dismutase (PSD) [122]; piperine [123]; curcumin [124]; L-phenylalanine; khellin; *Polypodium leucotomos*; ginkgo biloba; vitamin B12; folic acid; vitamins C, D [125] and E; alpha lipoic acid; and zinc have shown varying efficacy in the treatment of vitiligo, either as monotherapy or in combination with other treatments [31]. Topical basic fibroblast growth factor (bFGF)-related decapeptide is increasingly being used in augmenting repigmentation, though evidence regarding its efficacy is lacking. Low-dose oral administration of cytokines has been suggested as a newer therapeutic approach to normalise the melanocyte homeostasis in vitiligo [126]. However, larger randomised controlled trials are warranted before recommending them as primary agents in the treatment of vitiligo, and hence, to date, these agents are best regarded as adjuvants to primary agents during the active phase of the disease or as monotherapy during remission.

7. *Conventional steroid sparing agents*: Methotrexate can be used in patients with active vitiligo wherever corticosteroids are contraindicated as evidenced by a randomised study comparing oral mini-pulse corticosteroids and low-dose oral methotrexate (10 mg/week) [127]. Azathioprine has also found to be beneficial in enhancing repigmentation when used along with phototherapy [128]. Evidence for the beneficial effects of cyclosporine and cyclophosphamide in vitiligo is based on individual case reports [129, 130].

8. *Biologicals*: A phase 1 clinical trial is underway to ascertain the efficacy of abatacept, a soluble fusion protein consisting of human cytotoxic T-lymphocyte-associated antigen 4 (CTLA4), which prevents T-cell activation in active vitiligo [131]. Various anti-TNF alpha agents [132] as well as alefacept [133] have been found to be ineffective in treating vitiligo, though strength of evidence is less. Rituximab was found to be beneficial in active disseminated vitiligo [134]. Emergence or progression of vitiligo in patients treated with biological agents, especially TNF alpha inhib-

itors [135], understates the primary role of these targeted molecules in the pathogenesis of vitiligo and hence their usefulness in therapeutic targeting.

9. *Future trends*: Topical photocil, selectively filters solar radiation to deliver narrowband UVB to vitiligo lesions, obviating the need of phototherapy machines [136]. Transdermal protein transduction of melanocyte-lineage-specific genes is a possible modality for treatment of vitiligo [137]. Induction of melanogenesis even from glabrous vitiligo skin as demonstrated in an in vitro study [138] gives a glimmer of hope in the management of refractory acral vitiligo. Multilineage-differentiating stress-enduring (Muse) cells, a distinct stem cell type among human dermal fibroblasts, can be readily reprogrammed into functional melanocytes and can be a potential source of melanocytes for cell-based therapy in vitiligo [139].

Practical Approach to the Management of Vitiligo

The most recent Cochrane review on interventions in vitiligo concludes that cure for vitiligo and an effective method of limiting the spread of the disease are still an enigma [98]. Research for newer agents in the management raises new hopes in the vitiligo community. However, lack of evidence showing efficacy of these agents urges clinicians to use conventional modalities as the first lines of treatment. In 2013, the Vitiligo Guideline Subcommittee of the European Dermatology Forum developed a new treatment guideline for vitiligo, detailing first line to fourth line of therapy [67]. Here we would like to summarise briefly the approach to manage vitiligo based on the above guideline in the light of newer studies on vitiligo pathogenesis and medical modalities. In a patient with recent onset SV or NSV with fewer patches (<10–20% body surface area) topical modalities (corticosteroids or calcineurin inhibitors) or targeted phototherapies are preferred. Though there is no concrete evidence on clinical usefulness of antioxidants, clinicians are increasingly adopting various oral

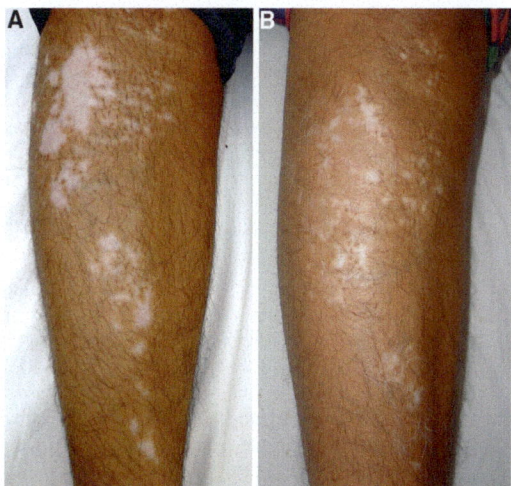

Fig. 8.7 Pre- and posttreatment photographs of a patient. A 14-year-old girl with depigmented patches of common vitiligo on both legs (**a**). Repigmentation of around 75% was attained after 4 months of morning application of topical mometasone furoate 0.1% cream and night application of topical tacrolimus 0.1% ointment along with daily oral folic acid and vitamin B12 supplements (**b**)

supplements with antioxidant property for stabilisation of disease at this stage, owing to recent emphasis on oxidant stress in vitiligo pathogenesis. A common approach is giving topical steroids in the morning and topical calcineurin inhibitors in the evening (Fig. 8.7). Topical calcineurin inhibitors are preferred for facial vitiligo (especially in children) and topical corticosteroids for other areas. Continuous administration of topical steroids should be restricted to 3 months, with alternate day or twice weekly regimen for another 3 months if needed, based on response. Potent steroids like mometasone furoate should be preferred over super potent steroids like clobetasol propionate owing to similar efficacy, lesser local side effects and minimal systemic absorption. Topical vitamin D analogues can be added if local side effects of steroids manifest or no further improvement is noted with topical steroids. Prostaglandin analogues and basic fibroblast-related decapeptide are other steroid sparing agents that can be used as first-line agents for facial vitiligo along with topical calcineurin inhibitors. Topical PUVA can be used for refractory acral vitiligo.

In patients with active widespread NSV (>10–20% body surface area), NBUVB is the treatment of choice. Stabilisation of disease with OMP before starting or during NBUVB therapy is a logical approach to prevent koebnerisation over photoexposed areas, when disease is rapidly spreading. Therapy can be stopped if no repigmentation occurs after 3 months or <25% repigmentation occurs after 6 months. If there is response, NBUVB should be maintained at least for a year. Topical modalities can be added to NBUVB to augment repigmentation. Oral PUVA can be tried as a second-line therapy. As with NBUVB, continuous treatment for 1–2 years is needed for maximal repigmentation. OMP, methotrexate or PUVA sol can be considered, if facility for phototherapy is not available and in the rapid spreading phase of SV. In stable vitiligo, immunosuppressants are not indicated as they are not beneficial in repigmentation. Use of newer agents like afamelanotide or tofacitinib should be restricted to refractory cases of active vitiligo as clinical trials only, since the long-term safety profile or sound evidence on the efficacy are not available at present. Depigmenting agents can be offered after proper counselling, if >50% body surface area is involved.

Surgical therapy can be offered to any individual lesion with more than 1 year clinical stability, and is an important treatment approach in SV. For all individual cases, psychological interventions and camouflaging options should be offered.

Acknowledgement Authors are indebted to Dr. Raihan Ashraf, MBBS and Dr. Rajsmita Bhattacharjee, MD for the English language editing.

References

1. Spritz RA. The genetics of generalized vitiligo and associated autoimmune diseases. Pigment Cell Res. 2007;20:271–8.
2. Sehgal VN, Srivastava G. Vitiligo: compendium of clinico-epidemiological features. Indian J Dermatol Venereol Leprol. 2007;73:149–56.
3. Parsad D, Pandhi R, Dogra S, Kanwar AJ, Kumar B. Dermatology life quality index score in vitiligo and its impact on the treatment outcome. Br J Dermatol. 2003;148:373–4.

4. Behl PN, Bhatia RK. 400 cases of vitiligo. A clinico-therapeutic analysis. Indian J Dermatol. 1972;17:51–6.

5. Picardo M, Dell'Anna ML, Ezzedine K, Hamzavi I, Harris JE, Parsad D, et al. Vitiligo. Nat Rev Dis Primers. 2015;1:15011.

6. Herane MI. Vitiligo and leukoderma in children. Clin Dermatol. 2003;21:283–95.

7. Nicolaidou E, Antoniou C, Miniati A, Lagogianni E, Matekovits A, Stratigos A, et al. Childhood- and later-onset vitiligo have diverse epidemiologic and clinical characteristics. J Am Acad Dermatol. 2012;66:954–8.

8. Ezzedine K, Lim HW, Suzuki T, Katayama I, Hamzavi I, Lan CC, et al. Revised classification/nomenclature of vitiligo and related issues: the vitiligo global issues consensus conference. Pigment Cell Melanoma Res. 2012;25:E1–13.

9. Hann SK, Lee HJ. Segmental vitiligo: clinical findings in 208 patients. J Am Acad Dermatol. 1996;35:671–4.

10. Koga M, Tango T. Clinical features and course of type a and type B vitiligo. Br J Dermatol. 1988;118:223–8.

11. van Geel N, De Lille S, Vandenhaute S, Gauthier Y, Mollet I, Brochez L, et al. Different phenotypes of segmental vitiligo based on a clinical observational study. J Eur Acad Dermatol Venereol. 2011;25:673–8.

12. van Geel NA, Mollet IG, De Schepper S, Tjin EP, Vermaelen K, Clark RA, et al. First histopathological and immunophenotypic analysis of early dynamic events in a patient with segmental vitiligo associated with halo nevi. Pigment Cell Melanoma Res. 2010;23:375–84.

13. Hann SK, Chang JH, Lee HS, Kim SM. The classification of segmental vitiligo on the face. Yonsei Med J. 2000;41:209–12.

14. van Geel N, Bosma S, Boone B, Speeckaert R. Classification of segmental vitiligo on the trunk. Br J Dermatol. 2014;170:322–7.

15. van Geel N, Mollet I, Brochez L, Dutre M, De Schepper S, Verhaeghe E, et al. New insights in segmental vitiligo: case report and review of theories. Br J Dermatol. 2012;166:240–6.

16. Ezzedine K, Gauthier Y, Leaute-Labreze C, Marquez S, Bouchtnei S, Jouary T, et al. Segmental vitiligo associated with generalized vitiligo (mixed vitiligo): a retrospective case series of 19 patients. J Am Acad Dermatol. 2011;65:965–71.

17. Ezzedine K, Mahe A, van Geel N, Cardot-Leccia N, Gauthier Y, Descamps V, et al. Hypochromic vitiligo: delineation of a new entity. Br J Dermatol. 2015;172:716–21.

18. Ezzedine K, Amazan E, Seneschal J, Cario-Andre M, Leaute-Labreze C, Vergier B, et al. Follicular vitiligo: a new form of vitiligo. Pigment Cell Melanoma Res. 2012;25:527–9.

19. Lommerts JE, Schilder Y, de Rie MA, Wolkerstorfer A, Bekkenk MW. Focal vitiligo: long-term follow-up of 52 cases. J Eur Acad Dermatol Venereol. 2016;30:1550–4.

20. Passeron T, Ortonne J-P. Generalized vitiligo. In: Picardo M, Taïeb A, editors. Vitiligo. Heidelberg: Springer; 2010. p. 35–9.

21. Le Poole IC, Das PK, van den Wijngaard RM, Bos JD, Westerhof W. Review of the etiopathomechanism of vitiligo: a convergence theory. Exp Dermatol. 1993;2:145–53.

22. Ongenae K, Van Geel N, Naeyaert JM. Evidence for an autoimmune pathogenesis of vitiligo. Pigment Cell Res. 2003;16:90–100.

23. Lerner AB. On the etiology of vitiligo and gray hair. Am J Med. 1971;51:141–7.

24. Spritz RA. Modern vitiligo genetics sheds new light on an ancient disease. J Dermatol. 2013;40:310–8.

25. Alkhateeb A, Fain PR, Thody A, Bennett DC, Spritz RA. Epidemiology of vitiligo and associated autoimmune diseases in Caucasian probands and their families. Pigment Cell Res. 2003;16:208–14.

26. Chen JX, Shi Q, Wang XW, Guo S, Dai W, Li K, et al. Genetic polymorphisms in the methylenetetrahydrofolate reductase gene (MTHFR) and risk of vitiligo in Han Chinese populations: a genotype-phenotype correlation study. Br J Dermatol. 2014;170:1092–9.

27. Jin Y, Andersen G, Yorgov D, Ferrara TM, Ben S, Brownson KM, et al. Genome-wide association studies of autoimmune vitiligo identify 23 new risk loci and highlight key pathways and regulatory variants. Nat Genet. 2016;48:1418–24.

28. Wang P, Li Y, Nie H, Zhang X, Shao Q, Hou X, et al. The changes of gene expression profiling between segmental vitiligo, generalized vitiligo and healthy individual. J Dermatol Sci. 2016;84:40–9.

29. Paradisi A, Tabolli S, Didona B, Sobrino L, Russo N, Abeni D. Markedly reduced incidence of melanoma and nonmelanoma skin cancer in a nonconcurrent cohort of 10,040 patients with vitiligo. J Am Acad Dermatol. 2014;71:1110–6.

30. Teulings HE, Limpens J, Jansen SN, Zwinderman AH, Reitsma JB, Spuls PI, et al. Vitiligo-like depigmentation in patients with stage III-IV melanoma receiving immunotherapy and its association with survival: a systematic review and meta-analysis. J Clin Oncol. 2015;33:773–81.

31. Manga P, Elbuluk N, Orlow SJ. Recent advances in understanding vitiligo. F1000Res. 2016;5 https://www.ncbi.nlm.nih.gov/pubmed/?term=Recent+advances+in+understanding+vitiligo.+F1000

32. Jin Y, Birlea SA, Fain PR, Gowan K, Riccardi SL, Holland PJ, et al. Variant of TYR and autoimmunity susceptibility loci in generalized vitiligo. N Engl J Med. 2010;362:1686–97.

33. Speeckaert R, Voet S, Hoste E, van Geel N. S100B is a potential disease activity marker in nonsegmental vitiligo. J Invest Dermatol. 2017;137:1445–53.

34. Richmond JM, Frisoli ML, Harris JE. Innate immune mechanisms in vitiligo: danger from within. Curr Opin Immunol. 2013;25:676–82.

35. Jacquemin C, Rambert J, Guillet S, Thiolat D, Boukhedouni N, Doutre MS, et al. HSP70 potentiates interferon-alpha production by plasmacytoid dendritic cells: relevance for cutaneous

lupus and vitiligo pathogenesis. Br J Dermatol. 2017;177(5):1367–1375.

36. Toosi S, Orlow SJ, Manga P. Vitiligo-inducing phenols activate the unfolded protein response in melanocytes resulting in upregulation of IL6 and IL8. J Invest Dermatol. 2012;132:2601–9.

37. Ogg GS, Rod Dunbar P, Romero P, Chen JL, Cerundolo V. High frequency of skin-homing melanocyte-specific cytotoxic T lymphocytes in autoimmune vitiligo. J Exp Med. 1998;188:1203–8.

38. Harris JE, Harris TH, Weninger W, Wherry EJ, Hunter CA, Turka LA. A mouse model of vitiligo with focused epidermal depigmentation requires IFN-gamma for autoreactive CD8(+) T-cell accumulation in the skin. J Invest Dermatol. 2012;132:1869–76.

39. Ferrari SM, Fallahi P, Santaguida G, Virili C, Ruffilli I, Ragusa F, et al. Circulating CXCL10 is increased in non-segmental vitiligo, in presence or absence of autoimmune thyroiditis. Autoimmun Rev. 2017;16:946–50.

40. Rezk AF, Kemp DM, El-Domyati M, El-Din WH, Lee JB, Uitto J, et al. Misbalanced CXCL12 and CCL5 chemotactic signals in vitiligo onset and progression. J Invest Dermatol. 2017;137:1126–34.

41. Lili Y, Yi W, Ji Y, Yue S, Weimin S, Ming L. Global activation of CD8+ cytotoxic T lymphocytes correlates with an impairment in regulatory T cells in patients with generalized vitiligo. PLoS One. 2012;7:e37513.

42. Zhou L, Li K, Shi YL, Hamzavi I, Gao TW, Henderson M, et al. Systemic analyses of immunophenotypes of peripheral T cells in non-segmental vitiligo: implication of defective natural killer T cells. Pigment Cell Melanoma Res. 2012;25:602–11.

43. Qiao Z, Wang X, Xiang L, Zhang C. Dysfunction of autophagy: a possible mechanism involved in the pathogenesis of vitiligo by breaking the redox balance of melanocytes. Oxidative Med Cell Longev. 2016;2016:7.

44. Boissy RE, Manga P. On the etiology of contact/occupational vitiligo. Pigment Cell Res. 2004;17:208–14.

45. Schallreuter KU, Elwary SM, Gibbons NC, Rokos H, Wood JM. Activation/deactivation of acetylcholinesterase by H2O2: more evidence for oxidative stress in vitiligo. Biochem Biophys Res Commun. 2004;315:502–8.

46. Regazzetti C, Joly F, Marty C, Rivier M, Mehul B, Reiniche P, et al. Transcriptional analysis of vitiligo skin reveals the alteration of WNT pathway: a promising target for repigmenting vitiligo patients. J Invest Dermatol. 2015;135:3105–14.

47. Vaccaro M, Bagnato G, Cristani M, Borgia F, Spatari G, Tigano V, et al. Oxidation products are increased in patients affected by non-segmental generalized vitiligo. Arch Dermatol Res. 2017;309:485–90.

48. Yang Y, Li S, Zhu G, Zhang Q, Wang G, Gao T, et al. A similar local immune and oxidative stress

phenotype in vitiligo and halo nevus. J Dermatol Sci. 2017;87:50–9.

49. Hasse S, Gibbons NC, Rokos H, Marles LK, Schallreuter KU. Perturbed 6-tetrahydrobiopterin recycling via decreased dihydropteridine reductase in vitiligo: more evidence for H2O2 stress. J Invest Dermatol. 2004;122:307–13.

50. Rokos H, Beazley WD, Schallreuter KU. Oxidative stress in vitiligo: photo-oxidation of pterins produces H(2)O(2) and pterin-6-carboxylic acid. Biochem Biophys Res Commun. 2002;292:805–11.

51. Dell'anna ML, Picardo M. A review and a new hypothesis for non-immunological pathogenetic mechanisms in vitiligo. Pigment Cell Res. 2006;19:406–11.

52. Kim J, Nakasaki M, Todorova D, Lake B, Yuan CY, Jamora C, et al. p53 Induces skin aging by depleting Blimp1+ sebaceous gland cells. Cell Death Dis. 2014;5:e1141.

53. Salem MM, Shalbaf M, Gibbons NC, Chavan B, Thornton JM, Schallreuter KU, Enhanced DNA. Binding capacity on up-regulated epidermal wild-type p53 in vitiligo by H2O2-mediated oxidation: a possible repair mechanism for DNA damage. FASEB J. 2009;23:3790–807.

54. Bondanza S, Maurelli R, Paterna P, Migliore E, Giacomo FD, Primavera G, et al. Keratinocyte cultures from involved skin in vitiligo patients show an impaired in vitro behaviour. Pigment Cell Res. 2007;20:288–300.

55. Fukunaga-Kalabis M, Hristova DM, Wang JX, Li L, Heppt MV, Wei Z, et al. UV-induced Wnt7a in the human skin microenvironment specifies the fate of neural crest-like cells via suppression of notch. J Invest Dermatol. 2015;135:1521–32.

56. Seleit I, Bakry OA, Abdou AG, Dawoud NM. Immunohistochemical expression of aberrant Notch-1 signaling in vitiligo: an implication for pathogenesis. Ann Diagn Pathol. 2014;18:117–24.

57. Rani S, Bhardwaj S, Srivastava N, Sharma VL, Parsad D, Kumar R. Senescence in the lesional fibroblasts of non-segmental vitiligo patients. Arch Dermatol Res. 2017;309:123–32.

58. Gauthier Y, Cario-Andre M, Lepreux S, Pain C, Taieb A. Melanocyte detachment after skin friction in non lesional skin of patients with generalized vitiligo. Br J Dermatol. 2003;148:95–101.

59. Wagner RY, Luciani F, Cario-Andre M, Rubod A, Petit V, Benzekri L, et al. Altered E-cadherin levels and distribution in melanocytes precede clinical manifestations of vitiligo. J Invest Dermatol. 2015;135:1810–9.

60. Kim NH, Lee AY. Reduced aquaporin3 expression and survival of keratinocytes in the depigmented epidermis of vitiligo. J Invest Dermatol. 2010;130:2231–9.

61. Li L, Wu Y, Li L, Sun Y, Qiu L, Gao XH, et al. Triple combination treatment with fractional CO2 laser plus topical betamethasone solution and narrowband

ultraviolet B for refractory vitiligo: a prospective, randomized half-body, comparative study. Dermatol Ther. 2015;28:131–4.

62. Bae JM, Yoo HJ, Kim H, Lee JH, Kim GM. Combination therapy with 308-nm excimer laser, topical tacrolimus, and short-term systemic corticosteroids for segmental vitiligo: a retrospective study of 159 patients. J Am Acad Dermatol. 2015;73:76–82.

63. Hossani-Madani AR, Halder RM. Topical treatment and combination approaches for vitiligo: new insights, new developments. G Ital Dermatol Venereol. 2010;145:57–78.

64. Abdel Latif AA, Ibrahim SM. Monochromatic excimer light versus combination of topical steroid with vitamin D3 analogue in the treatment of non-segmental vitiligo: a randomized blinded comparative study. Dermatol Ther. 2015;28:383–9.

65. Yazdani Abyaneh M, Griffith RD, Falto-Aizpurua L, Nouri K. Narrowband ultraviolet B phototherapy in combination with other therapies for vitiligo: mechanisms and efficacies. J Eur Acad Dermatol Venereol. 2014;28:1610–22.

66. Van Driessche F, Silverberg N. Current management of pediatric vitiligo. Paediatr Drugs. 2015;17:303–13.

67. Taieb A, Alomar A, Bohm M, Dell'anna ML, De Pase A, Eleftheriadou V, et al. Guidelines for the management of vitiligo: the European dermatology forum consensus. Br J Dermatol. 2013;168:5–19.

68. Bayoumi W, Fontas E, Sillard L, Le Duff F, Ortonne JP, Bahadoran P, et al. Effect of a preceding laser dermabrasion on the outcome of combined therapy with narrowband ultraviolet B and potent topical steroids for treating nonsegmental vitiligo in resistant localizations. Br J Dermatol. 2012;166:208–11.

69. Khurrum H, AlGhamdi KM, Osman E. Screening of glaucoma or cataract prevalence in vitiligo patients and its relationship with periorbital steroid use. J Cutan Med Surg. 2016;20:146–9.

70. Lan CC, CS W, Chen GS, Yu HS. FK506 (tacrolimus) and endothelin combined treatment induces mobility of melanoblasts: new insights into follicular vitiligo repigmentation induced by topical tacrolimus on sun-exposed skin. Br J Dermatol. 2011;164:490–6.

71. Radakovic S, Breier-Maly J, Konschitzky R, Kittler H, Sator P, Hoenigsmann H, et al. Response of vitiligo to once- vs. twice-daily topical tacrolimus: a controlled prospective, randomized, observer-blinded trial. J Eur Acad Dermatol Venereol. 2009;23:951–3.

72. Margolis DJ, Abuabara K, Hoffstad OJ, Wan J, Raimondo D, Bilker WB. Association between malignancy and topical use of pimecrolimus. JAMA Dermatol. 2015;151:594–9.

73. Siegfried EC, Jaworski JC, Hebert AA. Topical calcineurin inhibitors and lymphoma risk: evidence update with implications for daily practice. Am J Clin Dermatol. 2013;14:163–78.

74. Cavalie M, Ezzedine K, Fontas E, Montaudie H, Castela E, Bahadoran P, et al. Maintenance therapy of adult vitiligo with 0.1% tacrolimus ointment: a randomized, double blind, placebo-controlled study. J Invest Dermatol. 2015;135:970–4.

75. Li QL, YH W, Niu M, XJ L, Huang YH, He DH. Protective effects of tacalcitol against oxidative damage in human epidermal melanocytes. Int J Dermatol. 2017;56:232–8.

76. Xing C, Xu A. The effect of combined calcipotriol and betamethasone dipropionate ointment in the treatment of vitiligo: an open, uncontrolled trial. J Drugs Dermatol. 2012;11:e52–4.

77. Sahu P, Jain VK, Aggarwal K, Kaur S, Dayal S. Tacalcitol: a useful adjunct to narrow-band ultraviolet-B phototherapy in vitiligo. Photodermatol Photoimmunol Photomed. 2016;32:262–8.

78. Khullar G, Kanwar AJ, Singh S, Parsad D. Comparison of efficacy and safety profile of topical calcipotriol ointment in combination with NB-UVB vs. NB-UVB alone in the treatment of vitiligo: a 24-week prospective right-left comparative clinical trial. J Eur Acad Dermatol Venereol. 2015;29:925–32.

79. Kanwar AJ, Mahajan R, Parsad D. Low-dose oral mini-pulse dexamethasone therapy in progressive unstable vitiligo. J Cutan Med Surg. 2013;17:259–68.

80. Lee J, Chu H, Lee H, Kim M, Kim DS, Retrospective Study OSHA. Of methylprednisolone mini-pulse therapy combined with narrow-band UVB in nonsegmental vitiligo. Dermatology. 2016;232:224–9.

81. El Mofty M, Essmat S, Youssef R, Sobeih S, Mahgoub D, Ossama S, et al. The role of systemic steroids and phototherapy in the treatment of stable vitiligo: a randomized controlled trial. Dermatol Ther. 2016;29:406–12.

82. Shenoi SD, Prabhu S. Photochemotherapy (PUVA) in psoriasis and vitiligo. Indian J Dermatol Venereol Leprol. 2014;80:497–504.

83. Singh S, Khandpur S, Sharma VK, Ramam M. Comparison of efficacy and side-effect profile of oral PUVA vs. oral PUVA sol in the treatment of vitiligo: a 36-week prospective study. J Eur Acad Dermatol Venereol. 2013;27:1344–51.

84. Ibrahim ZA, El-Ashmawy AA, El-Tatawy RA, Sallam FA. The effect of platelet-rich plasma on the outcome of short-term narrowband-ultraviolet B phototherapy in the treatment of vitiligo: a pilot study. J Cosmet Dermatol. 2016;15:108–16.

85. Abdelghani R, Ahmed NA, Darwish HM. Combined treatment with fractional carbon dioxide laser, autologous platelet-rich plasma, and narrow band ultraviolet B for vitiligo in different body sites: a prospective, randomized comparative trial. J Cosmet Dermatol. 2017. http://doi: 10.1111/jocd.12397.

86. Xiao BH, Wu Y, Sun Y, Chen HD, Gao XH. Treatment of vitiligo with NB-UVB: a systematic review. J Dermatolog Treat. 2015;26:340–6.

87. Jo SJ, Kwon HH, Choi MR, Youn JI. No evidence for increased skin cancer risk in Koreans with skin phototypes III-V treated with narrowband UVB phototherapy. Acta Derm Venereol. 2011;91:40–3.

88. El Mofty M, Bosseila M, Mashaly HM, Gawdat H, Makaly H. Broadband ultraviolet A vs. psoralen ultraviolet A in the treatment of vitiligo: a randomized controlled trial. Clin Exp Dermatol. 2013;38:830–5.

89. Leone G, Tanew A. UVB total body and targeted phototherapies. In: Picardo M, Taïeb A, editors. Vitiligo. Heidelberg: Springer; 2010. p. 359–65.

90. Werfel T, Holiangu F, Niemann KH, Schmerling O, Lullau F, Zedler A, et al. Digital ultraviolet therapy: a novel therapeutic approach for the targeted treatment of psoriasis vulgaris. Br J Dermatol. 2015;172:746–53.

91. Reidel U, Bechstein S, Lange-Asschenfeldt B, Beyer M, Vandersee S. Treatment of localized mycosis fungoides with digital UV photochemotherapy. Photodermatol Photoimmunol Photomed. 2015;31:333–40.

92. Mysore V, Shashikumar BM. Targeted phototherapy. Indian J Dermatol Venereol Leprol. 2016;82:1–6.

93. Majid I, Imran S. Targeted ultraviolet B phototherapy in vitiligo: a comparison between once-weekly and twice-weekly treatment regimens. Indian J Dermatol Venereol Leprol. 2015;81:600–5.

94. Dillon JP, Ford C, Hynan LS, Pandya AG. A cross-sectional, comparative study of home vs in-office NB-UVB phototherapy for vitiligo. Photodermatol Photoimmunol Photomed. 2015;33:282–3.

95. Hossain C, Porto DA, Hamzavi I, Lim HW. Camouflaging agents for vitiligo patients. J Drugs Dermatol. 2016;15:384–7.

96. Solano F, Briganti S, Picardo M, Ghanem G. Hypopigmenting agents: an updated review on biological, chemical and clinical aspects. Pigment Cell Res. 2006;19:550–71.

97. AlGhamdi KM, Kumar A. Depigmentation therapies for normal skin in vitiligo universalis. J Eur Acad Dermatol Venereol. 2011;25:749–57.

98. Whitton ME, Pinart M, Batchelor J, Leonardi-Bee J, Gonzalez U, Jiyad Z, et al (2015) Interventions for vitiligo. Cochrane Database Syst Rev (2):CD003263.

99. Kruger C, Smythe JW, Spencer JD, Hasse S, Panske A, Chiuchiarelli G, et al. Significant immediate and long-term improvement in quality of life and disease coping in patients with vitiligo after group climatotherapy at the Dead Sea. Acta Derm Venereol. 2011;91:152–9.

100. Shah R, Hunt J, Webb TL, Thompson AR. Starting to develop self-help for social anxiety associated with vitiligo: using clinical significance to measure the potential effectiveness of enhanced psychological self-help. Br J Dermatol. 2014;171:332–7.

101. Jha A, Mehta M, Khaitan BK, Sharma VK, Ramam M. Cognitive behavior therapy for psychosocial stress in vitiligo. Indian J Dermatol Venereol Leprol. 2016;82:308–10.

102. Craiglow BG, King BA. Tofacitinib citrate for the treatment of vitiligo: a pathogenesis-directed therapy. JAMA Dermatol. 2015;151:1110–2.

103. Liu LY, Strassner JP, Refat MA, Harris JE, King BA. Repigmentation in vitiligo using the Janus kinase inhibitor tofacitinib may require concomitant light exposure. J Am Acad Dermatol. 2017;77:675.

104. Harris JE, Rashighi M, Nguyen N, Jabbari A, Ulerio G, Clynes R, et al. Rapid skin repigmentation on oral ruxolitinib in a patient with coexistent vitiligo and alopecia areata (AA). J Am Acad Dermatol. 2016;74:370–1.

105. Rothstein B, Joshipura D, Saraiya A, Abdat R, Ashkar H, Turkowski Y, et al. Treatment of vitiligo with the topical Janus kinase inhibitor ruxolitinib. J Am Acad Dermatol. 2017;76:1054–60.e1.

106. Agarwal P, Rashighi M, Essien KI, Richmond JM, Randall L, Pazoki-Toroudi H, et al. Simvastatin prevents and reverses depigmentation in a mouse model of vitiligo. J Invest Dermatol. 2015;135:1080–8.

107. Noel M, Gagne C, Bergeron J, Jobin J, Poirier P. Positive pleiotropic effects of HMG-CoA reductase inhibitor on vitiligo. Lipids Health Dis. 2004;3:7.

108. Vanderweil SG, Amano S, Ko WC, Richmond JM, Kelley M, Senna MM, et al. A double-blind, placebo-controlled, phase-II clinical trial to evaluate oral simvastatin as a treatment for vitiligo. J Am Acad Dermatol. 2017;76:150–1.e3.

109. Iraji F, Banihashemi SH, Faghihi G, Shahmoradi Z, Tajmirriahi N, Jazi SBA. Comparison of betamethasone Valerate 0.1% cream twice daily plus oral simvastatin versus betamethasone Valerate 0.1% cream alone in the treatment of vitiligo patients. Adv Biomed Res. 2017;6:34.

110. Lotti TM, Hercogova J, Schwartz RA, Tsampau D, Korobko I, Pietrzak A, et al. Treatments of vitiligo: what's new at the horizon. Dermatol Ther. 2012;25(Suppl 1):S32–40.

111. Lim HW, Grimes PE, Agbai O, Hamzavi I, Henderson M, Haddican M, et al. Afamelanotide and narrowband UV-B phototherapy for the treatment of vitiligo: a randomized multicenter trial. JAMA Dermatol. 2015;151:42–50.

112. Passeron T. Indications and limitations of afamelanotide for treating vitiligo. JAMA Dermatol. 2015;151:349–50.

113. Song X, Xu A, Pan W, Wallin B, Kivlin R, Lu S, et al. Minocycline protects melanocytes against H2O2-induced cell death via JNK and p38 MAPK pathways. Int J Mol Med. 2008;22:9–16.

114. Singh A, Kanwar AJ, Parsad D, Mahajan R. Randomized controlled study to evaluate the effectiveness of dexamethasone oral minipulse therapy versus oral minocycline in patients with active vitiligo vulgaris. Indian J Dermatol Venereol Leprol. 2014;80:29–35.

115. Siadat AH, Zeinali N, Iraji F, Abtahi-Naeini B, Nilforoushzadeh MA, Jamshidi K, et al. Narrowband ultraviolet B versus oral minocycline in treatment of unstable vitiligo: a prospective comparative trial. Dermatol Res Pract. 2014;2014:240856.

116. Chou SY, Chou CK, Kuang TM, Hsu WM. Incidence and severity of iris pigmentation on latanoprost-treated glaucoma eyes. Eye (Lond). 2005;19:784–7.

117. Anbar TS, El-Ammawi TS, Abdel-Rahman AT, Hanna MR. The effect of latanoprost on vitiligo: a preliminary comparative study. Int J Dermatol. 2015;54:587–93.

118. Korobko IV, Lomonosov KMA. Pilot comparative study of topical latanoprost and tacrolimus in combination with narrow-band ultraviolet B phototherapy and microneedling for the treatment of nonsegmental vitiligo. Dermatol Ther. 2016;29:437–41.

119. Tressler CS, Wiseman RL, Dombi TM, Jessen B, Huang K, Kwok KK, et al. Lack of evidence for a link between latanoprost use and malignant melanoma: an analysis of safety databases and a review of the literature. Br J Ophthalmol. 2011;95:1490–5.

120. Grimes PE. Bimatoprost 0.03% solution for the treatment of nonfacial vitiligo. J Drugs Dermatol. 2016;15:703–10.

121. Sehgal VN. Role of tacrolimus (FK506) 0.1% ointment WW in vitiligo in children and imperatives of combine therapy with Trioxsalen and Silymarin suspension in progressive vitiligo. J Eur Acad Dermatol Venereol. 2009;23:1218–9.

122. Naini FF, Shooshtari AV, Ebrahimi B, Molaei R. The effect of pseudocatalase/superoxide dismutase in the treatment of vitiligo: a pilot study. J Res Pharm Pract. 2012;1:77–80.

123. Faas L, Venkatasamy R, Hider RC, Young AR, Soumyanath A. Vivo evaluation of piperine and synthetic analogues as potential treatments for vitiligo using a sparsely pigmented mouse model. Br J Dermatol. 2008;158:941–50.

124. Asawanonda P, Klahan SO. Tetrahydrocurcuminoid cream plus targeted narrowband UVB phototherapy for vitiligo: a preliminary randomized controlled study. Photomed Laser Surg. 2010;28:679–84.

125. Karaguzel G, Sakarya NP, Bahadir S, Yaman S, Okten A. Vitamin D status and the effects of oral vitamin D treatment in children with vitiligo: a prospective study. Clin Nutr ESPEN. 2016;15:28–31.

126. Lotti T, Hercogova J, Fabrizi G. Advances in the treatment options for vitiligo: activated low-dose cytokines-based therapy. Expert Opin Pharmacother. 2015;16:2485–96.

127. Singh H, Kumaran MS, Bains A, Parsad DA. Randomized comparative study of oral corticosteroid Minipulse and low-dose oral methotrexate in the treatment of unstable vitiligo. Dermatology. 2015;231:286–90.

128. Radmanesh M, Saedi K. The efficacy of combined PUVA and low-dose azathioprine for early

and enhanced repigmentation in vitiligo patients. J Dermatolog Treat. 2006;17:151–3.

129. Gupta AK, Ellis CN, Nickoloff BJ, Goldfarb MT, Ho VC, Rocher LL, et al. Oral cyclosporine in the treatment of inflammatory and noninflammatory dermatoses. A clinical and immunopathologic analysis. Arch Dermatol. 1990;126:339–50.

130. Dogra S, Kumar B. Repigmentation in vitiligo universalis: role of melanocyte density, disease duration, and melanocytic reservoir. Dermatol Online J. 2005;11:30.

131. Open-label pilot study of abatacept for the treatment of vitiligo [Internet]. U.S. National Institutes of Health. 2016 [cited December 29, 2016]. Available from: https://clinicaltrials.gov/ct2/show/ NCT02281058.

132. Alghamdi KM, Khurrum H, Taieb A, Ezzedine K. Treatment of generalized vitiligo with anti-TNF-alpha agents. J Drugs Dermatol. 2012;11: 534–9.

133. Bin Dayel S, AlGhamdi K. Failure of alefacept in the treatment of vitiligo. J Drugs Dermatol. 2013;12: 159–61.

134. Ruiz-Arguelles A, Garcia-Carrasco M, Jimenez-Brito G, Sanchez-Sosa S, Perez-Romano B, Garces-Eisele J, et al. Treatment of vitiligo with a chimeric monoclonal antibody to CD20: a pilot study. Clin Exp Immunol. 2013;174:229–36.

135. Mery-Bossard L, Bagny K, Chaby G, Khemis A, Maccari F, Marotte H, et al. New-onset vitiligo and progression of pre-existing vitiligo during treatment with biological agents in chronic inflammatory diseases. J Eur Acad Dermatol Venereol. 2017;31:181–6.

136. Wang X, McCoy J, Lotti T, Goren A. Topical cream delivers NB-UVB from sunlight for the treatment of vitiligo. Expert Opin Pharmacother. 2014;15:2623–7.

137. Mou Y, Jiang X, Du Y, Xue L. Intelligent bioengineering in vitiligo treatment: transdermal protein transduction of melanocyte-lineage-specific genes. Med Hypotheses. 2012;79:786–9.

138. Kumar R, Parsad D, Rani S, Bhardwaj S, Srivastav N. Glabrous lesional stem cells differentiated into functional melanocytes: new hope for repigmentation. J Eur Acad Dermatol Venereol. 2016;30:1555–60.

139. Tsuchiyama K, Wakao S, Kuroda Y, Ogura F, Nojima M, Sawaya N, et al. Functional melanocytes are readily reprogrammable from multilineage-differentiating stress-enduring (muse) cells, distinct stem cells in human fibroblasts. J Invest Dermatol. 2013;133:2425–35.

Surgical Modalities in Management of Vitiligo

9

Sanjeev V. Mulekar

Introduction

Vitiligo is a common condition characterized by hypopigmented and/or depigmented spots on the skin. Clinically three distinct variants can be recognized: segmental, non-segmental, and unclassified. Non-segmental vitiligo is used as an umbrella term to describe different types such as acro-facial, generalized, mucosal, (multifocal), and universal [1].

Segmental vitiligo is unilateral and has a rapidly progressive but limited course; depigmentation spreads within the segment over a period of 6–24 months and then stops. Further extension is rare. In addition, in contrast to NSV, SV has an early involvement of hair follicle melanocytes, exhibiting poliosis with up to 50% of patients [2].

Until about 30 years ago, vitiligo was exclusively being treated with medical therapies, the aim of which was to prevent melanocyte destruction and stimulate residual melanocytes. However, there is no medical treatment, which can prevent melanocyte destruction for a prolonged period without significant side effects. In addition, medical therapies are highly dependent upon melanocyte reservoir to

S. V. Mulekar (✉)
National Center for Vitiligo & Psoriasis,
Riyadh, Saudi Arabia
e-mail: mulekar@gmail.com

be effective [3]. Surgical therapies replace missing melanocytes, obtained from normal appearing skin.

Surgical therapies can be divided into (1) tissue grafting, which uses tissues, and (2) cellular grafting methods, which uses cells separated from the epidermis as a source of melanocytes.

The earliest surgical interventions in the management of vitiligo can be traced to reports by Behl [4, 5] and Falabella [6].

Minigrafting or Punch Grafting

In this method, grafts are harvested with the help of biopsy punch preferably from the gluteal region and fixed into the pits created by similar instrument to the recipient area (Table 9.1). They are secured with "micropore tape" or "Steri-Strips." Dressing is removed after 7–14 days.

Several practitioners have modified the basic procedure in order to minimize the side effects, to increase the area to be treated, and to hasten and improve the pigmentation. The size of the grafts varies from 1 to 3 mm and are placed 3–10 mm apart, which may be determined by the skin type and graft size [7, 8]. The grafts obtained from dark skin individuals can be placed 5–10 mm apart due to the properties of melanocytes, which produce larger melanosomes. However, in Caucasian patients, it is advisable to transplant those 3–5 mm apart, as melanocytes obtained from Caucasian skin produce smaller

© Springer International Publishing AG, part of Springer Nature 2018
P. Kumarasinghe (ed.), *Pigmentary Skin Disorders*, Updates in Clinical Dermatology,
https://doi.org/10.1007/978-3-319-70419-7_9

Table 9.1 Minigrafting or punch grafting

Easiest and cheapest method
Acceptable cosmetic results
Cobblestoning and color mismatch are the most commonly reported side effects

Table 9.2 Epidermal grafting

Easy, safe, inexpensive, and effective method
Good color matching and scarless surgery
Time-consuming method and unsuitable for body folds

melanosomes [8]. Cobblestoning is the most commonly observed adverse effect of this procedure, which can be prevented by implanting grafts larger than the pits [9], trimming excess adipose tissue from the bottom of grafts [8], and punching the recipient pits 1 mm deeper than thickness of grafts [10]. Postoperative phototherapy is usually recommended to hasten the perigraft spread of pigment.

In a study to demonstrate usefulness of minigrafting in the treatment of localized vitiligo, 13 patients achieved 90–100% repigmentation, 2 had partial improvement, and 2 were not treated as they had negative minigraft test [11]. Twenty-three patients (36 lesions) were analyzed in a study to evaluate the efficacy of minigrafting in vitiligo vulgaris. Fourteen of 36 lesions showed 80–99% repigmentation, 10, 50, to 80%, and 12 showed 0–50% repigmentation [10]. Furthermore, in a prospective study by Malakar and Dhar of the 880 patients, 656 patients (74.55%) achieved 90–100% repigmentation. In 10.57% there was no spread of pigment, while in 2.39% patient's depigmentation of grafts was noticed. Polka dot appearance (43.98%) and color mismatch (34.32%) were the most frequent side effects [12].

This is the easiest and the most inexpensive method, which can be performed by any dermatologist in his/her office with cosmetically acceptable results. The repigmentation yield ratio varies from 1:10 to 1:20.

Recent trend is not to recommend mini-punch grafting due to high incidence of adverse effects [13].

Epidermal Grafting

Epidermal grafting involves obtaining pure viable epidermis bearing melanocytes in the form of blisters by applying negative pressure (300–500 mm Hg) to the normally pigmented skin (Table 9.2). The grafts thus obtained are transferred to the denuded recipient sites. They are held in place for 7 days with nonadherent dressing. This technique was first described by Kistala [14], but was used first to treat leukoderma/vitiligo by Falabella [15, 16]. Different custom-made devices, such as oil rotary vacuum connected to manometer [17], manually operated suction unit with transparent plastic cups [18], and disposable syringes attached to a three-way tap with latex rubber tube and 50 mL syringe [19] are used to produce blisters on the donor and recipient areas. The blisters on both the donor and recipient sites are produced simultaneously. The usual time to harvest blisters is about 2–3 h. However, this can be reduced by application of heat and by selecting the donor skin over bony prominences [19].

Thirty-one patients with segmental vitiligo and 14-nondermatomal types were treated by epidermal grafting and followed for more than 6 months postsurgically. In the segmental group, 25 patients regained normal pigmentation, 4 had partial improvement, and 2 did not respond to the treatment. In the nondermatomal group, 11 repigmented initially, but 3 of them lost the pigment subsequently [17]. Mutalik reported good repigmentation in 48 of 50 patients with localized long-standing stationary patches of vitiligo, treated by epidermal grafting within 3–4 months after transplantation [18]. In a retrospective, uncontrolled case series and literature review, the success rate for generalized and segmental/focal vitiligo was 53% (confidence interval 42–64) and 91% (CI 81–100), respectively, in 117 patients over a postoperative period of 6 months [20].

The significant advantage of this procedure is that this is a scarless surgery and gives very good cosmetic results. It is easy and inexpensive and can be performed on almost any anatomic site except body folds. However, it is quite time consuming and can treat only small areas in a single operative session. In addition, blister formation may be a painful procedure for many patients.

Split-Skin Grafting

Split-skin grafting is the first method used to treat vitiligo surgically (Table 9.3). This method uses skin grafts harvested with either handheld Humpy's knife or motorized Zimmer dermatome and placed directly on the recipient area prepared by laser ablation or motorized dermabrasion. They are secured with surgical dressing, which is removed after 1 week.

Behl reported excellent repigmentation in 70% of 107 treated patients with split-skin grafting [4]. All the 5 patients treated by grafts harvested with Zimmer dermatome repigmented completely during the follow-up period of 3.5–35.5 months. Though no scarring was observed, all the patients developed milia on the recipient site [21]. In another study by Kahn and Cohen, good to excellent repigmentation was observed in 88% of the 17 procedures performed on 12 patients using meshed grafts without scarring [22]. In another series of 21 patients with 32 stable refractory vitiligo patches, 100% repigmentation was achieved in 22 patches and 90–95% in 10 others [23].

The advantage of this method is that large areas can be treated in a single operative session. However, donor to recipient ratio remains 1:1, and hospital setting to treat larger areas increases the cost of therapy. Though scarring has been reported at donor and recipient site, it can be avoided at skilled hands and by use of instruments like Zimmer dermatome. Though, it gives excellent results, this is not a popular method with dermatologists and is mainly practiced and reported by surgeons.

Table 9.3 Split-skin grafting

This technique yields highest success rate and relatively large areas can be treated
Development of milia is the most common side effect
Scarring can be avoided in skilled hands and by using suitable instruments

Though tissue-grafting methods are easier and inexpensive and produce acceptable cosmetic results, they are time consuming, can treat smaller areas in one operative session, are not suitable for all anatomic locations due to technical difficulties, and are associated with several adverse effects [24].

Cellular Grafting: Non-cultured and Cultured Techniques

These techniques use separated cells in the form of suspension. These cellular suspensions are transplanted as with or without culturing them in vitro on to the recipient area.

Initial steps are common to both the techniques. They are as follows: A shave biopsy is taken with the help of Silver's skin grafting knife (E. Murray Co., UK) or a Goulian skin graft knife (E. Weck Co. Princeton, USA) from the gluteal area or upper thigh. The specimen is transferred to 0.25% trypsin with EDTA and incubated for a varying period of 15 min to 3 h [25–28]. After incubation, the skin sample is washed, trypsin is neutralized, and the epidermis is separated from the dermis mechanically, to obtain epidermal cells.

Non-cultured Melanocyte Keratinocyte Transplantation

This technique involves separation of epidermal cells as described earlier (section "Cellular Grafting: Non-cultured and Cultured Techniques"). The epidermal cells thus obtained are suspended in either normal saline [29], M2 melanocyte medium (PromoCell, Heidelberg, Germany) [30], Dulbecco modified essential medium [31], or sodium lactate [32]. Addition of hyaluronic acid to the cell suspension improves the viscosity and attachment of cells to recipient site [33]. Recipient area is denuded superficially, to dermo-epidermal junction. Clinically, the level of dermabrasion is determined by appearance of pinpoint bleeding. The cell suspension seeded on to the recipient area is first covered with collagen

Table 9.4 Non-cultured melanocytes-keratinocyte transplantation

Very large areas can be treated in one operative session
Good cosmetic results
Scarless surgery in skilled hands
Requires specialized instruments and trained personnel

dressing, which is held in place with sterile gauze pieces for 1 week. Absolute immobilization is not necessary. Table 9.4 summarizes the salient points of non-cultured melanocyte-keratinocyte cellular grafting.

The technique was first reported by Gauthier and Surleve-Bazeille [29], in which they injected the suspension in the blisters produced on the recipient area. Several modifications have been carried out over the years to make it more effective and simple. Olsson and Juhlin diluted the cell suspension to achieve donor to recipient ratio up to 1:10 and prepared the recipient area with motorized dermabrasion using diamond fraise wheel. This shortened the surgery time significantly, converting it into a day care procedure. They reported complete repigmentation in most vitiligo patients [30]. Mulekar simplified the procedure further, by using DMEM F12 medium (Invitrogen Corporation, Carlsbad, California) instead of different media at various stages of the procedure. The medium was not supplemented with penicillin, streptomycin, and basic fibroblast growth factor, and CO_2 incubator was replaced with an ordinary incubator. The cell separation was performed in the procedure room on a clean bench, thus eliminating the transfer of shave biopsy sample to a separate laboratory [31].

Some other modifications include incubation at 4^0 for about 18 h and using suspension obtained from hair follicle outer root sheath. Cold trypsinization: Incubation is done at 4^0 overnight [34]. Instead of epidermal cell suspension, Mohanty et al. used cells obtained from hair follicle outer root sheath to demonstrate that it was an effective and safe method to treat stable vitiligo [35]. Both the techniques were found to be of comparable efficacy [36]. In order to reduce or eliminate donor skin scarring and pigmentary changes, Gupta et al. suggested to obtain donor skin cells with manual dermabrader instead of thin split-skin graft [37].

In a long-term study over a period of 6 years with 142 patients with vitiligo vulgaris, 56% of patients showed excellent, 11% good, 9% fair, and 24% poor repigmentation [38]. In another long-term study over a period of 5 years, all the segmental vitiligo patients retained the repigmentation achieved at the end of respective follow-up period indicating the possibility of disease-free period for the rest of life [31].

There are several advantages of this technique. Extensive areas can be treated from small skin sample with cosmetic results comparable to those produced by cultured technique (Fig. 9.1a, b). This is a day care procedure, which can be completed in 45 min to 2 h. All the procedure steps can be performed in a clean procedure room. However, it requires specialized instruments such as dermabrader, incubator, and centrifuge. In addition, it requires adequately trained personnel to achieve desired results.

In Vitro Cultured Pure Melanocytes and Coculture of Keratinocytes/ Melanocytes or Cultured Epidermal Sheets

The initial steps to obtain the epidermal cells are described in section "Cellular Grafting: Non-cultured and Cultured Techniques". The cells obtained are transported to the cell culture laboratory for in vitro culture. Culturing process of melanocytes/epidermal sheets bearing melanocytes takes about 3 weeks to obtain the adequate yield required for transplantation. Thus, two visits are required to accomplish this treatment. In the first visit, a shave biopsy skin sample is harvested. The second visit is made after about 3 weeks for transplantation of cultured melanocytes/epidermal sheets. Recipient area is denuded with motorized dermabrasion, or with Er:YAG laser, cultured cell suspensions or epidermal sheets are transplanted on to the recipient area

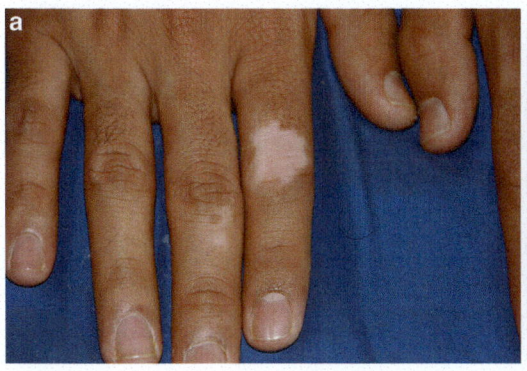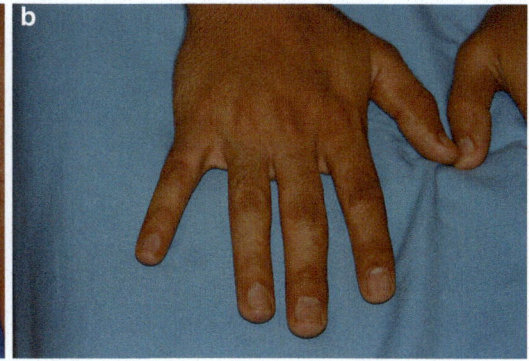

Fig. 9.1 (**a**) 26-year-old male, depigmented lesion on right index and middle finger before non-cultured cellular transplantation. (**b**) 2 years posttransplantation with good repigmentation

Table 9.5 In vitro cultured pure melanocytes and coculture of keratinocytes/melanocytes or cultured epidermal sheets

Excellent cosmetic results
Extensive areas can be treated
Complex, requires highly trained personnel and specialized equipment
Mainly restricted to research laboratories

and secured by suitable nonadherent dressing. Table 9.5 summarizes the salient points about this technique.

Olsson and Juhlin reported good cosmetic results in 9 of 10 patients treated with transplantation of autologous cultured melanocytes. Melanocytes were cultured using PC1 medium (Ventrex, Portland, ME) supplemented with 50 U/ml penicillin, 0.05 ng/ml streptomycin, 2 mM L-glutamine, and 5 ng/ml basic fibroblast growth factor. The melanocytes were seeded at the concentration of 1000–2000/mm² [26]. Melanocytes were isolated from donor skin sample obtained by producing suction blister and seeded into flasks containing modified melanocyte medium which consisted of Ham's F12 nutrient mixture (Gibco) supplemented with 50 µg/ml gentamicin, 20 ng/ml recombinant human basic fibroblast growth factor (Sigma), 10 ng/ml cholera toxin, and 20% fetal calf serum (Biological Industries, Kibbutz, Israel) for the culturing purpose. Adequate number of melanocytes was cultured after an average of 24.1 days. The epidermis of the affected area was removed superficially using SilkTouch flashscanner attached to Sharplan 1030 CO_2 laser. The melanocytes suspension was applied to laser-denuded area at the density of 70,000–100,000/cm². The repigmentation was classified as excellent 21 and good in 4 patients with segmental vitiligo patients in this study [39]. One hundred twenty patients were treated with transplantation of autologous pure melanocytes suspension. Cells were cultured in Hu16 medium with Ham F12 nutrient mixture (Gibco) supplemented with 50microg/ml gentamicin, 20 ng/ml recombinant human basic fibroblast growth factor (Sigma), 10 ng/ml cholera toxin, and 20% fetal calf serum (Biological Industries, Kibbutz, Israel). Cells were applied to laser-denuded area in the concentration of 60,000–100,000/cm². Excellent results were obtained in 84%, 54%, and 0% of the cases in stable localized group ($n = 80$), stable generalized group ($n = 26$), and active generalized group ($n = 14$), respectively [27]. A total of 2315.8 cm² of achromic surface in 21 patients was transplanted with autologous cultured epidermis, which was cultured in keratinocyte growth medium: Dulbecco-Vogt Eagle medium and Ham F12 media (2:1 mixture), containing 10% fetal calf serum, 0.1 nM cholera toxin, and 10 ng/mL of epidermal growth factor, in 5% carbon dioxide and humidified atmosphere. Recipient area was prepared using pulsed Er:Yag laser (Laser Smart 2940; DEKA Medical Electronics Laser Associated srl, Calenzano, Florence, Italy). The average percentage of repigmentation was 75.9%

at 6 months posttransplantation. Variation of the melanocyte concentration in cultured epidermis varied from 1:30 to 1:200 [40].

The significant advantage of this technique is the possibility to treat extensive areas with excellent cosmetic results. However, it is a very complex procedure requiring specialized instruments such as carbon dioxide incubator, laminar flow bench, and a cell culture laboratory. Due to these limitations, this technique is mainly limited to research facilities.

Comments

Until about 30 years ago, vitiligo was considered as a progressive disease in all the patients and was exclusively treated by medical therapies. Melanocytes destruction is the end result of incompletely understood pathological process in vitiligo leading to the development of achromic lesions. Aim of the medical therapies is to prevent destruction of melanocytes and stimulate proliferation and migration of residual melanocytes to achromic areas.

Surgical therapies have an important place in the management of vitiligo in the absence of any credible mechanism, which can prevent destruction of melanocytes for a prolonged period without side effects. The mesenchymal stem cell as a source of melanocytes in vivo is still hypothetical. Recent advances in the surgical methods have enabled the dermatologists to treat any anatomic site with acceptable cosmetic results at least temporarily in generalized type and almost permanently in the segmental type. Due to the high success rate, especially in the localized type, surgical options are being increasingly sought both by patients and physicians.

Any modification in surgical therapy will be successful provided it makes the procedure simpler and more effective with predictable outcome.

Non-cultured melanocyte-keratinocyte transplantation procedure (MKTP) combines all advantages of cultured technique while eliminating disadvantages of tissue grafting methods. Compared for parameters such as technique,

cost, cosmetically acceptable results, and adverse effects, it lies between cultured technique and tissue grafting techniques. Does it have a potential to become gold standard in the surgical management of vitiligo? More studies from different part of the world and comparative studies are required to establish this.

References

1. Ezzedine K, Lim HW, Suzuki T, et al. Revised classification/nomenclature of vitiligo and related issues: the Vitiligo global issues consensus conference. Pigment Cell Melanoma Res. 2012;25:E1–E13.
2. Hann SK, Lee JH. Segmental vitiligo: clinical findings in 208 patients. J Am Acad Dermatol. 1996;35:671–4.
3. Falabella R. Vitiligo and melanocyte reservoir. Indian J Dermatol. 2009;54:313–8.
4. Behl PN. Treatment of vitiligo with homologous thin Thiersch's skin grafts. Curr Med Pract. 1964;8:218–21.
5. Behl PN, Bhatia RK. Treatment of vitiligo with autologous thin Thiersch's graft. Int J Dermatol. 1973;12:329–31.
6. Falabella R. Repigmentation of segmental vitiligo by autologous minigrafting. J Am Acad Dermatol. 1983;9:514–21.
7. Falabella R, Barona MI. Update on skin repigmentation therapies in vitiligo. Pigment Cell Melanoma Res. 2008;22:42–65.
8. Mutalik S, Ginzberg A. Surgical management of stable vitiligo: a review with personal experience. Dermatol Surg. 2000;26:248–54.
9. Savant SS. Autologous miniature punch skin grafting in stable vitiligo. Indian J Dermatol Venereol Leprol. 1992;58:310–4.
10. Boersma B, Westerhof W, Bos JD. Repigmentation in vitiligo vulgaris by autologous minigrafting: results in nineteen patients. J Am Acad Dermatol. 1995;33:990–5.
11. Falabella R. Treatment of localized vitiligo by autologous Minigrafting. Arch Dermatol. 1988;124:1649–55.
12. Malakar S, Dhar S. Treatment of stable and recalcitrant vitiligo by autologous miniature punch grafting: a prospective study of 1000 patients. Dermatology. 1999;198:133–9.
13. Gawkrodger DJ, Ormerod AD, Shaw L, et al. Guidelines for the diagnosis and management of vitiligo. Br J Dermatol. 2008;159:1051–76.
14. Kistala U. Suction blister device for separation of viable epidermis from dermis. J Invest Dermatol. 1968;50:129–37.
15. Falabella R. Epidermal grafting. An original technique and its application in achromic and granulating areas. Arch Dermatol. 1971;104:592–600.

16. Falabella R. Repigmentation of leukoderma by autologous epidermal grafting. J Dermatol Surg Oncol. 1984;10:136–44.

17. Koga M. Epidermal grafting using the tops of suction blisters in the treatment of vitiligo. Arch Dermatol. 1988;124:1656–8.

18. Mutalik S. Transplantation of melanocytes by epidermal grafting- an Indian experience. J Dermatol Surg Oncol. 1993;19:231–4.

19. Gupta S, Shroff S. Modified technique of suction blistering for epidermal grafting in vitiligo. Int J Dermatol. 1999;38:306–9.

20. Gupta S, Kumar B. Epidermal grafting in vitiligo: influence of age, site of lesion, and type of disease on outcome. J Am Acad Dermatol. 2003;104:99–104.

21. Kahn AM, Cohen MJ. Vitiligo: treated by dermabrasion and epithelial sheet grafting. J Am Acad Deramatol. 1995;33:646–8.

22. Kahn AM, Cohen MJ. Repigmentation in vitiligo patients. Dermatol Surg. 1998;24:365–7.

23. Agarwal K, Agarwal A. Vitiligo: repigmentation with dermabrasion and thin split-thickness skin grafts. Dermatol Surg. 1995;43:273–4.

24. Njoo MD, Westerhof W, Bos JD, Bossuyt PMM. A systematic review of autologous transplantation methods in vitiligo. Arch Dermatol. 1998;134:1343–9.

25. Falabella R. Transplantation of in vitro-cultured epidermis bearing melanocytes for repigmenting vitiligo. J Am Acad Dermatol. 1989;21:257–64.

26. Olsson MJ, Juhlin L. Repigmentation of vitiligo by transplantation of cultured autologous melanocytes. Acta Derm Venereol. 1993;73:49–51.

27. Chen YF, Yang PY, Treatment HDN. Of vitiligo by transplantation of cultured pure melanocyte suspension: analysis of 120 cases. J Am Acad Dermatol. 2004;51:68–74.

28. Pianigiani E, Risulo M, Andrea A, Paolo T, Francesca I, Lucio A. Autologous epidermal cultures and narrow-band ultraviolet B in the surgical treatment of vitiligo. Dermatol Surg. 2005;31:155–9.

29. Gauthier Y, Surleve-Bazeille J-E. Autologous grafting with noncultured melanocytes: a simplified method for treatment of depigmented lesions. J Am Acad Dermatol. 1992;26:191–4.

30. Olsson MJ, Juhlin L. Leucoderma treated by transplantation of a basal layer enriched suspension. Br J Dermatol. 1998;138:644–8.

31. Mulekar SV. Long-term follow-up study of segmental and focal Vitiligo treated by autologous non-cultured melanocyte-keratinocyte cell transplantation. Arch Dermatol. 2004;140:1213–5.

32. Mulekar SV, Ghwish B, Al Issa A, Al Eisa A. Treatment of vitiligo lesions by ReCell vs conventional melanocyte-keratinocyte transplantation: a pilot study. Br J Dermatol. 2008;158:45–9.

33. Van Geel N, Ongenae K, De Mil M, Naeyaert JM. Modified technique of autologous noncultured epidermal cell transplantation for repigmenting vitiligo: a pilot study. Dermatol Surg. 2001;27:873–6.

34. Budania A, Prasad D, Kanwar AJ, Dogra S. Comparison between autologous noncultured epidermal cell suspension and suction blister epidermal grafting in stable vitiligo: a randomized study. Br J Dermatol. 2012;167:1295–301.

35. Mohanty S, Kumar A, Dhawan J, Sreenivas V, Gupta S. Extracted hair follicle outer root sheath cell suspension for transplantation in vitiligo. Br J Dermatol. 2011;164:1241–6.

36. Singh C, Prasad D, Kanwar AJ, et al. Comparison between autologous noncultured extracted outer root sheath cell suspension and autologous noncultured epidermal cell suspension in the treatment of stable vitiligo. Br J Dermatol. 2013;169:287–93.

37. Gupta S, Kumar A, Mahendra A, Gupta SA. Minimally invasive scarless technique of donor tissue harvesting for noncultured epidermal cell suspension transplantation in vitiligo. J Am Acad Dermatol. 2015;73:e213–5.

38. Mulekar SV. Melanocyte-keratinocyte cell transplantation for stable vitiligo. Int J Dermatol. 2003;42:132–6.

39. Chen YF, Chang JS, Yang PY, Hung CM, Huang MH, Transplant HDN. Of cultured autologous pure melanocytes after laser-abrasion for the treatment of segmental Vitiligo. J Dermatol. 2000;27:434–9.

40. Guerra L, Primavera G, Raskovic D, Pellegrini G, Golisano O, Bondanza S, et al. Erbium:YAG laser and cultured epidermis in the surgical therapy of stable vitiligo. Arch Dermatol. 2003;139:1303–10.

Progressive Macular Hypomelanosis

10

Germaine Nathalie Relyveld

Historical Background

Throughout the years the disorder has been given various names. The name "progressive macular hypomelanosis" was the first to be introduced in 1985 [1–3]. With this term a pigment disorder in people of mixed racial (Negroid and Caucasoid) ancestry, living in France, but originating from the French Caribbean islands was described. Since then, different authors from different parts in the world described similar skin disorders, however using different names: "nummular and confluent hypomelanosis of the trunk" in the Netherlands [4–6]; "cutis trunci variata" in Venezuela [7]; "creole dyschromia" in Martinique, West Indies [8]; and "idiopathic multiple large macular hypomelanosis" in the USA [9].

After many years it became obvious that all of the above mentioned names described similar skin lesions. Currently "progressive macular hypomelanosis" (PMH) is the most commonly used name and has been described in patients from many countries around the world [10, 11].

G. N. Relyveld (✉)
Antoni van Leeuwenhoek – Netherlands Cancer Institute, Amsterdam, The Netherlands

Mauritskliniek Amsterdam, Amsterdam, The Netherlands
e-mail: g.relyveld@nki.nl;
grelyveld@mauritsklinieken.nl

Clinical Characteristics

PMH is primarily a morphologic entity characterized by ill-defined, nummular, hypopigmented macules, symmetrically localized, and predominantly on the trunk, but sometimes progressing to the neck and the face, the buttocks, and the proximal parts of the extremities. In the majority of patients, a rather well-defined hypopigmented area that appears to originate from confluence of macules can be recognized on the front and back of the trunk [3, 5, 7, 8, 12]. The width of this confluent region varies from patient to patient; sometimes this region is absent, showing hypopigmented macules mainly in the flanks (Fig. 10.1a–c). A red follicular fluorescence can be observed in the hypopigmented spots, which is not present in normal adjacent skin, when patients are examined in a dark room using a Wood's lamp (Fig. 10.2a, b). Anaerobic culture on blood agar plates of biopsy specimens from PMH patients shows growth of colonies compatible with *Propionibacterium acnes* (*P. acnes*) bacteria [13].

Additional laboratory tests (ESR, complete blood count, blood glucose, liver enzymes, and urea) and urine analysis are within normal limits, and potassium-hydroxide tests of skin scrapings are negative for fungal elements [5]. Usually there is no history of pruritus, pain, or a preceding inflammatory dermatosis.

P. Kumarasinghe (ed.), *Pigmentary Skin Disorders*, Updates in Clinical Dermatology,
https://doi.org/10.1007/978-3-319-70419-7_10

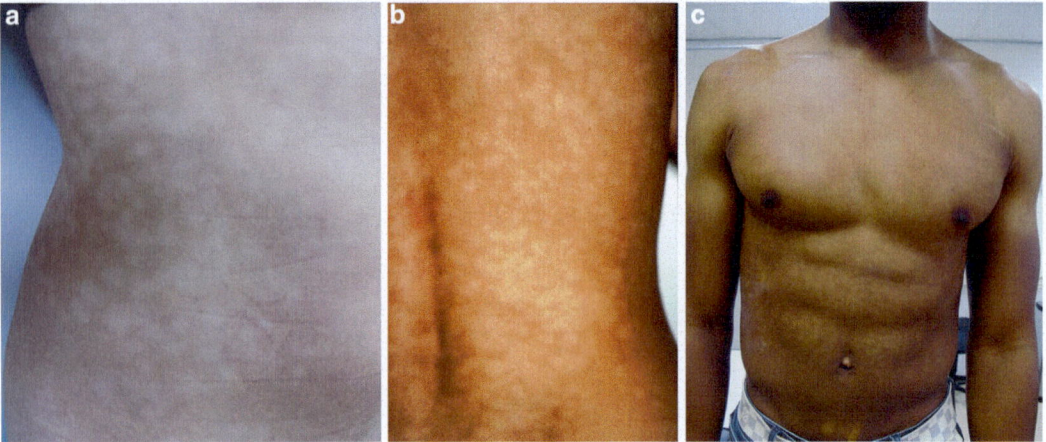

Fig. 10.1 (**a**) 34-year-old woman with skin type III showing a hypopigmented area in the midline on the front of the trunk and hypopigmented macules in the flanks. (**b**) 28-year-old woman with skin type IV showing a broad area in the midline of the back with symmetrically distrib-uted hypopigmented macules. (**c**) 32-year-old man with skin type VI showing hypopigmented macules toward the flanks and a confluent hypopigmented region in the midline of the front of the trunk

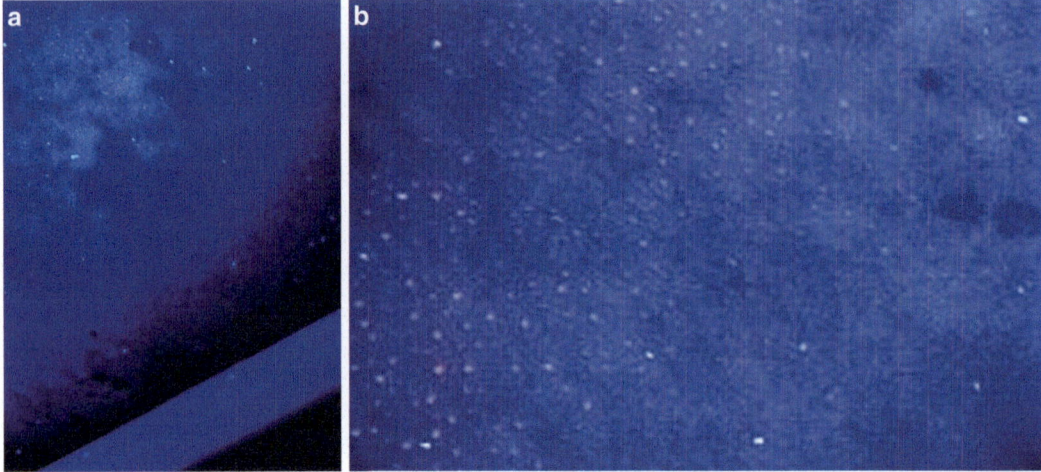

Fig. 10.2 (**a**, **b**) Red follicular fluorescence in hypopigmented macules, which is absent in adjacent, non-lesional skin

Epidemiology

PMH is mostly observed in adolescents and young adults between the ages of 13 and 45 years, with a mean age of 20,8–26,5 years [5, 8, 9, 11, 12, 14, 15]. Although the true prevalence of PMH is unknown, it seems to be a common disorder [8, 12]. The disorder is mostly seen in patients with darker skin types (III–VI); however, it has been described in patients of all skin types. In lighter skin types, the hypopigmented macules are much less obvious, and therefore patients often do not notice the lesions or do not find it worth visiting a doctor. The distribution among the sexes is unknown. In earlier years, it was mostly described in women [1–3]; however lately PMH has been described equally in both sexes [7].

Etiology and Pathogenesis

PMH is mainly a cosmetically disturbing disorder. However, especially in tropical countries where leprosy is endemic, patients may worry about the probability of having leprosy when they see the hypopigmented spots on their skin.

There is accumulating evidence for a correlation between *P. acnes* bacteria and PMH. The red follicular fluorescence that is observed in the hypopigmented spots is due to *P. acnes* bacteria residing in pilosebaceous ducts [13]. *P. acnes* is considered to be commensal flora and related to acne vulgaris. It accounts for approximately half of the total skin microbiota [16]. However, there does not seem to be a relation between PMH and acne. 16S rDNA analysis of cultured *P. acnes* strains from PMH lesions actually shows genetically and phenotypically distinct type III *P. acnes* strains [13, 17–19]. These type III strains have been isolated solely in PMH patients, and not in acne patients [13], suggesting a relationship between PMH and these bacteria.

Histology and Electron Microscopy

Hematoxylin-eosin staining of the skin of hypopigmented spots shows only a subtle decrease in melanin content in the epidermis compared with that in normal adjacent skin. There is no significant inflammatory infiltrate or epidermotropism of leukocytes. Fontana-Masson-staining shows overall reduction in melanization of the basal cell layer of lesional skin. Melanocytes stain negative for HMB 45 and Melan A stains. S100 staining does not show any differences in the number of melanocytes, Langerhans cells, or other dermal dendritic cells. Occasional melanophages are present in the dermis of both lesional and normal skin on hematoxylin-eosin and CD68 staining [3, 8]. In both the lesional and the non-lesional skin of PMH patients, the melanocyte cell bodies contain melanosome precursors in all stages of development. In lesional skin, however, mature melanosomes are distinctly smaller and less melanized than those in non-lesional skin. This can best be observed in the melanocytic dendrites in the lesional skin of patients with skin types V and VI, containing smaller, less melanized melanosomes than those in non-lesional skin (Fig. 10.3a, b). In patients with skin types III and IV, this phenomenon is less obvious, due to the fact that in these skin types, the melanosomes in normal skin are already smaller and less melanized [20].

Differential Diagnosis

PMH is most often misdiagnosed as pityriasis versicolor (PV) or pityriasis alba (PA). Many patients have been previously treated with antimycotic or anti-inflammatory therapy, without any effect before the diagnosis PMH is given. Other disorders with hypopigmentation that should be considered are post-inflammatory hypopigmentation, for instance, after atopic dermatitis, seborrheic dermatitis or superficial scaly dermatitis, leprosy especially in endemic countries, and hypopigmentation caused by proliferative neoplastic disorders, i.e., mycosis fungoides. In dark-skinned patients, hypopigmented mycosis fungoides (HMF) can mimic PMH. In such situations, skin biopsy becomes useful. In regions where there is visceral leishmaniasis, hypopigmented lesions of post-kala-azar dermal leishmaniasis (PKDL) too can be considered in the differential diagnosis [10]. Table 10.1 summarizes the important differences between PMH, PV, PA, HMF, and PKDL.

Treatment

Although PMH seems to be self-limiting, it may take years before lesions disappear. Therefore, many patients prefer treatment instead of waiting. The hypothetical overgrowth of *P. acnes* being the cause of PMH leads to various studies in which the eradication of these bacteria with antibacterial agents was the goal. The topical combination therapy of benzoyl peroxide 5% hydrogel at night and clindamycin 1% lotion in the morning during 3 months combined with UVA phototherapy three times a week with an

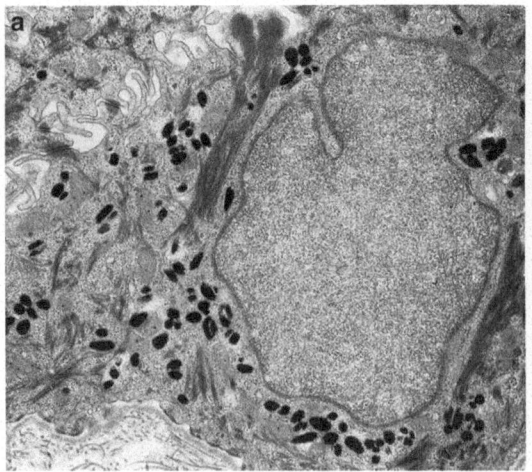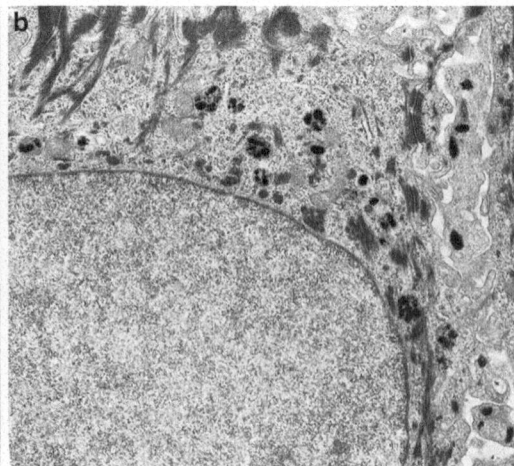

Fig. 10.3 (**a**) Keratinocyte of normal skin in a PMH patient with skin type V showing numerous, single, large, intensely melanocytic melanosomes. (**b**) Keratinocyte in lesional skin of the same patient, showing smaller, less dense melanosomes, clustered in membrane-bound groups

Table 10.1 Most important differences between PMH, PV, PA, HMF, and PKDL

Disorder	Patient characteristics	Diagnostic features	Clinical course
PMH	Adolescents and young adults Possibly a genetic component	Symmetrical, hypopigmented macules, mainly on the trunk, mostly no other objective or subjective symptoms Red follicular fluorescence in hypopigmented macules under Wood's light Gram-positive rodlike bacteria in sebaceous ducts and glands of lesional skin, but absent in normal (perilesional) skin [3]	Progression on the trunk, face, and proximal extremities No response to antimycotic or anti-inflammatory treatment If lesions resolve, recurrence in same areas
PV	Adolescents and young adults No genetic component	Asymmetrical hypopigmented, scaly macules on the trunk, sometimes the proximal arms Yellow fluorescence of macules under Wood's light KOH preparation: + (spores and mycelia)	Can progress further on trunk or proximal arms Good effect of antimycotic treatment Recurrence usually on different parts of the trunk and proximal arms
PA	Children Certainly a genetical component (often seen in atopic patients)	Starts with erythematous asymmetrical macules; evolves in hypopigmented, scaly macules on the trunk, proximal arms, and face No fluorescence under Wood's light	Usually resolving in adolescent years Good effect of anti-inflammatory treatment Recurrence usually on different parts of the trunk, face, and proximal arms
HMF		Asymmetrical distribution. Usually in buttocks area, sometimes on upper limbs and trunk. Eczematous changes of skin, early lesions atrophic, later infiltrated plaque lesions	Progresses in time, becoming tumors and ulcerations
PKDL		Asymmetrical distribution. Macular, maculopapular, and nodular rash. Usually starts around the mouth and later spreads to other parts of the body. Endemic area, past history of visceral leishmaniasis. Diagnosis mainly clinical, but parasites can be seen in smears	May act as a reservoir for parasites and therefore may play an important role in inter-epidemic periods of visceral leishmaniasis

PMH progressive macular hypomelanosis, *PV* pityriasis versicolor, *PA* pityriasis alba, *HMF* hypopigmented mycosis fungoides, *PKDL* post-kala-azar dermal leishmaniasis

effective flux of 233 J/m^2 during 20 min showed total repigmentation in 62% of patients [21].

Another well-documented treatment for PMH seems to be narrowband ultraviolet B phototherapy (NB UVB) [22]. NB UVB has been shown to exhibit excellent antibacterial properties and also promotes the synthesis of melanin by stimulating residual melanocytes while also increasing the melanization in melanosomes [22]. More than 90% of patients treated with an average of 22 sessions of NB UVB showed more than 80% repigmentation.

At present, the benzoyl peroxide/clindamycin alone or combined with NB UVB twice a week seems to be the most effective. NB UVB has the fastest result; however benzoyl peroxide/clindamycin shows considerably less to no relapses in a 2-year period [21–25].

Conclusion

PMH seems to be a common skin disorder in patients of all skin types. Especially in fair-skinned people, it may be difficult to recognize. These patients usually complain after sun exposure, when the hypopigmented macules become more obvious. It may be merely a cosmetic problem; however sometimes it leads to psychological stress. It is important to differentiate PMH from other more serious hypopigmented skin disorders like mycosis fungoides or certain forms of leishmaniasis. Unfortunately, it is often misdiagnosed. Various studies show very promising treatment results leading to complete repigmentation; however relapses can occur. Since it concerns a rather novel diagnosis, further research into the pathogenesis and other treatment modalities are of great importance.

References

1. Guillet G, Gauthier Y, Helenon R. Hypomélanose maculaire progressive du tronc (hypopigmentation primitive acquise des Antilles) Soc Fr Dermatol (Paris), mars 1985.
2. Guillet G, Helenon R, Gauthier Y, Surleve-Bazeille JE, Plantin P, Sassolas B. Progressive macu-
lar hypomelanosis of the trunk: primary acquired hypopigmentation. J Cutan Pathol. 1988;15:286–9.
3. Guillet G, Helenon R, Guillet MH, Gauthier Y, Menard N. Hypomelanose maculeuse confluente et progressive du metis melanoderme. Ann Dermatol Venereol. 1992;119(1):19–24.
4. Menke HE, Doornweerd S, Zaal J, Roggeveen C, Dingemans KP, van der Bergh Weerman M, Westerhof W. Acquired nummular and confluent hypomelanosis of the trunk. Paper presented at: second annual meeting of the European Society for Pigment Cell Research; June 18-21 1989; Uppsala, Sweden.
5. Menke HE, Ossekoppele R, Dekker SK, v Praag MCG, Zaal J, Noordhoek-Hegt V, Westerhof W. Nummulaire en confluerende hypomelanosis van de romp. Ned Tijdsch Dermatol Venereol. 1997;7:117–22.
6. Menke HE, Relyveld G, Njoo D, Westerhof W. Progressive macular hypomelanosis. In: Nordlund JJ, et al., editors. The pigmentary system. 2nd ed. Malden: Blackwell Publishing; 2006. p. 748–51.
7. Borelli D. Cutis trunci variata: nueva genodermatosis. Med Cutan Ibero-Lat-Am. 1987;15:317–9.
8. Lesueur A, Garcia-Granel V, Helenon R, Cales-Quist D. Hypomélanose maculeuse confluente et progressive du métis mélanoderme: etude epidemiologique sur 511 subjets. Ann Dermatol Venereol. 1994;121:880–3.
9. Sober AJ, Fitzpatrick TB, editors. Yearbook of dermatology. St Louis: Mosby-Year Book; 1996. p. 416–7.
10. Kumarasinghe P, Thng S. Progressive macular hypomelanosis. In: Lahiri K, Chatterjee M, Sarkar R, editors. Pigmentary disorders: a comprehensive compendium. 1st ed. New Delhi: Jaypee Brothers Medical Publishers (P) Ltd; 2014. p. 386–92.
11. Relyveld GN, Menke HE, Westerhof W. Progressive macular hypomelanosis: an overview. Am J Clin Dermatol. 2007;8(1):13–9.
12. Kumarasinghe SP, Tan SH, Thng S, Thamboo TP, Liang S, Lee YS. Progressive macular hypomelanosis in Singapore: a clinico-pathological study. Int J Dermatol. 2006;45(6):737–42.
13. Westerhof W, Relyveld GN, Kingswijk MM, de Man P, Menke HE. Propionibacterium acnes and the pathogenesis of progressive macular hypomelanosis. Arch Dermatol. 2004;140(2):210–4.
14. Hwang SW, Hong SK, Kim SH, Park JH, Seo JK, Sung HS, Lee D. Progressive macular hypomelanosis in korean patients: a clinicopathologic study. Ann Dermatol. 2009 Aug;21(3):261–7.
15. Duarte I, Nina BI, Gordiano MC, Buense R, Lazzarini R. Progressive macular hypomelanosis: an epidemiological study and therapeutic response to phototherapy. An Bras Dermatol. 2010;85(5):621–4.
16. Tancrede C. Role of human microbiota in health and disease. Eur. J. Clin Microbiol. Infect Dis. 1992;11:1012–5.
17. Relybeld GN, Westerhof W, Woudenberg J, Kingswijk M, Langenberg M, Vandenbroucke-Grauls CM, et al. Progressive macular hypomelanosis is associated

with a putative Propionibacterium species. J Invest Dermatol. 2010 Apr;130(4):1182–4.

18. Petersen R, Lomholt HB, Scholz CFP, Brüggemann H. Draft genome sequences of two Propionibacterium acnes strains isolated from progressive macular hypomelanosis lesions of human skin. Genome Announc. 2015;3(6):e01250–15.

19. Barnard E, Liu J, Yankova E, Cavalcanti SM, Magalhães M, Li H, et al. Strains of Propionibacterium acnes type III lineage are associated with the skin condition progressive macular hypomelanosis. Sci Rep. 2016;6:31968.

20. Relyveld GN, Dingemans KP, Menke HE, Bos JD, Westerhof W. Ultrastructural findings in progressive macular hypomelanosis indicate decreased melanin production. J Eur Acad Dermatol Venereol. 2008;22(5):568–74.

21. Relyveld GN, Kingswijk MM, Reitsma JB, Menke HE, Bos JD, Westerhof W. Benzoyl peroxide/clindamycin/UVA is more effective than fluticasone/UVA in

progressive macular hypomelanosis: a randomized study. J Am Acad Dermatol. 2006;55(5):836–43.

22. Thng ST, Long VS, Chuah SY, Tan VW. Efficacy and relapse rates of different treatment modalities for progressive macular hypomelanosis. Indian J Dermatol Venereol Leprol. 2016;82(6):673–6.

23. Fluhr JW, Gloor M. The antimicrobial effect of narrow-band UVB (313 nm) and UVA1 (345-440 nm) radiation in vitro. Photodermatol Photoimmunol Photomed. 1997;13:197–201.

24. Santos JB, Almeida OL, Silva LM, Barreto ER. Efficacy of topical combination of benzoyl peroxide 5% and clindamycin 1% for the treatment of progressive macular hypomelanosis: a randomized, double blind, placebo-controlled trial. An Bras Dermatol. 2011;86(1):50–4.18.

25. Kim MB, Kim GW, Cho HH, Park HJ, Kim HS, Kim SH, et al. Narrowband UVB treatment of progressive macular hypomelanosis. J Am Acad Dermatol. 2012;66(4):598–605.

Guttate Leukoderma

11

Nisansala Mahenthi Nagodavithana and Prasad Kumarasinghe

Introduction

Originating from the Latin term "gutta" (a drop) and "guttatus" (speckled), guttate leukoderma refers to "drop-like" hypopigmentation. The degree of hypopigmentation can vary from hypo- to depigmentation depending on the underlying pathology.

In general when a patient presents with guttate hypomelanosis, first it has to be ascertained whether it is present from birth or acquired later in life. Then the lesions should be carefully examined to evaluate whether there is a textural change of the lesions or not. A careful history is important to establish relevant family history, preceding history of infection, injury, pruritus, inflammation, exposure to toxins, as well as associated other comorbidities. (Please refer to Chap. 1 of this book for a comprehensive classification of pigmentary disorders.)

The differential diagnosis for guttate leukoderma is vast ranging from inherited to acquired disorders, while idiopathic guttate hypomelanosis (IGH) is the commonest. This chapter mainly focuses on IGH with brief descriptions of other important guttate hypomelanoses (Table 11.1).

N. M. Nagodavithana (✉)
Department of Dermatology, Sir Charles Gairdner Hospital, Nedlands, WA, Australia

P. Kumarasinghe
Department of Dermatology, Fiona Stanley Hospital and University of Western Australia, Perth, WA, Australia

Idiopathic Guttate Hypomelanosis (IGH)

IGH is a benign acquired hypopigmentary disorder characterized by multiple discrete hypopigmented and porcelain-white macules commonly distributed over extensor limbs. Typically they occur in older age, and postulated pathophysiological mechanisms include UV radiation, hereditary factors, aging, trauma, autoimmunity, and melanocyte inhibition.

Few researchers have delineated clinical, dermoscopic, histopathologic and ultrastructural findings of this entity. IGH can be of great cosmetic concern for patients with darker skin. The treatment is very challenging, particularly when they are numerous. Current treatment options include cryotherapy, topical retinoids, topical calcineurin inhibitors, intralesional steroids, chemical peeling, dermabrasion, fractional CO_2 laser, non-ablasive photothermolysis, and skin grafting.

Epidemiology

Cumming and Cotel first introduced the term "idiopathic guttate hypomelanosis" in 1966 [1]. However, Costa was the first to report a similar entity under "symmetrical progressive leukopathy" in 1951 [2]. "Angular depigmented macules" and "senile depigmented (hypopigmented)

© Springer International Publishing AG, part of Springer Nature 2018
P. Kumarasinghe (ed.), *Pigmentary Skin Disorders*, Updates in Clinical Dermatology,
https://doi.org/10.1007/978-3-319-70419-7_11

Table 11.1 Differential diagnosis for guttate leukoderma (guttate hypochromia)

Conditions with textural change	Conditions without textural change
Achromic verruca plana	Bier's spots (psuedoleukoderma angiospasticum)
Clear cell papulosis	Chronic arsenic poisoning
Cutaneous papular mucinosis	Cole disease
Epidermodysplasia verruciformis – pityriasis versicolor-like lesions	Confetti-like lesions in tuberous sclerosis
Hypopigmented mycosis fungoides	Darier's disease
Lymphomatoid papulosis	Generalized Dowling Degos disease
Sarcoidosis	Dyschromatosis symmterica hereditaria
Tumor of follicular infundibulum	Dyschromatosis universalis hereditaria
White fibrous papulosis	Dyschromic amyloidosis
	Exogenous ochronosis
	Familial white lentiginosis
	Grover's disease
	Idiopathic guttate hypomelanosis
	Lichen sclerosus et atrophicus
	Multiple halo nevi
	Pityriasis alba
	Pityriasis lichenoides chronica
	Pityriasis versicolor
	Post-inflammatory hypopigmentation
	Progressive macular hypomelanosis
	Vitiligo ponctue
	Xeroderma pigmentosum

spots" described by Whitehead and Hamada et al. respectively resemble IGH closely and possibly the same entity [3, 4].

The earliest reported incidence of IGH varies from 47% [1] to 68% [3]. Shin et al. in 2011 reported a prevalence of 55% in a sample of 1174 dermatology outpatients [5]. The same study revealed almost a similar prevalence of the disease among females and males: 56% and 54%, respectively. Earlier studies have revealed a slightly high female preponderance [6].

IGH is seen more commonly on aging skin, with a prevalence of 87% among the subjects over 40 years [5]. However, the earliest onset reported has been at 3 years [7].

Falabella reported a familial aggregation, suggesting a genetic basis for the disease [6]. HLA-DQ3 has been associated with IGH in a group of renal transplant patients [8].

Clinical Features

IGH presents as discrete sharply demarcated macules with variable pigment loss ranging from 0.2 to 2 cm [1]. Shin et al. found the established lesions can grow in size, contrary to previous reports [5]. Lesion number can vary from 1 to 134 [5] (Fig 11.1a).

Lesion distribution favors sun-exposed areas, distal legs being the most commonly affected, closely followed by distal upper extremities. The face and neck are the least commonly involved sites. Some authors have noted a tendency for women to develop lesions over the anterior lower legs, while men develop lesions more on upper limbs [9].

Kumarasinghe has described four clinical types of IGH [10]:

1. Multiple hypopigmented or porcelain-white lesions on sun-damaged skin (geronto-actinic)
2. Solitary or multiple porcelain-white lesions irrespective of areas of sun damage (non-actinic)
3. Relatively smaller punctate leukoderma-like lesions with or without a history of ultraviolet treatment for other conditions (punctate)
4. Hypopigmented macules with a thin keratinous layer on top (hyperkeratotic) (Fig. 11.1b)

Etiology and Pathogenesis

IGH is probably a multifactorial disease. So far, senile degeneration, chronic UV exposure,

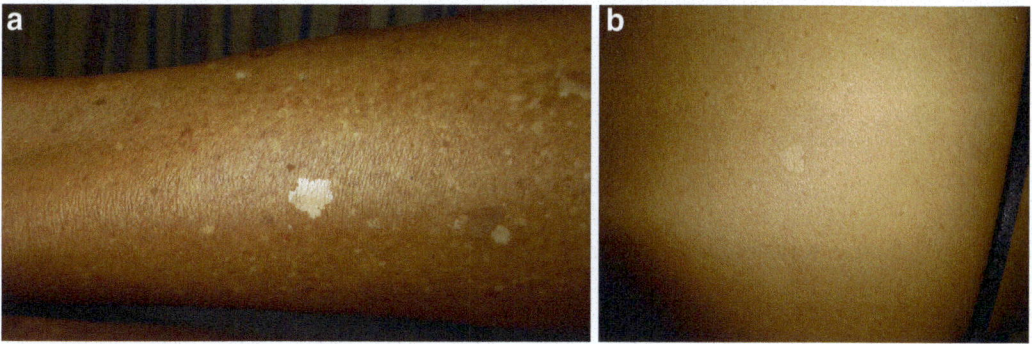

Fig. 11.1 (**a**) IGH lesions on a lower leg of a Sri Lankan female (**b**) An IGH lesion with a keratotic top, in a Sri Lankan woman (Photographs courtesy: Dr. Chamila Ariyaratne)

genetics, trauma, autoimmunity, and local inhibition of melanogenesis have been implicated [11].

Dermoscopy

Bambroo et al. appreciated four patterns in dermoscopy of IGH, namely, nebuloid, petalloid, feathery, and amoeboid [12]. Nebuloid pattern of IGH was observed in lesions of recent onset and also among older patients. Feathery, amoeboid, and petalloid patterns were more commonly seen in older lesions of IGH [13].

Pathology

Histopathology of IGH lesions has revealed changes in both pigmentary and epidermal changes. Amount of melanin in the basal layer is significantly decreased in IGH, while the melanocytes are smaller, less in number, and weaker in Dopa reaction [4]. Skip areas of retained melanin in a flat depigmented epidermis have been proposed as a clue to the diagnosis by Joshi et al. in 2014 [14].

When the lesional skin was compared with adjacent perilesional normal skin, hyperkeratosis, flattened rete ridges, epidermal atrophy, and acanthosis have been observed [6].

Epidermal atrophy was more significant in sun-exposed areas compared to non-sun-exposed areas.

Electron Microscopy

Melanocyte number is reduced in lesional skin, while the residual melanocytes show degenerative changes with decreased number of melanosomes. However, a recent study failed to demonstrate any structural changes to melanocytes and melanosomes, while some areas showed reduced uptake of melanosomes by keratinocytes suggesting a functional defect in transfer of melanosomes from melanocytes to keratinocytes [7, 15, 16].

Culture of IGH Melanocytes

In an ongoing collaborative study, Parsad, Kumarasinghe, and Kumar et al. have shown that IGH melanocytes can produce melanin on cell culture, but they express more senescence markers such as p21, Ki67, and SAHF than controls (unpublished data).

Treatment

Despite being a benign asymptomatic dermatosis, many patients seek medical attention to exclude vitiligo and due to cosmetic disfigurement. However, once they are reassured about the benign nature of the condition and vitiligo has been excluded, most patients do not insist on treatment. Counseling together with treatment of lesions for 3 months has shown significant improvement of DLQI in a group of Indian patients with IGH [17].

Various medical and surgical treatment options are available for IGH with varying degrees of success.

Topical retinoids have been claimed to show a greater response rate of repigmentation [18], followed by 1% pimecrolimus cream (75%) [19], 88% phenol peeling (64%) [20], and monthly intralesional steroids (47%) [6] in individual studies. 0.1% tacrolimus cream has shown a low response rate of 11% [21]. A recent study using 88% phenol spot peeling followed by regular local application of placental extract failed to demonstrate a significant benefit than phenol alone [22].

Cryotherapy is reported to be effective in IGH [23, 24]. We find that a single 3–5 s short burst is sufficient, particularly discrete lesions [23]. The other surgical modalities described are single application of 10s cryoprobe (91% showed repigmentation) [24], single session of dermabrasion (80% success rate) [25], single session of fractional CO_2 laser (43–48% showed >75% improvement) [26], and fractional 1550 nm ytterbium/erbium laser (60% showing >50% improvement) [27]. In our experience topical tretinoin is not very effective in treatment of IGH. A recent pilot study on six patients has shown excimer laser is another safe and effective treatment for IGH [28]. Normal autologous skin graft on depigmented lesions showed only a minimal response [6].

Overall, it appears that IGH lesions resist pigmentation by the surrounding active melanocytes by an active pigment inhibitory mechanism [23]. Removal of the epidermis of the IGH lesions in some form appears to remove or minimize that inhibitory effect, facilitating repigmentation [10].

Darier's Disease (DD)

In addition to the classic clinical features of Darier's disease, guttate leukoderma is seen over the abdomen, trunk, limbs, hands, and feet on patients with pigmented skin. Its course is stable over time (Fig. 11.2).

Various hypotheses have been proposed regarding the pathogenesis of these macules including impaired melanin transfer, melanocytic apoptosis due to perturbed cell-cell adhesion and occurring as a subclinical form of brown papules as well as post-inflammatory [29–33].

Acantholysis and dyskeratosis due to DD, low melanin levels, and reduced melanocyte number are the most frequently reported histological features [34].

Familial White Lentiginosis

This is a relatively newly described entity with only four cases described so far [35–37]. It is clinically characterized by lenticular white macules occurring most frequently in dark-colored individuals of phototype IV–V with a typical distribution on the trunk, décolleté, neck, and hands and on the extensor surface of the upper arms. It is an acquired disorder with a chronic course and characterized by peculiar histopathologic features of lentiginous epidermal hyperplasia with elongated club-shaped rete ridges and an unusual loss of pigmentation. An autosomal dominant or X-linked inheritance is speculated.

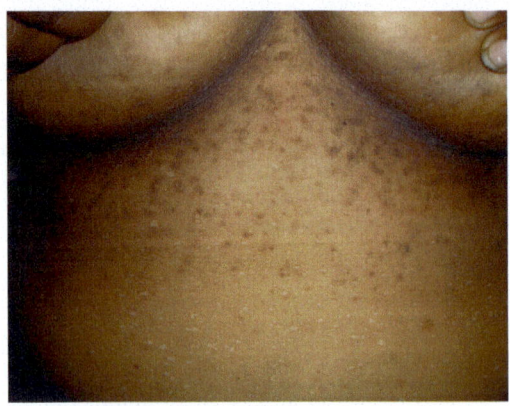

Fig. 11.2 Guttate leukoderma on the abdomen of a Sri Lankan patient with Darier's disease

Cole Disease

Cole disease is a rare autosomal dominant geno-dermatosis characterized by congenital or early-onset punctate keratoderma associated with irregularly shaped hypopigmented macules, which are typically found over the arms and legs, but not the trunk or acral regions.

Hypopigmented areas of the skin demonstrate hyperkeratosis and normal melanocyte density with a reduction in melanin content in keratino-cytes, but not in melanocytes. The ultrastructural changes of melanocytes showing a dispropor-tionately large number of melanosomes in the cytoplasm and dendrites but that keratinocytes showing a paucity of these organelles suggest a defect in melanin transfer [38–41].

Mutations in ENPP1, encoding ectonucleotide pyrophosphatase/phosphodiesterase 1, have been implicated [42, 43].

Clear Cell Papulosis

This relatively recently described entity is char-acterized by asymptomatic hypopigmented mac-ules or flat-topped papules distributed mainly on the lower aspect of the abdomen or along the milk lines in young children [44, 45]. The num-ber of skin lesions increases over the first few months or years. Thus, there may be numerous lesions by the time of diagnosis. Clear cell papu-losis is more common among the Oriental ethnic groups. Histopathologically, clear cells with a benign appearance are scattered among basal keratinocytes. Clear cells are mucin stain positive and S100 negative. They also often stain positive with carcinoembryonic antigen, AE 1 + 3, epithe-lial membrane antigen, cell adhesion molecule 5.2, gross cystic disease fluid protein (GCDFP-15), and cytokeratin 7 [46, 47].

Usually no treatment is required. With a median follow-up duration of 11.5 years, regres-sion of skin lesions was observed in 85.7% of patients by Tseng et al. [48].

Lichen Sclerosus et Atrophicus (LSA)

Guttate leukoderma in LSA presents as small, ivory, or porcelain-white, shiny, round macules or papules, a few millimeters in diameter. However, occasionally, they are semitranslucent and resemble mother of pearl. They may be very extensive, involving most of the trunk. Lesions may follow Blaschko's lines [49] (Fig. 11.3).

Tumor of Follicular Infundibulum (TFI)

TFI are benign adnexal tumors that can present as common solitary form or rare eruptive form. The solitary form does not show any distinctive clini-cal features and frequently misdiagnosed as seb-orrhoeic keratosis or basal cell carcinoma [50]. However, the eruptive form has been described in most reports as symmetrically distributed tumors of variable scaling, hypopigmented mac-ules, and papules with irregular or angulated borders confined to the face, neck, and upper trunk [51]. Rarely, the tumors occur on the extremities and buttocks.

Histology shows platelike anastomosing cords of cytologically bland, pale, squamoid, and basa-loid epithelium extending from the undersurface

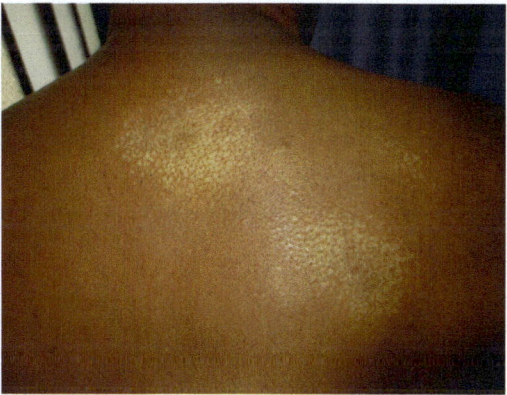

Fig. 11.3 Lichen sclerosus on the back of a Sri Lankan male

of the epidermis. The bulk of the tumor cells show isthmic differentiation. Decreased melanin pigmentation in the tumor cells seen in eruptive form [51]. TFI also shows a unique brush-like network of elastin fibers when stained for elastin fibers.

Chronic Arsenic Poisoning

The earliest symptoms of chronic arsenic toxicity are the pigmentary changes and the palmar plantar keratosis. Generally, the pigmentary changes start as finely freckled hyperpigmentation and hypopigmentation of the upper chest, arms, and legs described as "raindrops on a dusty road." More specifically, this raindrop pattern consists of less pigmented, round spots that are several millimeters in diameter on a background of diffuse hyperpigmentation [52]. Patients with chronic arsenic poisoning may also develop multiple malignancies especially squamous cell carcinoma (Fig. 11.4).

Furthermore, Unicef Endemic Arsenicosis Diagnostic Manual has graded the degree of hypopigmentation (as well as hyperpigmentation and hyperkeratoses) in order to form clinical criteria for diagnosis of arsenicosis [53].

Grade I
Hypopigmentation that appears on unexposed areas of the body, mainly on the trunk, as symmetrically scattered pale spots the size of pinheads

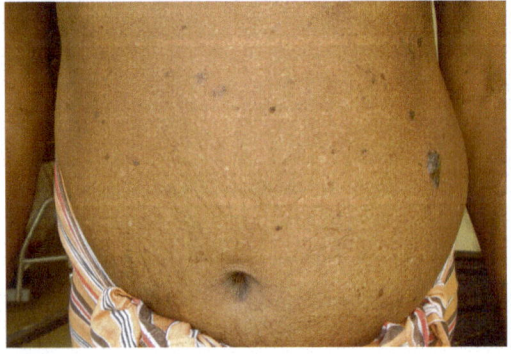

Fig. 11.4 Guttate leukoderma due to chronic arsenic poisoning in a Sri Lankan male

Grade II
Hypopigmentation that is accentuated on unexposed areas of the body, mainly on the trunk, as hypopigmented spots
Grade III
Hypopigmentation that occurs on unexposed areas of the body, mainly on the trunk, in an extensive and confluent manner

Tuberous Sclerosis (TSC)

Hypomelanotic macules are the commonest and earliest cutaneous finding in TSC, often presenting at birth or in infancy. Although the classic presentation is that of an "ash-leaf spot" with a lanceolate shape, they may take on several different forms, including polygonal or round to oval "thumb print" macules.

"Confetti skin lesions" present as a localized area of guttate, hypopigmented, small macules and are a minor criterion for the diagnosis of TSC [54]. The prevalence of confetti-like macules has varied widely among studies (2.8–58%) [55–58]. Clues to the diagnosis of confetti skin lesions include appearance in childhood, lack of scale or preceding rash, and asymmetric involvement [59].

Sarcoidosis

Hypopigmented macules are a very rare form of chronic cutaneous sarcoidosis [60]. Hypopigmented macules have been reported mostly in patients with darker skin [61]. Demonstration of granulomas on biopsy is more elusive in these macular lesions than in other cutaneous forms of sarcoidosis, so a high suspicion and repeat biopsies may aid the diagnosis [62].

Exogenous Ochronosis Secondary to Bleaching Agents

Classical features of exogenous ochronosis are asymptomatic blue-black macules with textural coarsening and sooty tipped papules on the malar area, temples, inferior cheeks, and neck reported mainly in Asian and African patients [63–66]. "Confetti-like" hypopigmented macules interspersed between pigmented macules have been reported in the literature, possibly a side effect from other coexisting bleaching agents such as phenolic or mercurial products in unapproved preparations [65].

Vitiligo Ponctue

Vitiligo ponctue is a rare, unusual variant of vitiligo that presents as discrete, confetti-like amelanotic macules that occur on normal or hyperpigmented skin. However, on its own, arguably, this may not be an actual type of vitiligo, but a form of punctate leukoderma. When punctate vitiligo coexists with classical vitiligo macules, it is best classified as nonsegmental vitiligo. Confetti-like depigmentation has also been reported after psoralen plus ultraviolet A (PUVA) therapy in patients with more classic vitiligo, as an adverse effect of PUVA therapy [67].

Pityriasis Alba

It is characterized by multiple ill-defined hypopigmented macules and patches (usually 0.5–2 cm in diameter) with fine scaling, typically located on the face but occasionally on the shoulders and arms. These lesions are most obvious in individuals with darkly pigmented skin and/or following sun exposure. Hypopigmentation is thought to result from a low-grade eczematous dermatitis that disrupts the transfer of melanosomes from melanocytes to keratinocytes. Similar hypopigmented lesions can appear upon resolution of more overtly inflamed, erythematous lesions of atopic dermatitis [68].

Pityriasis Versicolor

Proposed mechanisms for hypopigmentation in PV include [69]:

- Indole derivatives produced by *Malassezia furfur* – Malassezin

Malassezin was initially isolated from ethyl acetate extracts of *M. furfur* cultures [70].
Malassezin induces apoptosis of melanocytes and reduces biosynthesis of melanin.
Hypopigmentation seems to be enhanced by the inhibition of melanin transportation from melanocytes to keratinocytes due to the breakdown of the actin cytoskeleton [71].

- Pityriacitrin

It is proposed that fungal cells produce pityriacitrin as an agent that protects against UV light [72, 73]. Although the presence of pityriacitrin on human skin was initially proposed to convey UV protection to the hypopigmented lesions of pityriasis versicolor and prevent the skin from the development of sunburn [74], it was not confirmed by subsequent in vitro experiments [75], and the substances produced by *Malassezia* yeasts that protect against UV in vivo are still under investigation [69].

- Azelaic acid

Hypopigmentation in pityriasis versicolor is also attributed to competitive inhibition of tyrosinase activity by *Malassezia*-produced azelaic acid [76].

Progressive Macular Hypomelanosis

Progressive macular hypomelanosis (PMH) is characterized by ill-defined nummular, non-scaly hypopigmented asymptomatic spots on the trunk, often confluent in and around the midline, and rarely extending to the proximal extremities and the neck (Fig. 11.5).

Hypopigmentation in PMH has been linked to decreased production of melanosomes, transfer of less melanized melanosomes, and aggregated melanosomes instead of single melanosomes in lesional skin of type V and VI patients [77]. It is

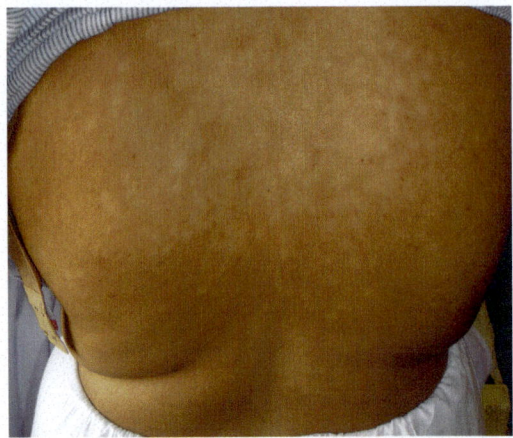

Fig. 11.5 Progressive macular hypomelanosis lesions on the back of a Sri Lankan young female

thought to be due to a subspecies of *Propionibacterium acnes*. Chapter 10 of this book gives further details of this condition.

Bier Spots (Psuedoleukoderma Angiospasticum)

These were first described by Bier in 1898 and represent a pattern of vascular mottling consisting of 3–6 mm white macular areas surrounded by a red to occasionally blue cyanotic background usually over arms and legs of young adults.

The causative mechanism leading to Bier spots is the exaggerated vasoconstrictive response of arterioles to tissue hypoxia. This could be induced by physiological venous stasis and the lack of venoarteriolar reflex in dermal ascending arterioles in response to venous filling, venous and lymphatic hypertension, or hyperviscosity [78].

Generalized Dowling Degos Disease

Classic Dowling Degos disease (DDD) is characterized by a triad of reticular pigmentation in the flexures, comedo-like lesions, and pitted acneiform scars.

Rarely, hypopigmented macules or papules resembling dychromatosis symmetrica hereditaria

(DSH) or dyschromatosis universalis hereditaria (DUH) have been reported [79–83]. Wu et al. described a family with autosomal dominant inheritance of a skin disorder with clinical features of both DDD and DUH, and they coined the term "generalized DDD." They also divided these disorders with overlapping features into two main groups [84].

The first is the DDD group, with reticulated pigmentation confined to flexural areas "classic DDD" or generalized with multiple hypopigmented macules and papules "generalized DDD." The characteristic histologic findings include increased pigmentation of the basal layer and finger-like rete ridges with thinning of the suprapapillary epithelium. This results in an "antler-like" pattern arising from the under surface of the epidermis and hair follicles [85]. The hypopigmented lesions show elongation of rete ridges, basal hypopigmentation with pigment in the tip of rete ridges [84].

The second major group is dyschromatosis, including DUH and DSH. Clinically, both have hyperpigmented and hypopigmented lesions and histopathologic findings that are similar to each other but that differ from the DDD group. The histopathologic findings in hypopigmented DSH and DUH macules are of normal skin structure aside from the hypopigmentation.

Dyschromic Amyloidosis

A rare variant of cutaneous amyloidosis, amyloidosis cutis dyschromica, is characterized by (i) dotted, reticular hyperpigmentation with hypopigmented macules distributed extensively, (ii) no or little itch, (iii) onset before puberty, and (iv) focal subepidermal amyloid deposition [86].

Ho et al. reported three cases of primary cutaneous amyloidosis with hypopigmentation as a predominant feature with or without reticular hyperpigmentation, no itching, adult onset, and dermal papillary amyloid deposition [87].

The mechanism for hypopigmentation could be pigmentary incontinence rather than the amyloid deposition [88].

Dyschromatosis Symmetrica Hereditaria (DSH)

DSH is an autosomal dominant disorder characterized by early-onset hypo- and hypopigmented macules over the dorsal aspects of extremities sparing palm, soles, and mucous membrane [85]. It is due to a mutation in the DSRAD (double-stranded RNA-specific adenosine deaminase) gene on chromosome 1q21.

Dyschromatosis Universalis Hereditaria (DUH)

DUH is a rare autosomal dominant or recessive disorder that presents with widespread hypo- and hyperpigmented macules involving the head, neck, trunk, and limbs including extremities [85]. They can involve palms and soles but spare mucous membranes. Over 80% of DUH patients develop dyschromia by 6 years of age, and approximately 20% have dyspigmentation at birth. The relationship to DSH is unclear [85].

The histopathology of hypopigmented macules reveal decreased melanin content in the basal layer [89].

Xeroderma Pigmentosum (XP)

XP is a rare autosomal recessive disease characterized by photosensitivity, pigmentary changes, premature skin aging, neoplasia, and abnormal DNA repair. Some patients with XP also have neurological complications [90]. Hypopigmented lesions in XP manifest as small, round or irregular, white, atrophic macules following either crusted vesiculobullous lesions or independently [91]. Photoprotection and surveillance for skin malignancies is very important in patients with XP.

Epidermodysplasia Verruciformis (EV)

EV is a rare genetic disorder that leads to increased susceptibility to cutaneous infections with HPV types in the genus β [92]. It is characterized by polymorphic skin lesions that include widespread, discrete, or confluent papules that resemble flat warts and scaly, pinkish, or hypopigmented guttate macules and thin plaques that resemble pityriasis versicolor. In addition seborrhoeic keratosis-like lesions and premalignant lesions like actinic keratoses that may slowly transform into invasive squamous cell carcinomas develop over the photo-exposed areas.

White Fibrous Papulosis (WFP)

WFP is characterized by multiple, confluent, 2–3-mm-sized, well-demarcated, smooth-topped, ivory-colored non-follicular papules on the neck and back [93]. It is a disease of the elderly, and these changes have been attributed to aging or photoaging. Clinical similarities exist between WFP and a number of dermatological conditions such as pseudoxanthoma elasticum-like papillary dermal elastosis and mid-dermal elastosis, but can be differentiated histologically by intact elastic fibers and focal increase of collagen in the mid-reticular dermis in the former.

Cutaneous Papular Mucinosis

This localized form of mucinosis presents with small, firm, waxy, ivory-or flesh-colored papules (or nodules and plaques produced by the confluence of papules) confined to few sites only (usually upper and lower limbs and trunk). This entity has been further divided into five subtypes: a discrete form, acral persistent papular mucinosis, self-healing papular mucinosis, papular mucinosis of infancy, and a pure nodular form [94].

Histopathologic examination reveals mucin deposition with variable fibroblast proliferation.

Leukoderma Acquisitum Centrifugum (Halo Nevi)

This refers to development of a halo of hypomelanosis around a central cutaneous tumor. This tumor is usually a benign melanocytic nevus but may be a neuroid nevus, a blue nevus, a neurofibroma, or a primary or secondary malignant melanoma [95]. Halo phenomenon commonly occurs in children and young adults and often on the back of the trunk. Halos can occur around multiple lesions either simultaneously or at intervals, involving many but not all nevi. These range from 0.5 to 1.0 cm in width [96]. Following the appearance of the halo, the central melanocytic lesion disappears gradually, and the remaining hypopigmented macule may persist for years before it gets repigmented (Fig. 11.6).

Hypopigmented Mycosis Fungoides (MF)

Hypopigmented mycosis fungoides presents asymptomatic or slightly pruritic ill-demarcated macules and patches with a centripetal distribution more frequently in patients with dark skin [97]. It presents at a younger age than classical MF (Fig. 11.7).

Pityriasis Lichenoides Chronica (PLC)

PLC presents as erythematous, brownish lichenoid papules with adherent "mica-like" scale that resolve with hypopigmented macules mainly over the trunk and the proximal limbs. Sometimes, these hypopigmented macules are the presenting complaint [98] (Fig. 11.8).

In summary, guttate leukoderma encompass a wide range of differential diagnoses ranging from idiopathic to infections to malignancy. It can cause considerable distress and anxiety in many patients however benign, especially in pigmented ethnic groups. A careful history and a thorough examination, appropriately complemented by microbiology/histopathology/immunohistochemistry, will aid the diagnosis in many cases.

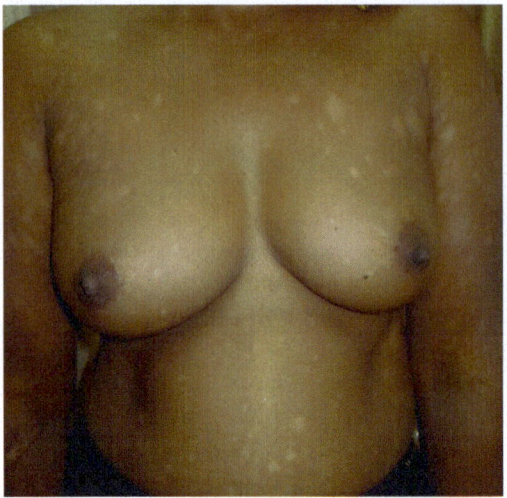

Fig. 11.7 Hypopigmented MF in a Sri Lankan female

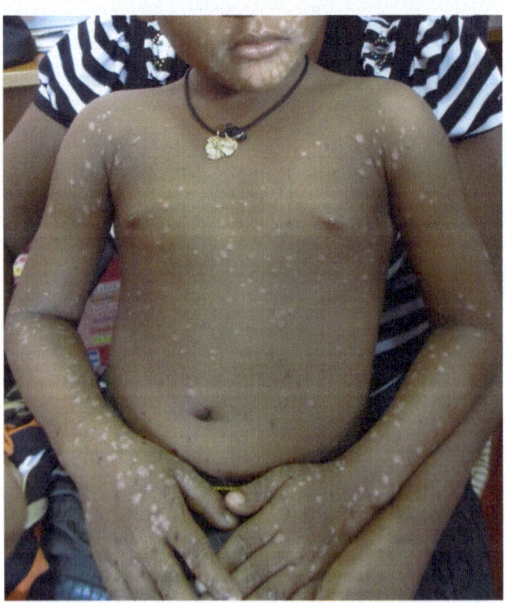

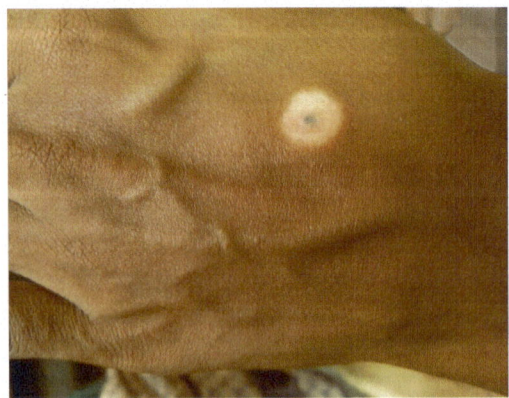

Fig. 11.6 Halo nevus

Fig. 11.8 PLC in a Sri Lankan boy

References

1. Cummings KI, Cottel WI. Idiopathic guttate hypomelanosis. Arch Dermatol. 1966;93(2):184–6.
2. Costa OG. Progressive symmetrical leukopathia of the extremities. Ann Dermatol Syphiligr (Paris). 1951;78(4):452–4.
3. Whitehead WJ, Moyer DG, Vander Ploeg DE. Idiopathic guttate hypomelanosis. Arch Dermatol. 1966;94(3):279–81.
4. Hamada T, Saito T. Senile depigmented spots (idiopathic guttate hypomelanosis) . Arch Dermatol. 1967;95(665).
5. Shin MK, Jeong KH, Oh IH, Choe BK, Lee MH. Clinical features of idiopathic guttate hypomelanosis in 646 subjects and association with other aspects of photoaging. Int J Dermatol. 2011;50(7):798–805.
6. Falabella R, Escobar C, Giraldo N, Rovetto P, Gil J, Barona MI, et al. On the pathogenesis of idiopathic guttate hypomelanosis. J Am Acad Dermatol. 1987;16(1 Pt 1):35–44.
7. Kim SK, Kim EH, Kang HY, Lee ES, Sohn S, Kim YC. Comprehensive understanding of idiopathic guttate hypomelanosis: clinical and histopathological correlation. Int J Dermatol. 2010;49(2):162–6.
8. Arrunategui A, Trujillo RA, Marulanda MP, Sandoval F, Wagner A, Alzate A, et al. HLA-DQ3 is associated with idiopathic guttate hypomelanosis, whereas HLA-DR8 is not, in a group of renal transplant patients. Int J Dermatol. 2002;41(11):744–7.
9. McDaniel WE, Richfield DF. Macular hypopigmentation on legs of women. Dermatol Digest. 1965;4:59–66.
10. Kumarasinghe P. Idiopathic guttate hypomelanosis. In: Dermatological cryosurgery and cryotherapy. London: Springer; 2016. p. 407–11.
11. Juntongjin P, Laosakul K. Idiopathic guttate hypomelanosis: a review of its etiology, pathogenesis, findings, and treatments. Am J Clin Dermatol. 2016;17(4):403–11.
12. Bambroo MP, Pande S, Khopkar U. Dermoscopy in the differentiation of idiopathic guttate hypomelanosis (IGH) and Guttate vitiligo. In: Khopkar S, editor. Dermoscopy and trichoscopy in diseases of the brown skin atlas and short text. 1st ed. New Delhi: Jaypee Brothers Ltd; 2012. p. 97–103.
13. Ankad BS, Beergouder SL. Dermoscopic evaluation of idiopathic guttate hypomelanosis: a preliminary observation. Indian Dermatol Online J. 2015;6(3):164–7.
14. Joshi R. Skip areas of retained melanin: a clue to the histopathological diagnosis of idiopathic guttate hypomelanosis. Indian J Dermatol. 2014;59(6):571–4.
15. Wilson PD, Lavker RM, Kligman AM. On the nature of idiopathic guttate hypomelanosis. Acta Derm Venereol. 1982;62(4):301–6.
16. Kakepis M, Havaki S, Katoulis A, Katsambas A, Stavrianeas N, Troupis TG. Idiopathic guttate hypomelanosis: an electron microscopy study. J Eur Acad Dermatol Venereol. 2015;29(7):1435–8.
17. Joshipura S, editor. Idiopathic guttate hypopigmentation. 45th national conference of Indian Association of Dermatologists, Venereologists & Leprologists, DERMACON 2017, 12–15 Jan 2017, Kolkata, India.
18. Pagnoni A, Kligman AM, Sadiq I, Stoudemayer T. Hypopigmented macules of photodamaged skin and their treatment with topical tretinoin. Acta Derm Venereol Stockholm. 1999;79:305–10.
19. Asawanonda P, Sutthipong T, Prejawai N. Pimecrolimus for idiopathic guttate hypomelanosis. J Drugs Dermatol. 2010;9(3):238–9.
20. Ravikiran SP, Sacchidanand S, Leelavathy B. Therapeutic wounding – 88% phenol in idiopathic guttate hypomelanosis. Indian Dermatol Online J. 2014;5(1):14–8.
21. Rerknimitr P, Disphanurat W, Achariyakul M. Topical tacrolimus significantly promotes repigmentation in idiopathic guttate hypomelanosis: a double-blind, randomized, placebo-controlled study. J Eur Acad Dermatol Venereol. 2013;27(4):460–4.
22. Gupta K, Tripathi S, Kaur M. Evaluation of placental extracts as an adjuvant therapy to phenol in treatment of idiopathic guttate hypomelanosis. J Clin Diagn Res. 2016;10(8):WC01.
23. Kumarasinghe SP. 3-5 second cryotherapy is effective in idiopathic guttate hypomelanosis. J Dermatol. 2004;31(5):437–9.
24. Ploysangam T, Dee-Ananlap S, Suvanprakorn P. Treatment of idiopathic guttate hypomelanosis with liquid nitrogen: light and electron microscopic studies. J Am Acad Dermatol. 1990;23(4 Pt 1):681–4.
25. Hexsel DM. Treatment of idiopathic guttate hypomelanosis by localized superficial dermabrasion. Dermatol Surg. 1999;25(11):917–8.
26. Shin J, Kim M, Park SH, Oh SH. The effect of fractional carbon dioxide lasers on idiopathic guttate hypomelanosis: a preliminary study. J Eur Acad Dermatol Venereol. 2013;27(2):e243–6.
27. Rerknimitr P, Chitvanich S, Pongprutthipan M, Panchaprateep R, Asawanonda P. Non-ablative fractional photothermolysis in treatment of idiopathic guttate hypomelanosis. J Eur Acad Dermatol Venereol. 2015;29(11):2238–42.
28. Gordon JR, Reed KE, Sebastian KR, Ahmed AM. Excimer light treatment for idiopathic guttate hypomelanosis: a pilot study. Dermatol Surg. 2017;43(4):553–7.
29. Cattano AN. An unusual case of keratosis follicularis. Arch Dermatol. 1968;98(2):168–74.
30. Berth-Jones J, Hutchinson P. Darier's disease with peri-follicular depigmentation. Br J Dermatol. 1989;120(6):827–30.
31. Hakuno M, Shimizu H, Akiyama M, Amagai M, Wahl J, Wheelock M, et al. Dissociation of intra-and extracellular domains of desmosomal cadherins and E-cadherin in Hailey–Hailey disease and Darier's disease. Br J Dermatol. 2000;142(4):702–11.

32. Goh B, Kumarasinghe S, Ng S. Two Singaporean cases of guttate leucoderma in Darier's disease. Clin Exp Dermatol. 2004;29(3):313–4.
33. Goh B, Kumarasinghe P, Lee Y. Loss of melanosome transfer accounts for guttate leucoderma in Darier's disease. Pigment Cell Res. 2005;18:48.
34. Terrom M, Dhaille F, Baltazard T, Dadban A, Sevestre H, Lok C, et al. Guttate leukoderma in Darier disease: case report and review. J Eur Acad Dermatol Venereol. 2016;30(12):e205–e9.
35. Grosshans E, Sengel D, Heid E. White lentiginosis. Annales de dermatologie et de venereologie. 1994;121(1):7–10.
36. Moulinas C, Banea S, De Cambourg G, Bochaton H, Tortel M, Cribier B, et al. A second case of white lentiginosis. Annales de dermatologie et de venereologie. 2015;142(4):281–4.
37. Neri I, Bassi A, Misciali C, Bagni A, Patrizi A. Familial white lentiginosis. British Journal of Dermatology. 2017;177(2):535–7.
38. Cole LA. Hypopigmentation with punctate keratosis of the palms and soles. Arch Dermatol. 1976;112(7):998–1000.
39. Moore MM, Orlow SJ, Kamino H, Wang N, Schaffer JV. Cole disease: guttate hypopigmentation and punctate palmoplantar keratoderma. Arch Dermatol. 2009;145(4):495–7.
40. Schmieder A, Hausser I, Schneider SW, Goerdt S, Peitsch WK. Palmoplantar hyperkeratoses and hypopigmentation. Cole disease. Acta Derm Venereol. 2011;91(6):737–8.
41. Vignale R, Yusin A, Panuncio A, Abulafia J, Reyno Z, Vaglio A. Cole disease: hypopigmentation with punctate keratosis of the palms and soles. Pediatr Dermatol. 2002;19(4):302–6.
42. Goldfine ID, Maddux BA, Youngren JF, Reaven G, Accili D, Trischitta V, et al. The role of membrane glycoprotein plasma cell antigen 1/ectonucleotide pyrophosphatase phosphodiesterase 1 in the pathogenesis of insulin resistance and related abnormalities. Endocr Rev. 2008;29(1):62–75.
43. Eytan O, Morice-Picard F, Sarig O, Ezzedine K, Isakov O, Li Q, et al. Cole disease results from mutations in ENPP1. Am J Hum Genet. 2013;93(4):752–7.
44. Wysong A, Sundram U, Benjamin L. Clear-cell papulosis: a rare entity that may be misconstrued pathologically as normal skin. Pediatr Dermatol. 2012;29(2):195–8.
45. Kuo TT, Chan HL, Hsueh S. Clear cell papulosis of the skin. A new entity with histogenetic implications for cutaneous Paget's disease. Am J Surg Pathol. 1987;11(11):827–34.
46. Kumarasinghe SPW, Chin GY, Kumarasinghe MP. Clear cell papulosis of the skin: a case report from Singapore. Arch Pathol Lab Med. 2004;128(11):e149–e52.
47. Kuo T-T, Huang C-L, Chan H-L, Yang L-J, Chen M-J. Clear cell papulosis: report of three cases of a newly recognized disease. J Am Acad Dermatol. 1995;33(2):230–3.
48. Tseng FW, Kuo TT, Lu PH, Chan HL, Chan MJ, Hui RC. Long-term follow-up study of clear cell papulosis. J Am Acad Dermatol. 2010;63(2):266–73.
49. Goodfield M, Jones S, Veale D. The 'connective tissue diseases'. In: Burns T, Breathnach S, Cox N, Griffiths C, editors. Rook's textbook of dermatology, vol. 3. 8th ed. Hoboken: Wiley-Blackwell; 2010. p. 51.112–51.8.
50. Suchonwanit P, Ruangchainikom P, Apibal Y. Eruptive tumors of the follicular infundibulum: an unexpected diagnosis of Hypopigmented macules. Dermatol Ther (Heidelb). 2015;5(3):207–11.
51. Alomari A, Subtil A, Owen CE, McNiff JM. Solitary and multiple tumors of follicular infundibulum: a review of 168 cases with emphasis on staining patterns and clinical variants. J Cutan Pathol. 2013;40(6):532–7.
52. Matveev N, Kile M. Pigmentation changes resulting from chronic arsenic exposure. In: Zhai H, Wilhelm K, Maibach H, editors. Marzulli and Maibach's dermatotoxicology. 7th ed. Boca Raton: CRC Press/ Taylor and Francis Group; 2008. p. 873–80.
53. Guifan S, Jiayi L, Luong T, Dianjun S, Liying W. In: Guifan S, editor. Endemic arsenicosis: A clinical diagnostic manual with photo illustrations. UNICEF East Asia and Pacific Regional Office: Bangkok; 2004. 59 p.
54. Northrup H, Krueger DA, Group ITSCC. Tuberous sclerosis complex diagnostic criteria update: recommendations of the 2012 international tuberous sclerosis complex consensus conference. Key Points of the Chinese Guidelines for Clinical Diagnostic of arsenicosis. Pediatr Neurol. 2013;49(4):243–54.
55. Jozwiak S, Schwartz RA, Janniger CK, Michałowicz R, Chmielik J. Skin lesions in children with tuberous sclerosis complex: their prevalence, natural course, and diagnostic significance. Int J Dermatol. 1998;37(12):911–7.
56. Webb D, Carke A, Fyer A, Osborne J. The cutaneous features of tuberous sclerosis: a population study. Br J Dermatol. 1996;135(1):1–5.
57. Au KS, Williams AT, Roach ES, Batchelor L, Sparagana SP, Delgado MR, et al. Genotype/phenotype correlation in 325 individuals referred for a diagnosis of tuberous sclerosis complex in the United States. Genet Med. 2007;9(2):88–100.
58. Seibert D, Hong C-H, Takeuchi F, Olsen C, Hathaway O, Moss J, et al. Recognition of tuberous sclerosis in adult women: delayed presentation with life-threatening consequences. Ann Intern Med. 2011;154(12):806–13.
59. Jacks SK, Witman PM. Tuberous sclerosis complex: an update for dermatologists. Pediatr Dermatol. 2015;32(5):563–70.
60. Marchell RM, Judson MA. Chronic cutaneous lesions of sarcoidosis. Clin Dermatol. 2007;25(3):295–302.

61. Thomas RH, McKee PH, Black MM. Hypopigmented sarcoidosis. J R Soc Med. 1981;74(12):921–3.
62. Hall RS, Floro JF, King LE Jr. Hypopigmented lesions in sarcoidosis. J Am Acad Dermatol. 1984;11(6):1163–4.
63. Tan SK, Sim CS, Goh CL. Hydroquinone-induced exogenous ochronosis in Chinese – two case reports and a review. Int J Dermatol. 2008;47(6):639–40.
64. Tan SK. Exogenous ochronosis in ethnic Chinese Asians: a clinicopathological study, diagnosis and treatment. J Eur Acad Dermatol Venereol. 2011;25(7):842–50.
65. Liu WC, Tey HL, Lee JS, Goh BK. Exogenous ochronosis in a Chinese patient: use of dermoscopy aids early diagnosis and selection of biopsy site. Singap Med J. 2014;55(1):e1–3.
66. Simmons BJ, Griffith RD, Bray FN, Falto-Aizpurua LA, Nouri K. Exogenous ochronosis: a comprehensive review of the diagnosis, epidemiology, causes, and treatments. Am J Clin Dermatol. 2015;16(3):205–12.
67. Arunprasath P, Reji S, Srivenkateswaran K. Vitiligo ponctue. Pigment Int. 2015;2(2):103.
68. Bieber T, Bussmann C. Atopic Dermatitis. In: Bolognia J, Joseph L, Shaffer J, editors. Dermatology. 1. 3 ed: Elsevier Saunders; 2012. p. 203–17.
69. Gaitanis G, Magiatis P, Hantschke M, Bassukas ID, Velegraki A. The Malassezia genus in skin and systemic diseases. Elsevier Saunders, Philadelphia. Clin Microbiol Rev. 2012;25(1):106–41.
70. Wille G, Mayser P, Thoma W, Monsees T, Baumgart A, Schmitz HJ, et al. Malassezin – a novel agonist of the arylhydrocarbon receptor from the yeast Malassezia furfur. Bioorg Med Chem. 2001;9(4):955–60.
71. Kramer HJ, Kessler D, Hipler UC, Irlinger B, Hort W, Bodeker RH, et al. Pityriarubins, novel highly selective inhibitors of respiratory burst from cultures of the yeast Malassezia furfur: comparison with the bisindolylmaleimide arcyriarubin A. Chembiochem. 2005;6(12):2290–7.
72. Machowinski A, Kramer HJ, Hort W, Mayser P. Pityriacitrin – a potent UV filter produced by Malassezia furfur and its effect on human skin microflora. Mycoses. 2006;49(5):388–92.
73. Mayser P, Schafer U, Kramer HJ, Irlinger B, Steglich W. Pityriacitrin – an ultraviolet-absorbing indole alkaloid from the yeast Malassezia furfur. Arch Dermatol Res. 2002;294(3):131–4.
74. Larangeira de Almeida H, Mayser P. Absence of sunburn in lesions of pityriasis versicolor alba. Mycoses. 2006;49(6):516.
75. Gambichler T, Kramer HJ, Boms S, Skrygan M, Tomi NS, Altmeyer P, et al. Quantification of ultraviolet protective effects of pityriacitrin in humans. Arch Dermatol Res. 2007;299(10):517–20.
76. Nazzaro-Porro M, Passi S. Identification of tyrosinase inhibitors in cultures of Pityrosporum. J Invest Dermatol. 1978;71(3):205–8.
77. Relyveld GN, Menke HE, Westerhof W. Progressive macular hypomelanosis. Am J Clin Dermatol. 2007;8(1):13–9.
78. Bessis D, Jeziorski É, Rigau V, Pralong P, Pallure V. Bier anaemic spots, cyanosis with urticaria-like eruption (BASCULE) syndrome: a new entity? Br J Dermatol. 2016;175(1):218–20.
79. Lestringant GG, Masouyé I, Frossard P, Adeghate E, Galadari I. Co-existence of leukoderma with features of Dowling-Degos disease: reticulate acropigmentation of Kitamura spectrum in five unrelated patients. Dermatology. 1997;195(4):337–43.
80. Lee SJ, Lee HJ, Kim DW, Jun JB, Chung SL, Bae HI. A case of Dowling-Degos disease suggesting an evolutional sequence. J Dermatol. 2000;27(9):591–7.
81. Sandhu K, Saraswat A, Kanwar A. Dowling–Degos disease with dyschromatosis universalis hereditaria-like pigmentation in a family. J Eur Acad Dermatol Venereol. 2004;18(6):702–4.
82. Thami G, Jaswal R, Kanwar A, Radotra B, Singh I. Overlap of reticulate acropigmentation of Kitamura, acropigmentation of Dohi and Dowling-Degos disease in four generations. Dermatology. 1998;196(3):350–1.
83. Nirmal B, Dongre AM, Khopkar US. Dermatoscopic features of hyper and hypopigmented lesions of Dowling-Degos disease. Indian J Dermatol. 2016;61(1):125.
84. Wu Y-H, Lin Y-C. Generalized Dowling-Degos disease. J Am Acad Dermatol. 2007;57(2):327–34.
85. Chang MW. Disorders of Hyperpigmentation. In: Bolognia J, Joseph L, Shaffer J, editors. Dermatology. 1. 3 ed. Philadelphia: Elsevier Saunders; 2012. p. 1049–74.
86. Morishima T. A clinical variety of primary localized cutaneous amyloidosis characterized by dyschromia (amyloidosis cutis dyschromica). Jpn J Dermatol Ser B. 1970;80(1):43–52.
87. Ho MS, Ho J, Tan SH. Hypopigmented macular amyloidosis with or without hyperpigmentation. Clin Exp Dermatol. 2009;34(8):e547–51.
88. Eng AM, Cogan L, Gunnar RM, Blekys I. Familial generalized dyschromic amyloidosis cutis. J Cutan Pathol. 1976;3(2):102–8.
89. Al Hawsawi K, Al Aboud K, Ramesh V, Al Aboud D. Dyschromatosis universalis hereditaria: report of a case and review of the literature. Pediatr Dermatol. 2002;19(6):523–6.
90. Pawsey SA, Magnus IA, Ramsay CA, Benson PF, Giannelli F. Clinical, genetic and DNA repair studies on a consecutive series of patients with xeroderma pigmentosum. Q J Med. 1979;48(190):179–210.
91. Irvine A, Mellerio J. Genetics and Genodermatoses. In: Burns T, Breathnach S, Cox N, Griffiths C, editors. Rook's textbook of Dermatology, 1. 8 ed. Hoboken, NJ: Wiley-Blackwell; 2010. p. 15.1–.97.
92. Kirnbauer R, Lenz P. Human Papillomaviruses. In: Bolognia J, Joseph L, Shaffer J, editors. Dermatolgy. 2. 3 ed. Philadelphia: Elsevier Saunders; 2012. p. 1303–18.

93. Kim HS, DS Y, Kim JW. White fibrous papulosis of the neck. J Eur Acad Dermatol Venereol. 2007;21(3):419–20.
94. Rongioletti F, Rebora A. Updated classification of papular mucinosis, lichen myxedematosus, and scleromyxedema. J Am Acad Dermatol. 2001;44(2, Part 1):273–81.
95. Kopf AW, Morrill S, Silberberg I. Broad spectrum of leukoderma acquisitum centrifugum. Arch Dermatol. 1965;92(1):14–35.
96. Anstey A. Disorders of Skin Colour. In: Burns T, Breathnach S, Cox N, Griffiths C, editors. Rook's textbook of Dermatology. 3. Hoboken, NJ: Wiley-Blackwell; 2010. p. 58. 49–50.
97. Kazakov D, Burg G, Kempf W. Clinicopathological spectrum of mycosis fungoides. J Eur Acad Dermatol Venereol. 2004;18(4):397–415.
98. Bowers S, Warshaw EM. Pityriasis Lichenoides and its subtypes. J Am Acad Dermatol. 2006;55(4): 557–72.

Current Views on Melasma

12

Kyoung-Chan Park and Hee Young Kang

Epidemiology

Melasma is a common acquired hyperpigmentary disorder that occurs more frequently in women and in those with darker skin types, such as Hispanics and Asians. The prevalence of melasma was reported to range from 8.8% among Latino women in the Southern United States to as high as 40% in Southeast Asia [1]. Ten to fifteen percent of pregnant women develop melasma, and 10–25% of women taking oral contraceptives report having melasma [2, 3]. Men represent approximately 10% of patients, though researchers have found a rate as high as 20% among Indian melasma patients [4].

Chronic sun exposure, genetic influences, and female sex hormones have been posited as major etiological factors [5–8]. A large global survey with 324 women with melasma showed that combinations of triggering factors can affect the onset of melasma [5]. In that study, the most common time of onset was after pregnancy (42%), with 26% during pregnancy. Only 25%

of patients taking oral contraceptives experienced the onset of melasma after starting to take the contraceptive. It has also been suggested that melasma which first appears during a pregnancy is more likely to resolve spontaneously [1]. The study concluded that a combination of factors, including UV exposure, family history, and hormonal disturbances, likely plays a role in the development of melasma. An epidemiologic study with 302 Brazilian melasma patients found that melasma was also common in middle-aged woman with intermediate skin phototypes, in this case Fitzpatrick skin phototypes III and IV [6]. A high familial incidence in more than half of the patients was reported, supporting the contention that genetic factors are important in the development of melasma. It was noted that patients who had a positive family history had longer disease durations. The most commonly reported precipitating factors were pregnancy (36.4%), taking oral contraceptives (16.2%), and sun exposure (27.2%). It was noted that pregnancy-associated melasma had an earlier onset and was more common in those who had multiple pregnancies. In another multicenter study involving 953 Brazilian melasma patients [7], the findings suggested that the age at the onset of melasma is related to skin phototypes and family history; i.e., Fitzpatrick skin phototypes II and III and a positive family history of melasma were associated with early onsets of melasma when compared to skin phototypes IV, V, and VI

K. -C. Park
Department of Dermatology, Seoul National
University Bundang Hospital, Seongnam, Korea

H. Y. Kang (✉)
Department of Dermatology, Ajou University
School of Medicine, Suwon, Korea
e-mail: hykang@ajou.ac.kr

© Springer International Publishing AG, part of Springer Nature 2018
P. Kumarasinghe (ed.), *Pigmentary Skin Disorders*, Updates in Clinical Dermatology,
https://doi.org/10.1007/978-3-319-70419-7_12

or an absence of family history. Extrafacial melasma was more frequent in postmenopausal women. In an Indian study of 312 cases, a positive family history was observed in 33.3%, and approximately 55.1% reported intense sun exposure [8]. Also in this Indian study, only 22.4% of patients reported pregnancy as a triggering or aggravating factor, and only 18.4% of them were taking oral contraceptives when they contracted the disease.

The studies mentioned above suggest that sun exposure and/or hormonal stimuli trigger melasma development in patients who have intrinsic sensitivity to such stimuli. The high incidence of family history in melasma patients suggests a genetic component as well. Sun exposure and hormonal stimuli are commonly reported triggering factors in those studies. Prolonged sun exposure could stimulate the upregulation of certain melanogenic factors in melasma skin. The presence of local hormones in the skin may play a role in the development of melasma, although the exact mechanism remains unclear. It is likely that certain effects induced by sex hormones in patients require additional synergistic events such as UV exposure before melasma develops.

Clinical Features and Classification

Melasma is characterized by light-to-dark-brown macules and patches occurring in sun-exposed areas of the face. Clinically, melasma has been described as centrofacial, malar, and mandibular patterns, and many patients have a mixture of these patterns [9]. The centrofacial pattern is most common, consisting of lesions on the forehead, cheeks, nose, upper lip, and/or chin (Fig. 12.1a). The malar pattern describes lesions located primarily on the cheeks and nose. The mandibular pattern consists of lesions on the ramus of the mandible. This clinical classification of melasma may not be meaningful, as it does not affect therapeutic plan or outcomes. Cases of extrafacial melasma occurring on the forearms have also been described [10].

Traditionally, the categorization of melasma relies on the depth of the melanin pigment in epidermal melasma, in dermal melasma, and in the mixed type. At present, researchers consider the dermal type of melasma to be the most resistant to treatments. Current clinical practices rely on examinations using a Wood's light to ascertain the depth of the melanin pigment present. Epidermal melasma is associated with color enhancements of the lesions, whereas this is not the case with dermal melasma. However, more recent work posits a poor correlation between classifications based on assessments using a Wood's light and biopsy skin samples analyzed via light microscopy [11, 12]. In a clinical study, Wood's light examinations could not increase the accuracy of treatment responses of melasma [13]. This indicates that the clinical use of this type of light for assessment purposes is not effective when attempting to determine the level or depth of melanin pigment. A skin biopsy is a better option when seeking a more accurate measurement of the pigment depth in melasma cases. However, other findings have called into question the comprehensiveness of earlier histological classifications from single skin biopsies [14]. Upon an examination of a complete melasma lesion with in vivo reflectance confocal microscopy (RCM), high heterogeneousness was found in the topographic distribution of melanophages from certain areas of the melasma lesion to others. This was also the case within specific regions of the melasma lesion. Another consideration is that dermal melanophages commonly exist in skin exposed to the sun while normal facial skin also contains pigments in the dermis. Kang et al. [15] doubted that a true dermal type exists for melasma. For Korean patients, melanophages exist in both melasma lesional and perilesional normal skin in 36% of cases [15]. A study by Grimes et al. found as well that the lesional and nonlesional skin of normal melasma patients in general contains melanophages [11]. In one study involving 26 cases of melasma, epidermal hyperpigmentation was detected using RCM in all patients, lending support to the contention of the

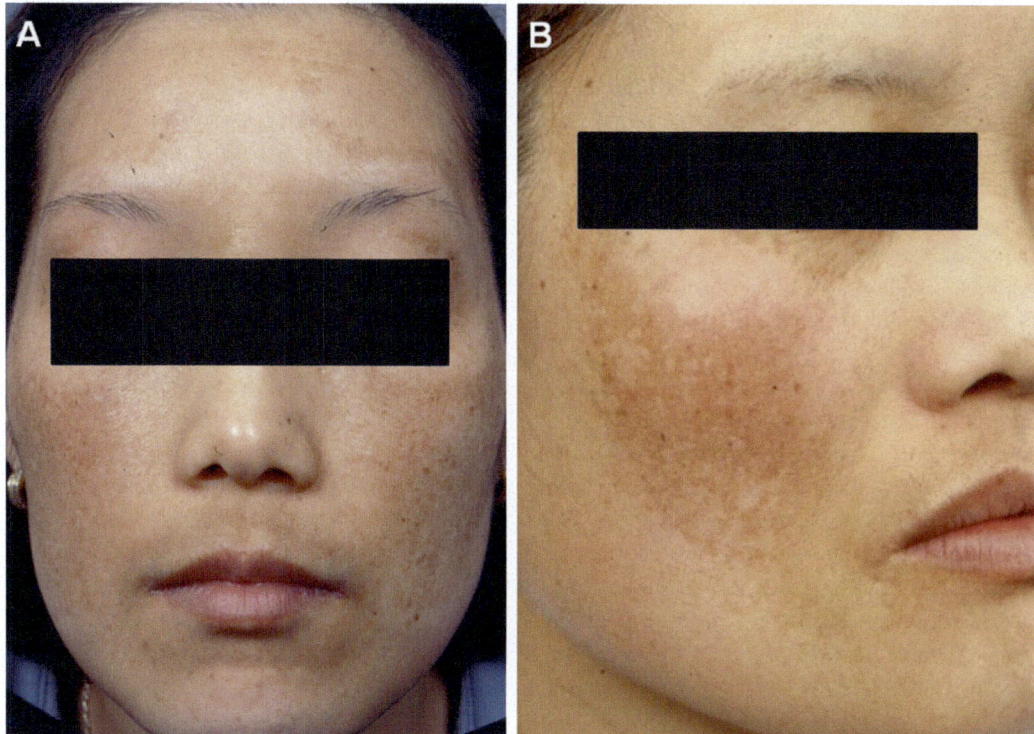

Fig. 12.1 (a) Centrofacial pattern of melasma. (b) Melasma with increased vasculature

absence of a true dermal type of melasma [14]. There were no statistically significant differences in the amount of dermal melanin in lesional skin compared to those of perilesional normal skin, although relatively more lesions were found [11, 15]. Therefore, further studies are needed to determine if this small amount of dermal melanin in melasma lesional skin does in fact affect the therapeutic outcomes of treatments and if classification according to pigment depth is meaningful with regard to treatments.

A major clinical feature of melasma is the hyperpigmented patches, but melasma patients have additional distinguishing features such as pronounced telangiectatic erythema confined to melasma lesional skin (Fig. 12.1b). Recent data has shown that melasma lesions have more vascularization as compared to perilesional normal skin [14, 16]. In this regard, some investigators have classified melasma into four types on the basis of Wood's light and glass compression examinations. These are the melanin type, vascular type, mela-

nin-dominant type, and vascular-dominant type. Dermoscopic examinations of melasma could be useful to reveal the capillary vessels in some parts of the lesions. The vascular type of melasma with, as the name suggests, vascularization, could be considered as a type suitable for vascular-targeted treatments such as a vascular laser.

Recent work has divided melasma into the "noninflammatory" and "inflammatory" types [17]. Among 197 subjects, 50 patients (25.4%) were categorized into the inflammatory group. This group comprised cases that had inflammatory symptoms including itching/tingling, dryness, and erythema/telangiectasia and events that triggered melasma lesions. The lesional dermis contained more CD68+ melanophages, CD117+ mast cells, and LCA+ leukocytes in the inflammatory group than in the noninflammatory group. This study suggested that subtypes of melasma may be used as a clinical parameter to assess and predict the clinical profile of melasma and its response to treatment.

Pathogenesis

The pathogenesis of melasma is not fully understood, but current studies suggest that endogenous or exogenous stimuli or both may stimulate the microenvironment, leading to the release of various mediators that activate melanocytes during the development of melasma. In melasma skin, in addition to melanocytes, other factors most likely affect the development and relapse of melasma.

Effect of Sun Exposure

Melasma occurs in sun-exposed areas, and many patients report aggravated melasma upon sun exposure. While sunscreens alone for the treatment of melasma have never been studied, their use is recommended based on clinical experience. The regular use of broad-spectrum sunscreens is effective for both preventing melasma and enhancing the efficacy of other topical therapies once melasma has developed [18, 19]. Immunohistochemical studies have shown that melasma skin shows the features of mainly solar-damaged skin [15, 20]. Increased solar elastosis in lesional skin has been noted, suggesting that the process of solar damage may influence the development of hyperpigmentation in melasma skin. During sun exposure, ultraviolet (UV) irradiation is one possible main triggering or exacerbating factor in the development of melasma. It is commonly known that UV radiation induces melanocyte proliferation, migration, and melanogenesis. In addition, UV irradiation serves to increase the production of multiple cytokines, including alpha-MSH and ACTH derived from POMC in keratinocytes. These cytokines then upregulate melanocyte proliferation and increase melanin synthesis via the stimulation of tyrosinase activity and TRP-1 [21]. When comparing biopsies of lesional and perilesional normal skin in ten melasma cases, lesional skin showed a statistically significant increase in the expression of alpha-MSH [22]. These findings suggest that the sustained overexpression of MSH in lesional skin after UV exposure may be a significant factor in the development of melasma.

Interestingly, it was recently suggested that visible light can also induce hyperpigmentation, at least on types IV–VI skin [22]. For those with dark skin types, both UVA and visible light induced pigmentation, but the pigmentation was more intense and more stable after visible light exposure as compared with UVA exposure. Therefore, it is emphasized that broad-spectrum UVA- and UVB-protective sunscreen, along with a physical block such as titanium dioxide or zinc oxide, should be used by patients with melasma and should be reapplied frequently.

The Epidermal-Dermal Interplay in the Development of Melasma

Pigmentation of melasma is confined to the epidermis, but dermal factors are suspected to be the main causes behind the recurrent and refractory nature of this disorder. Indeed, melasma dermal skin differs from perilesional normal skin and shows features of prominent solar-damaged skin. During exposure to the sun, the network of cellular interactions between fibroblasts and perhaps the vasculature as well as keratinocytes and melanocytes may play important roles in epidermal hyperpigmentation in relation to melasma.

Role of Fibroblasts

Fibroblasts in the dermis may play a role in the development of melasma. As was recently suggested, during UV irradiation, fibroblasts are senescent and produce multiple skin-aging-associated secreted proteins (SAASP) compared to normal fibroblasts, which include differently expressed secreted factors controlling melanogenesis. Examples include the KIT ligand, hepatocyte growth factor, and/or keratinocyte growth factor [23, 24]. Immunohistochemical staining with the p16 antibody demonstrated that melasma skin contains more senescent fibroblasts in melasma pigmented skin (Fig. 12.2). It was reported that the protein expression levels of both the stem cell factor (SCF) from fibroblasts and c-kit were significantly increased in melasma

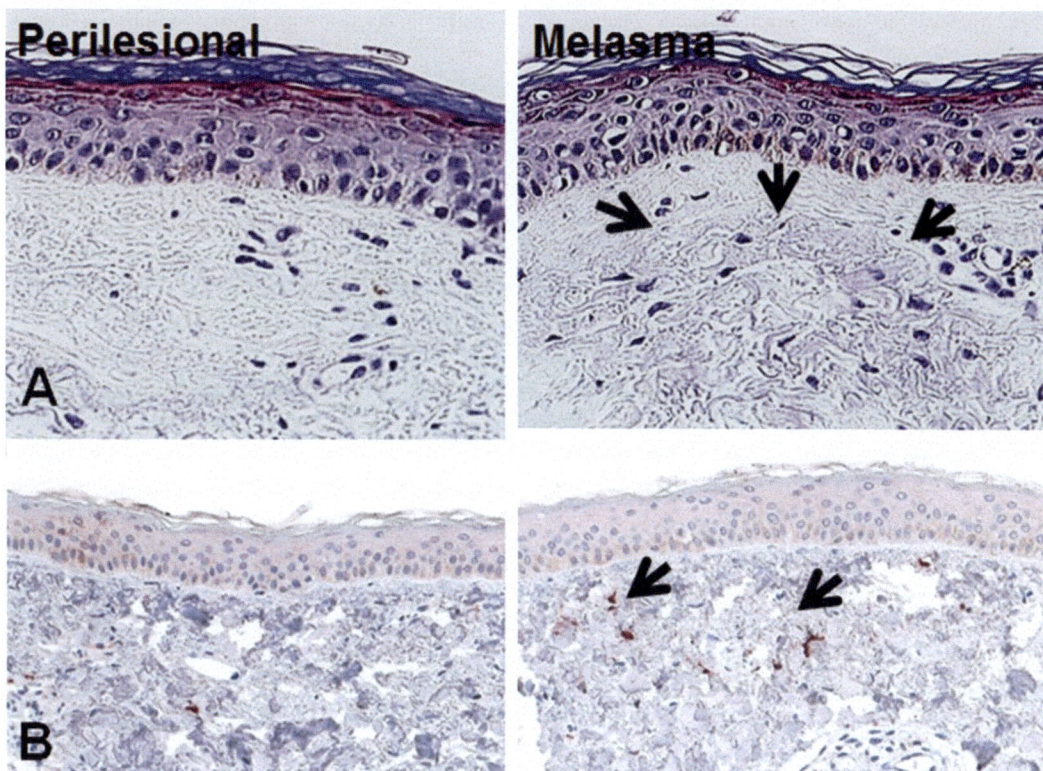

Fig. 12.2 (**a**) Increased solar elastosis in lesional skin of melasma compared to perilesional skin (arrow). (**b**) p16 immunostaining showed melasma skin contains more senescent fibroblasts (arrow) in melasma pigmented skin suggesting a role of photoaged fibroblasts

lesional skin [25]. The mRNA expressions of SCF and c-kit were also increased in melasma. Fibroblast-derived cytokines were found to stimulate the proliferation and melanogenesis of melanocytes in cell culture studies [26]. A clinical case also supported the role of dermal SCF in epidermal pigmentation [27]. The accumulation of the melanogenic factor KGF in the lesional epidermis has also been observed [28]. Very recently, the upregulation of secreted frizzled-related protein 2 (sFRP2) was uncovered in melasma skin, solar lentigo, and acutely UV-irradiated skin. This overexpression leads to increased melanogenesis through the activation of the β-catenin signaling and thus the upregulation of MITF and tyrosinase in melanocytes. Interestingly, strong expression of sFRP2 was detected in lesional fibroblasts, further demonstrating the crucial role of the epithelial-mesenchymal interplay in the control of the

physiological and pathological processes of skin pigmentation [29]. For this reason, dermal inflammation as caused by accumulated UV irradiation has been surmised as associated with photoaged changes of fibroblasts, possibly leading to the upregulation of SAASP in the dermis of melasma patients and thus increased melanogenesis.

Role of Blood Vessels

In cases of melasma, a prominent clinical feature is the presence of hyperpigmented patches. However, other distinguishing features can also be found. Examples include distinct telangiectatic erythema mainly found in lesional skin in melasma cases (Fig. 12.1). Greater vascularization has been found in melasma lesions compared to that in perilesional normal skin [14, 16]. Moreover, lesional skin displays a considerably higher erythema index as compared to perilesional normal skin, and a positive correlation was also found between the melanin index and erythema index. Other reports imply that the severity of the disease can be estimated by "erythema" in melasma, with deeper erythema and less pigmentation in melasma possibly associated with poorer responses to laser treatments [30]. Immunohistochemistry for vascular markers revealed increased numbers of vessels in the upper dermis [15]. The number of vessels was positively correlated with epidermal pigmentation in melasma lesional skin. Chronic sun exposure stimulates vascular endothelial growth factor (VEGF) secretion from keratinocytes. The increased expression of VEGF in keratinocytes has been suggested as a major angiogenic factor behind the altered vessels found in melasma [15].

Endothelial cells produce prostaglandins, nitric oxide, and EDN1, a factor shown to induce pigmentation [31]. Dermal endothelial cells play an inhibitory role during the process of skin pigmentation, possibly doing so by secreting ample amounts of TGFβ1 [32]. Hence, endothelial cells may play a role in regulating constitutive human skin color and perhaps its dysfunction in pigmentary diseases. Nevertheless, it was suggested that stimulated cells under pathological conditions respond differently compared to those under normal physiological conditions. Regazzetti et al. reported that endothelial cells play a stimulating role during pigmentation through EDN1 signaling [31].

Possible Role of the Disrupted Basement Membrane

Recent histological studies of melasma have described changes in the basement membrane in melasma lesional skin [33, 34]. The basement membrane structure in lesional skin is not intact and appears disrupted. Type IV collagen expression overall was significantly reduced in lesional skin compared to perilesional normal skin [33]. This feature was more evident at the margin of

some melanocytes, with protrusion into the dermis in cases known as pendulous melanocytes. The MMP2 protein and mRNA expression levels were markedly increased in lesional skin compared to perilesional normal skin. It was suggested that chronic UV irradiation is responsible for the loosening of the basement membrane through the upregulation of MMP2 expression in melasma because MMP2 immunoreactivity was co-localized with elastotic materials.

What role does the impaired basement membrane have in melasma pathogenesis? It is speculated that the changes facilitate interaction between dermal structures and epidermal melanocytes. In pigmented areas, certain types of melanogenesis-stimulating factors, such as SCF or factors related to the vasculature, easily penetrate from the dermis into the epidermis through a loosened basement membrane. This suggests that heparanase in the epidermis, activated by UVB exposure, degrades heparan sulfate at the DEJ. The degradation of HS in the basement membrane allows the transfer of these growth factors from the dermis to melanocytes, leading to the promotion of melanogenesis in solar lentigo [35].

It has also been surmised that the loosening of the basement membrane facilitates a pendulous change in melanocytes. Pendulous cells appear to be vulnerable to traumatic events, including a laser treatment. They can easily drop into the dermis or become destroyed and would thus leave heavy pigmentation in the dermis, resulting in hyperpigmentation during treatment. It was suggested that pendulous melanocytes with disrupted basement membranes are associated with the aggravation of melasma after a fractional laser treatment [36]. The protrusion of melanocytes was aggravated after the fractional laser treatment, and the total absence of the basement membrane was observed. Therefore, a gentle treatment which does not affect the basement membrane or a treatment supporting the basement membrane is mandatory for a satisfactory and safe outcome during the treatment of melasma.

Role of Sex Hormones

The more common incidence of melasma in women during their reproductive years and the link between melasma and oral contraceptives suggest female sex hormones as an important precipitating factor influencing its development and intensification. Immunohistochemistry has revealed an increased degree of estrogen receptor (ER) expression in affected skin [37], signifying a prospective role of estrogen in cases of melasma. Estrogens were found to stimulate melanogenesis in cultured human melanocytes through the synthesis of melanogenic enzymes such as tyrosinase, TRP-1, TRP-2, and MITF [38–40]. Melanocytes express ERs [39, 41], linked to estrogen-induced melanogenesis, and ER inhibition by its antagonist diminishes melanogenesis [39]. The upregulated expression of PDZ domain protein kidney 1 (PDZK1) in hyperpigmented skin in cases of melasma has been found [39]. Estrogen has also been shown to enhance PDZK1 with tyrosinase expression in melanocyte-keratinocyte co-cultures as well as in melanocyte monocultures. Moreover, estrogen-stimulated tyrosinase expression levels and melanosome transfer with ER-alpha and ER-beta expression are also increased by PDZK1 overexpression [39].

Wnt Pathway and MicroRNAs

A transcriptional analysis was conducted in melasma skin samples for a comparison with the surrounding healthy skin [42]. A total of 279 genes were found to be differentially expressed in lesional and perilesional skin. As was expected, the mRNA levels of a number of known melanogenesis-associated genes, such as TYR, MITF, SILV, and TYRP1, were found to be elevated in lesional skin. Interestingly, several genes involved in other biological processes and/or expressed by cells other than melanocytes were found to be differentially expressed as compared with the surrounding unaffected skin. The increased expressions of a subset of genes modulating the Wnt pathway, such as WIF1, SFRP2,

and Wnt5a, were noted in melasma lesions, and WIF1 was one of the 20 most upregulated genes. Wnt signaling plays a role in the differentiation as well as the development of melanocytes. The hyperpigmentary skin of melasma expresses high levels of frizzled-related protein 2 (sFRP2) and Wnt inhibitory factor-1 (WIF-1) compared to perilesional normal skin. sFRP2 and WIF-1 are expressed in both the melanocytes of normal human skin and in cultured melanocytes, suggesting that these molecules have physiologic functions in melanocytes as an autocrine or paracrine modulator of Wnt signaling. Moreover, the upregulation of sFRP2 and WIF-1 in cultured normal human melanocytes significantly stimulates melanogenesis through the increased expression levels of MITF and tyrosinase. Ex vivo human skin was maintained in the presence of recombinant human sFRP2 or WIF-1. In the presence of rsFRP2 or rWIF-1, the skin showed significantly increased pigmentation compared to control skin samples, as shown by Fontana-Masson staining. These findings suggest that UV irradiation stimulates sFRP2 and WIF-1 secretion in the skin, which functions as a melanogenic stimulator. The Wnt signaling pathway may play an important role in the development of melasma [29, 43].

A potential role of miRNAs has been presented in melasma. Melasma skin shows H19 noncoding RNA downregulation. Moreover, expression levels of the H19 RNA-derived miRNA miR-675 are lessened in the hyperpigmented skin of melasma cases [44]. The overexpression of miR-675 also decreases the degrees to which tyrosinase, TRP-1, and TRP-2 are expressed, and the knockdown of miR-675 increases these expression levels. Increased cadherin 11 (CDH11) expression as another target of miR-675 has also been assessed in hyperpigmented skin in melasma cases, signifying that CDH11 acts in melasma. While the expression of CDH11 cannot be found in melanocytes, it, when it exists in fibroblasts or keratinocytes, can stimulate melanogenesis by means of the established Wnt and apoptosis signal-regulating kinase (AKT) activation pathways in cases of co-cultured melanocytes via the induction of N-cadherin.

Evaluation of Melasma

Clinical Evaluation of Melasma

Melasma area and severity index (MASI) is developed for the assessment of melasma. The severity of the melasma in each of the four regions (forehead, right malar region, left malar region, and chin) is assessed based on three variables: percentage of the total area involved (A), darkness (D), and homogeneity (H). A numerical value is calculated for the corresponding percentage area. To calculate the MASI score, the sum of the severity grade for darkness (D) and homogeneity (H) is multiplied by the numerical value of the areas (A) involved and by the percentages of the four facial areas (10–30%). Although MASI is known as a standard way of evaluation in melasma, modified version of MASI (mMASI) was developed to evaluate melasma more objectively and easily [45]. Of course, global assessment of melasma can be done based on standard photograph [46].

Instrumental Evaluation of Melasma

The Mexameter® MX18 is a simple, easy, and quick tool to measure the two components responsible for the color of the skin: melanin and hemoglobin. The measurement is based on absorption/reflection, and the melanin is measured by specific wavelengths chosen to correspond to different absorption rates by the pigments. For the erythema measurement, the same principle is applied to avoid other color influences. It has been used in many studies and may be one standard method to evaluate the pigmentary changes. However, it has some disadvantage that it can measure only a small area at one time [47]. We have used Mexameter® MX18 to measure the pigmentation changes in several studies. Interestingly, erythema changes are also consistently associated with changes of pigmentation. Mexameter® MX18 can measure the melanin index and erythema index simultaneously. Chromameter or colorimeter is a portable,

battery-powered, and handheld instrument. This instrument has the ability to measure precise color difference expressed in L*a*b*. Value of L is usually used to measure pigmentation changes and has been used in many studies [48]. However, it has the same disadvantage that it can measure only a small area at one time.

Image Analysis

There have been several studies which utilize new methods to evaluate melasma severity by image analysis. mMASI is a method to simplify MASI in the evaluation of melasma. Tay et al. suggested a method to determine mMASI by using a novel image analysis software through analyzing whole-face digital photographs [49]. In addition, digital image and ultraviolet computerized image analysis can be used in the evaluation of melasma [50]. Otherwise, a novel photography-based system has been reported which integrates a consistent photography setting and image processing diagnostic algorithms [51].

Treatment of Melasma

Melasma is an acquired hypermelanosis characterized by symmetrical, irregular light-to-dark-brown macules and patches on sun-exposed area. It is common during their third and fourth decades of life [52]. A genetic predisposition, chronic exposure to ultraviolet (UV) radiation, and female sex hormones are considered to be important in its pathogenesis [53, 54]. Histologically, epidermal hyperpigmentation is accompanied by an increased number of melanocytes, overexpression of melanogenic enzymes, and underlying dermal changes [15]. Treatment of melasma is difficult because it is recalcitrant to therapy and it frequently recurs even after successful clearance. There are various treatment options including topical hypopigmentation agents, laser or light therapies, systemic tranexamic acid (TXA), and chemical peels.

Topical Treatment Agents

Hydroquinone (Dihydroxybenzene) and Triple Combination Cream

Hydroquinone (HQ) is the most commonly used anti-melanogenic agent. It inhibits the conversion of l-3,4-dihydroxyphenylalanine to melanin by the competitive inhibition of tyrosinase. HQ's oxidative products also cause oxidative damage to membrane lipids and proteins. In a randomized, double-blind, placebo-controlled trial, it was demonstrated that 38% of patients showed good response with 4% HQ in 12 weeks compared with only 8% of patients in the control group. There is a safety issue in the use of HQ. In Europe, the use of HQ is prohibited in cosmetics because of possible long-term complications, such as exogenous ochronosis and permanent depigmentation. Especially, accumulation of homogentisic acid causes degeneration of collagen and elastic fibers, followed by the deposition of ocher-colored fibers. This condition is extremely difficult to treat. Westerhof et al. further warned the potential carcinogenic risk of HQ due to its metabolite, p-benzoquinone, formed in the liver [55]. On the other hand, Nordlund et al. reviewed the evidence for the safety of HQ and concluded that it is reasonable to use HQ in the treatment of hyperpigmentation [56].

It is reported that triple combination cream (TCC) containing 4% HQ, 0.05% tretinoin, and 0.01% fluocinolone acetonide is the most effective in the treatment of melasma, and it is approved by the US Food and Drug Administration (FDA) for the treatment of melasma [56]. Especially, topical tretinoin exhibits the well-known anti-wrinkle effect, but it also has a hypopigmentation effect [57]. Included steroids can suppress melanogenic cytokines, such as endothelin-1 (ET-1) and granulocyte-macrophage colony-stimulating factor (GM-CSF), which mediate UV-induced melanogenesis.

Cestari et al. demonstrated that TCC was more effective than 4% HQ in an 8-week trial [58]. In this study, clearance of melasma lesions was observed in 35% of the patients in the TCC group compared with 5% of the patients in the HQ group, while the incidence of adverse events, including erythema, burning sensations, and desquamation, was similar in both groups. In a multicenter comparison study involving Asian patients, TCC exhibited superior efficacy in the treatment of melasma than 4% HQ cream, with 64.2% of the patients treated with TCC showing "none" or "mild" melasma at 8 weeks compared with 39.4% of patients in the HQ group. Despite more adverse events occurring in the TCC group than in the HQ group in this study (48.8% versus 13.7%), most of them were mild [46]. However, the use of TCC should be limited to twice daily for 6 months because of the possibility of steroid-induced atrophy, which disqualifies it from use as a maintenance therapy for melasma.

Other Tyrosinase Inhibitors

Arbutin, a naturally occurring hydroquinone β-D-glucopyranoside derived from the bearberry plant, shows anti-melanogenic properties. It has been known to inhibit tyrosinase activity, without affecting its mRNA expression, and 5,6-dihydroxyindole-2-carboxylic acid (DHICA) polymerase activity [59]. In a clinical study, a significant decrease in the melanin index was observed in ten patients treated with 1% arbutin for 6 months ($p < 0.05$) [60].

Kojic acid (5-hydroxy-2-[hydroxymethyl]-4H–pyran-4-one), an antibiotic produced by species of *Aspergillus* and *Penicillium* bacteria, chelates the copper in tyrosinase and inhibits NF-κB in keratinocytes, thereby showing bleaching activity.

Azelaic acid, a naturally derived dicarboxylic acid synthesized by *Malassezia furfur*, weakly inhibits tyrosinase, which leads to the hypopigmented macules commonly observed in tinea versicolor [61]. In a 24-week trial, 20% azelaic acid produced "good" or "excellent" results in 65% of patients, while 72% of patients treated with 4% HQ reported the same result. However, there was no significant difference between the two groups.

A novel anti-melanogenic compound, 4-n-butylresorcinol, has recently been shown to inhibit the activities of tyrosinase and tyrosinase-related protein-1 (TRP-1) in vitro [62]. In a randomized, double-blind, vehicle-controlled, split-face study that investigated liposome-encapsulated 4-n-butylresorcinol, the melanin index, determined using a Mexameter®, showed a significant reduction on the treated side of the face compared with the control side after 8 weeks of treatment (−7.5% versus −3.3%, $p < 0.05$), without any occurrence of adverse events [63].

Ascorbic Acid (Vitamin C) and Antioxidants

Antioxidant may interact with copper at the active sites of tyrosinase. Thus, antioxidant can inhibit tyrosinase activity and prevent oxidative polymerization in melanin intermediates. Ascorbic acid, a well-known antioxidant agent, interferes with melanogenesis by chelating the copper ions in tyrosinase [64]. In our clinic, the effects of ascorbic acid were studied through iontophoresis. In a randomized, double-blind, placebo-controlled, split-face study, colorimeter measurements demonstrated a significant effect with iontophoresis with ascorbic acid [65]. Other oxidant compounds, including α-tocopherol, hydrocoumarins (6-hydroxy-3,4-dihydrocoumarins), and thioctic acid (α-lipoic acid), also display anti-melanogenic properties by inhibiting lipid peroxidation, accelerating glutathione synthesis, and downregulating NF-κB activation, respectively [66–68]. In an animal model, methimazole displayed regulatory activity toward peroxidase, thereby reducing the polymerization rate of eumelanin [69, 70].

We performed a clinical trial to evaluate the efficacy of a whitening agent containing 0.05% resveratrol, a natural extract derived from the roots of the Japanese knotweed, in the treatment of melasma. Its antioxidant activity has been proved by a 14-fold increase in the action of superoxide dismutase 2 (SOD2) in cells treated with resveratrol [71]. A total of 30 patients applied the agent twice daily and demonstrated a significant improvement in melanin index measured by a Mexameter® and clinical photographic assessment after 8 weeks ($p < 0.05$).

Niacinamide (Vitamin B3) and Melanosome Transfer Inhibitors

A reduction in melanosome transfer results in hypopigmentation by blocking the dispersion of pigment to the keratinocytes. A serine protease inhibitor has been reported to modulate the activation of the protease-activated receptor 2, resulting in the accumulation of melanosomes within melanocytes in vitro [72, 73]. Lectins and neo-glycoproteins have also been shown to reduce melanosome transfer in vitro. Hakozaki et al., in a split-face trial, showed that 5% niacinamide cream significantly reduced hyperpigmentation and lightened basal skin color in 8 weeks ($p < 0.05$) [74].

Other Compounds

Topical application of linolenic acid, linoleic acid, oleic acid, and phospholipase D2 resulted in hypopigmentation of the skin of guinea pigs after UV irradiation via the stimulation of tyrosinase ubiquitination and proteasomal degradation [75].

Several compounds that modify tyrosinase structures at glycosylation sites have been found to induce hypopigmentation in vitro, including glucosamine, tunicamycin, and calcium D-pantetheine-S-sulfonate [76, 77].

Laser and Light Therapies

Intense-Pulsed Light Therapy

Intense-pulsed light (IPL) emits a broad spectrum of wavelengths and may provide selective photothermolysis by use of filter. Li et al. evaluated the effects of IPL treatment in Chinese melasma patients [78]. They reported that there were significant reductions in the mean melasma area and severity index (MASI) score after four treatment sessions [78]. In this study, transient erythema and edema were the most common adverse events, and three patients experienced PIH.

Although IPL may be a good therapeutic option for melasma, melasma-like pigmentation can develop after IPL treatment, which is even more intensely pigmented. Because laser energy induces hyperactive melanocytes through inflammation and prostaglandin and cytokine production, a mixture of PIH and aggravated melasma can develop. Since subtle melasma is clinically invisible to the naked eye but is detected by UV photography in 28.3% of Asian patients, IPL treatment must be performed very cautiously [79].

Fractional 1550-nm Non-ablative Laser Therapy

Fractional photothermolysis creates numerous microthermal zones (MTZ) of thermal injury in the skin while leaving the areas between them unaffected. Theoretically, transepidermal elimination could effectively remove dermal melanophages like an enhanced drug delivery into the dermis [80]. In contrast, the unaffected areas may recover rapidly. Thus, there is a low risk of subsequent inflammation and PIH.

In a small clinical trial involving four-to-six sessions of fractional non-ablative laser treatment, six out of ten patients achieved 75–100% clearance of the lesion, with PIH occurring in one patient [81]. In contrast, a split-face study showed a significant worsening of pigmentation and a higher incidence of PIH (31%) in the laser-treated group. However, in a similar trial by the same investigators, the study groups treated with either fractional non-ablative laser or TCC showed significant improvements in the investigator's global assessment scores [82].

Although fractional non-ablative laser is the only laser device approved by the FDA for melasma, the results are not consistent, and there are high risks of PIH, especially in Asian patients. To lower the risk of PIH, treatment with lower fluences, variable pulses, and pretreatment with HQ are recommended, particularly in patients who have a history of PIH.

Q-Switched Neodymium-Doped Yttrium Aluminum Garnet Laser Treatment

Since high-fluence laser has the risk of adverse events, the concept of using collimated, low-fluence, 1064-nm QSNYL treatment has been suggested. This "laser-toning" technique is especially popular in East Asian countries and has become one of the first-line therapies for melasma. While its action mechanism is unclear, several studies have found that "laser toning" removes the melanosomes but not the melanocytes. Furthermore, it damages the dendrites of the melanocytes without killing the cells, thereby functionally downregulating the melanocytes in a process called "subcellular selective photothermolysis" [83]. Recently, reductions in the expression of proteins associated with melanogenesis, including TRP-1, tyrosinase-related protein-2, nerve growth factor, α-melanocyte-stimulating hormone, and tyrosinase, were also demonstrated after "laser toning."

In an 8-week trial, 58.8% of the patients who received "laser toning" weekly, administered at 1.6–2.5 J/cm^2, demonstrated an improvement of 50–75% in investigator's global assessment scores. In this study, transient pain, erythema, and edema were commonly reported, while partially hypopigmented macules and diffuse hyperpigmentation rarely occurred. Wattanakrai et al. undertook a split-face trial to compare "laser toning" with 2% HQ treatment [84]. They found that the side of face that received "laser toning" weekly, administered at 3.0–3.8 J/cm^2 for five sessions, achieved marked improvements in the lightness index (L*) score (92.5%), and in the modified MASI score (75.9%), compared with 19.7% and 24%, respectively, for the side of face which had 2% HQ. The investigators also reported that mottled hypopigmentation developed in three patients and melasma lesions recurred in all patients during follow-up.

Pulsed-Dye Laser Treatment

Pulsed-dye laser (PDL) treatment is the gold standard therapy for vascular lesions. However, evidence showed that there is increased vascularization in melasma lesions, which may play a role in the recurrence of the disease [85]. An increase in the expression of vascular endothelial growth factor (VEGF) has led to the suggestion that they may act in vessels, because functioning VEGF receptors were demonstrated in melanocytes in vitro. Elevations in the levels of expression of c-kit, stem cell factor (SCF), and inducible nitric oxide synthase have also been observed, which could affect vascularization [25].

In a split-face trial, Passeron et al. compared TCC plus PDL with TCC alone in melasma [85]. At the end of treatment, the MASI scores were significantly lowered in both groups ($p < 0.05$). However, while the improvement was sustained at the 2-month follow-up assessment in the group that received combination treatment, it was not sustained in the group that received TCC alone.

Copper Bromide Laser Treatment

Copper bromide lasers emit two wavelengths of light either separately or simultaneously: the 511-nm green beam for the treatment of pigmented lesions and the 578-nm yellow beam for the treatment of vascular lesions. In a recent pilot study, 10 Korean patients were treated with copper bromide laser at 2-week intervals for 8 weeks to evaluate its efficacy and safety [86]. At the 1-month posttreatment follow-up, the mean MASI score decreased modestly from 12.3 to 9.5. L*, and the erythema index (a*), measured using a Chromameter®, showed significant improvements ($p < 0.05$).

Systemic Tranexamic Acid

Pathogenesis of melasma is poorly understood. It includes disruptions and thinning of the basement membrane; prominent solar elastosis; increases in vascularization; elevations in the expression of VEGF, c-kit, and SCF; and

increases in the number of mast cells. TXA inhibits plasmin, a key molecule in angiogenesis that converts extracellular matrix-bound VEGF into its free forms [87]. TXA has also been reported to suppress neovascularization induced by basic fibroblast growth factor [88]. Therefore, TXA could reverse melasma-related dermal changes.

In a recent clinical trial that evaluated the efficacy of systemic TXA in the treatment of melasma, we demonstrated a decrease in the lesional melanin index and a* (erythema index) after 250 mg TXA was administered orally to 25 female study participants three times daily for 8 weeks [47]. Histological analysis showed significant reductions in epidermal pigmentation, vessel numbers, and mast cell counts. In another trial, 64.8% of the patients who were administered 250 mg TXA orally twice daily for 6 months showed "excellent" or "good" outcomes 6 months after the treatment had ceased. In this study, gastrointestinal discomfort (5.4%) and hypomenorrhea (8.1%) were commonly reported, but no severe adverse events occurred.

Chemical Peels

Chemicals peels are often recommended in the treatment of melasma in patients with pale skins. However, the result is not consistent with the high risk of adverse effects, especially PIH. Nowadays, chemical peels are not preferred in Asian patients.

References

1. Sheth VM, Pandya AG. Melasma: a comprehensive update: part I. J Am Acad Dermatol. 2011;65(4):689–97.
2. Hexsel D, Rodrigues T, Dal'forno T, Zechmeister-Prado D, Lima M. Melasma and pregnancy in southern Brazil. J Eur Acad Dermatol Venereol. 2009;23(3):367–8.
3. Moin A, Jabery Z, Fallah N. Prevalence and awareness of melasma during pregnancy. Int J Dermatol. 2006;45(3):285–8.
4. Sarkar R, Puri P, Jain RK, Singh A, Desai A. Melasma in men: a clinical, aetiological and histological study. J Eur Acad Dermatol Venereol. 2010;24(7):768–72.
5. Ortonne JP, Arellano I, Berneburg M, Cestari T, Chan H, Grimes P, et al. A global survey of the role of ultra-

violet radiation and hormonal influences in the development of melasma. J Eur Acad Dermatol Venereol. 2009;23(11):1254–62.

6. Tamega AA, Miot LD, Bonfietti C, Gige TC, Marques ME, Miot HA. Clinical patterns and epidemiological characteristics of facial melasma in Brazilian women. J Eur Acad Dermatol Venereol. 2013;27(2):151–6.

7. Hexsel D, Lacerda DA, Cavalcante AS, Filho CA, Kalil CL, Ayres EL, et al. Epidemiology of melasma in Brazilian patients: a multicenter study. Int J Dermatol. 2014;53(4):440–4.

8. Achar A, Rathi SK. Melasma: a clinico-epidemiological study of 312 cases. Indian J Dermatol. 2011;56(4):380–2.

9. Sanchez NP, Pathak MA, Sato S, Fitzpatrick TB, Sanchez JL, Mihm MC Jr. Melasma: a clinical, light microscopic, ultrastructural, and immunofluorescence study. J Am Acad Dermatol. 1981;4(6):698–710.

10. Madke B, Kar S, Yadav N, Bonde P. Extrafacial melasma over forearms. Indian Dermatol Online J. 2016;7(4):344–5.

11. Grimes PE, Yamada N, Bhawan J. Light microscopic, immunohistochemical, and ultrastructural alterations in patients with melasma. Am J Dermatopathol. 2005;27(2):96–101.

12. Sarvjot V, Sharma S, Mishra S, Singh A. Melasma: a clinicopathological study of 43 cases. Indian J Pathol Microbiol. 2009;52(3):357–9.

13. Lawrence N, Cox SE, Brody HJ. Treatment of melasma with Jessner's solution versus glycolic acid: a comparison of clinical efficacy and evaluation of the predictive ability of Wood's light examination. J Am Acad Dermatol. 1997;36(4):589–93.

14. Kang HY, Bahadoran P, Suzuki I, Zugaj D, Khemis A, Passeron T, et al. Vivo reflectance confocal microscopy detects pigmentary changes in melasma at a cellular level resolution. Exp Dermatol. 2010;19(8):e228–33.

15. Kang WH, Yoon KH, Lee ES, Kim J, Lee KB, Yim H, et al. Melasma: histopathological characteristics in 56 Korean patients. Br J Dermatol. 2002;146(2):228–37.

16. Kim EH, Kim YC, Lee ES, Kang HY. The vascular characteristics of melasma. J Dermatol Sci. 2007;46(2):111–6.

17. Noh TK, Choi SJ, Chung BY, Kang JS, Lee JH, Lee MW, et al. Inflammatory features of melasma lesions in Asian skin. J Dermatol. 2014;41(9):788–94.

18. Lakhdar H, Zouhair K, Khadir K, Essari A, Richard A, Seite S, et al. Evaluation of the effectiveness of broad-spectrum sunscreen in the prevention of chloasma in pregnant women. J Eur Acad Dermatol Venereol. 2007;21(6):738–42.

19. V_azquez M, S_anchez JL. The efficacy of a broad-spectrum sunscreen in the treatment of melasma. Cutis 1983;32(1):92, 95–6.

20. Hernández-Barrera R, Torres-Alvarez B, Castanedo-Cazares JP, Oros-Ovalle C, Moncada B. Solar elastosis and presence of mast cells as key features in the pathogenesis of melasma. Clin Exp Dermatol. 2008;33(3):305–8.

21. Suzuki I, Kato T, Motokawa T, Tomita Y, Nakamura E, Katagiri T. Increase of pro-opiomelanocortin mRNA prior to tyrosinase, tyrosinase-related protein 1, dopachrome tautomerase, Pmel-17/gp100, and P-protein mRNA in human skin after ultraviolet B irradiation. J Invest Dermatol. 2002;118(1):73–8.

22. Im S, Kim J. On WY, Kang WH. Increased expression of alpha-melanocyte-stimulating hormone in the lesional skin of melasma. Br J Dermatol. 2002;146(1):165–7.

23. Kovacs D, Cardinali G, Aspite N, Cota C, Luzi F, Bellei B, et al. Role of fibroblast-derived growth factors in regulating hyperpigmentation of solar lentigo. Br J Dermatol. 2010;163(5):1020–7.

24. Chen N, Hu Y, Li WH, Eisinger M, Seiberg M, Lin CB. The role of keratinocyte growth factor in melanogenesis: a possible mechanism for the initiation of solar lentigines. Exp Dermatol 2010;19(10):865–872.

25. Kang HY, Hwang JS, Lee JY, Ahn JH, Kim JY, Lee ES, et al. The dermal stem cell factor and c-kit are overexpressed in melasma. Br J Dermatol. 2006;154(6):1094–9.

26. Imokawa G. Autocrine and paracrine regulation of melanocytes in human skin and in pigmentary disorders. Pigment Cell Res. 2004;17(2):96–110.

27. Kim YJ, Kang HY. Pigmentation after using topical tacrolimus to treat lichen sclerosus: possible role of stem cell factor. J Am Acad Dermatol. 2007;57(5 Suppl):S125–7.

28. Hasegawa K, Fujiwara R, Sato K, Shin J, Kim SJ, Kim M, et al. Possible involvement of keratinocyte growth factor in the persistence of hyperpigmentation in both human facial solar lentigines and melasma. Ann Dermatol. 2015;27(5):626–9.

29. Kim M, Han JH, Kim JH, Park TJ, Kang HY. Secreted frizzled-related protein 2 (sFRP2) functions as a Melanogenic stimulator; the role of sFRP2 in UV-induced Hyperpigmentary disorders. J Invest Dermatol. 2016;136(1):236–44.

30. Choi JR, Won CH, ES O, An J, Chang SE. The degree of erythema in melasma lesion is associated with the severity of disease and the response to the low-fluence Q-switched 1064-nm Nd:YAG laser treatment. J Dermatolog Treat. 2013;24(4):297–9.

31. Regazzetti C, De Donatis GM, Ghorbel HH, Cardot-Leccia N, Ambrosetti D, Bahadoran P, et al. Endothelial cells promote pigmentation through Endothelin receptor B activation. J Invest Dermatol. 2015;135(12):3096–104.

32. Park JY, Kim M, Park TJ, Kang HY. TGFβ1 derived from endothelial cells inhibits melanogenesis. Pigment Cell Melanoma Res. 2016;29(4):477–80.

33. Lee DJ, Park KC, Ortonne JP, Kang HY. Pendulous melanocytes: a characteristic feature of melasma and how it may occur. Br J Dermatol. 2012;166(3):684–6.

34. Torres-Álvarez B, Mesa-Garza IG, Castanedo-Cázares JP, Fuentes-Ahumada C, Oros Ovalle C, Navarrete-Solis J, et al. Histochemical and immunohistochemical study in melasma: evidence of damage in the basal membrane. Am J Dermatopathol. 2011;33(3):291–5.

35. Iriyama S, Ono T, Aoki H, Amano S. Hyperpigmentation in human solar lentigo is promoted by heparanase-induced loss of heparan sulfate chains at the dermal–epidermal junction. J Dermatol Sci. 2011;64(3):223–8.

36. Park GH, Lee JH, Choi JR, Chang SE. Does altered basement membrane of melasma lesion affect treatment outcome in Asian skin? Am J Dermatopathol. 2013;35(1):137–8.

37. Lieberman R, Moy L. Estrogen receptor expression in melasma: results from facial skin of affected patients. J Drugs Dermatol. 2008;7(5):463–5.

38. Jian D, Jiang D, Su J, Chen W, Hu X, Kuang Y, et al. Diethylstilbestrol enhances melanogenesis via cAMP-PKA-mediating upregulation of tyrosinase and MITF in mouse B16 melanoma cells. Steroids. 2011;76(12):1297–304.

39. Kim NH, Cheong KA, Lee TR, Lee AY. PDZK1 upregulation in estrogen-related hyperpigmentation in melasma. J Invest Dermatol. 2012;132(11):2622–31.

40. Kippenberger S, Loitsch S, Solano F, Bernd A, Kaufmann R. Quantification of tyrosinase, TRP-1, and Trp-2 transcripts in human melanocytes by reverse transcriptase-competitive multiplex PCR--regulation by steroid hormones. J Invest Dermatol. 1998;110(4):364–7.

41. Jee SH, Lee SY, Chiu HC, Chang CC, Chen TJ. Effects of estrogen and estrogen receptor in normal human melanocytes. Biochem Biophys Res Commun. 1994;199(3):1407–12.

42. Kang HY, Suzuki I, Lee DJ, Ha J, Reiniche P, Aubert J, et al. Transcriptional profiling shows altered expression of wnt pathway- and lipid metabolism-related genes as well as melanogenesis-related genes in melasma. J Invest Dermatol. 2011;131(8):1692–700.

43. Park TJ, Kim M, Kim H, Park SY, Park KC, Ortonne JP, et al. Wnt inhibitory factor (WIF)-1 promotes melanogenesis in normal human melanocytes. Pigment Cell Melanoma Res. 2014;27(1):72–81.

44. Kim NH, Choi SH, Kim CH, Lee CH, Lee TR, Lee AY. Reduced MiR-675 in exosome in H19 RNA-related melanogenesis via MITF as a direct target. J Invest Dermatol. 2014;134(4):1075–82.

45. Kang WH, Chun SC, Lee S. Intermittent therapy for melasma in Asian patients with combined topical agents (retinoic acid, hydroquinone and hydrocortisone): clinical and histological studies. J Dermatol. 1998;25(9):587–9.

46. Chan R, Park KC, Lee MH, Lee ES, Chang SE, Leow YH, et al. A randomized controlled trial of the efficacy and safety of a fixed triple combination (fluocinolone acetonide 0.01%, hydroquinone 4%, tretinoin 0.05%) compared with hydroquinone 4% cream in Asian patients with moderate to severe melasma. Br J Dermatol. 2008;159(3):697–703.

47. Na JI, Choi SY, Yang SH, Choi HR, Kang HY, Park KC. Effect of tranexamic acid on melasma: a clinical trial with histological evaluation. J Eur Acad Dermatol Venereol. 2013;27(8):1035–9.

48. Kim SJ, Park JY, Shibata T, Fujiwara R, Kang HY. Efficacy and possible mechanisms of topical tranexamic acid in melasma. Clin Exp Dermatol. 2016;41(5):480–5.

49. Tay EY, Gan EY, Tan VW, Lin Z, Liang Y, Lin F, et al. Pilot study of an automated method to determine Melasma area and severity index. Br J Dermatol. 2015;172(6):1535–40.

50. Cameli N, Abril E, Agozzino M, Mariano M. Clinical and instrumental evaluation of the efficacy of a new depigmenting agent containing a combination of a retinoid, a phenolic agent and an antioxidant for the treatment of solar lentigines. Dermatology. 2015;230(4):360–6.

51. Cho M, Lee DH, Kim Y, Koh W, Chung JH, Kim HC, et al. Development and clinical validation of a novel photography-based skin pigmentation evaluation system: a comparison with the calculated consensus of dermatologists. Int J Cosmet Sci. 2016;38(4):399–408.

52. Newcomer VD, Lindberg MC, Sternberg THA. Melanosis of the face ("chloasma"). Arch Dermatol. 1961;83:284–99.

53. Pathak MA, Riley FC, Fitzpatrick TB. Melanogenesis in human skin following exposure to long-wave ultraviolet and visible light. J Invest Dermatol. 1962;39:435–43.

54. Grimes PE. Melasma. Etiologic and therapeutic considerations. Arch Dermatol. 1995;131(12):1453–7.

55. Westerhof W, Kooyers TJ. Hydroquinone and its analogues in dermatology - a potential health risk. J Cosmet Dermatol. 2005;4(2):55–9.

56. Nordlund JJ, Grimes PE, Ortonne JP. The safety of hydroquinone. J Eur Acad Dermatol Venereol. 2006;20(7):781–7.

57. Kang HY, Valerio L, Bahadoran P, Ortonne JP. The role of topical retinoids in the treatment of pigmentary disorders: an evidence-based review. Am J Clin Dermatol. 2009;10(4):251–60.

58. Ferreira Cestari T, Hassun K, Sittart A, de Lourdes Viegas MA. Comparison of triple combination cream and hydroquinone 4% cream for the treatment of moderate to severe facial melasma. J Cosmet Dermatol. 2007;6(1):36–9.

59. Chakraborty AK, Funasaka Y, Komoto M, Ichihashi M. Effect of arbutin on melanogenic proteins in human melanocytes. Pigment Cell Res. 1998;11(4):206–12.

60. Ertam I, Mutlu B, Unal I, Alper S, Kivcak B, Ozer O. Efficiency of ellagic acid and arbutin in melasma: a randomized, prospective, open-label study. J Dermatol. 2008;35(9):570–4.

61. Nazzaro-Porro M, Passi S. Identification of tyrosinase inhibitors in cultures of Pityrosporum. J Invest Dermatol. 1978;71(3):205–8.

62. Kim DS, Kim SY, Park SH, Choi YG, Kwon SB, Kim MK, et al. Inhibitory effects of 4-n-butylresorcinol on tyrosinase activity and melanin synthesis. Biol Pharm Bull. 2005;28(12):2216–9.

63. Huh SY, Shin JW, Na JI, Huh CH, Youn SW, Park KC. Efficacy and safety of liposome-encapsulated 4-n-butylresorcinol 0.1% cream for the treatment of melasma: a randomized controlled split-face trial. J Dermatol. 2010;37(4):311–5.

64. Ros JR, Rodriguez-Lopez JN, Garcia-Canovas F. Effect of L-ascorbic acid on the monophenolase activity of tyrosinase. Biochem J. 1993;295(Pt 1):309–12.

65. Huh CH, Seo KI, Park JY, Lim JG, Eun HC, Park KCA. Randomized, double-blind, placebo-controlled trial of vitamin C iontophoresis in melasma. Dermatology. 2003;206(4):316–20.

66. Ichihashi M, Funasaka Y, Ohashi A, Chacraborty A, Ahmed NU, Ueda M, et al. The inhibitory effect of DL-alpha-tocopheryl ferulate in lecithin on melanogenesis. Anticancer Res. 1999;19(5A):3769–74.

67. Yamamura T, Onishi J, Nishiyama T. Antimelanogenic activity of hydrocoumarins in cultured normal human melanocytes by stimulating intracellular glutathione synthesis. Arch Dermatol Res. 2002;294(8): 349–54.

68. Saliou C, Kitazawa M, McLaughlin L, Yang JP, Lodge JK, Tetsuka T, et al. Antioxidants modulate acute solar ultraviolet radiation-induced NF-kappa-B activation in a human keratinocyte cell line. Free Radic Biol Med. 1999;26(1–2):174–83.

69. Kasraee B. Depigmentation of brown Guinea pig skin by topical application of methimazole. J Invest Dermatol. 2002;118(1):205–7.

70. Kasraee B. Peroxidase-mediated mechanisms are involved in the melanocytotoxic and melanogenesis-inhibiting effects of chemical agents. Dermatology. 2002;205(4):329–39.

71. Robb EL, Page MM, Wiens BE, Stuart JA. Molecular mechanisms of oxidative stress resistance induced by resveratrol: specific and progressive induction of MnSOD. Biochem Biophys Res Commun. 2008;367(2):406–12.

72. Seiberg M, Paine C, Sharlow E, Andrade-Gordon P, Costanzo M, Eisinger M, et al. Inhibition of melanosome transfer results in skin lightening. J Invest Dermatol. 2000;115(2):162–7.

73. Seiberg M, Paine C, Sharlow E, Andrade-Gordon P, Costanzo M, Eisinger M, et al. The protease-activated receptor 2 regulates pigmentation via keratinocyte-melanocyte interactions. Exp Cell Res. 2000;254(1):25–32.

74. Hakozaki T, Minwalla L, Zhuang J, Chhoa M, Matsubara A, Miyamoto K, et al. The effect of niacinamide on reducing cutaneous pigmentation and suppression of melanosome transfer. Br J Dermatol. 2002;147(1):20–31.

75. Ando H, Ryu A, Hashimoto A, Oka M, Ichihashi M. Linoleic acid and alpha-linolenic acid lightens ultraviolet-induced hyperpigmentation of the skin. Arch Dermatol Res. 1998;290(7):375–81.

76. Mishima Y, Imokawa G. Selective aberration and pigment loss in melanosomes of malignant melanoma cells in vitro by glycosylation inhibitors: premelanosomes as glycoprotein. J Invest Dermatol. 1983;81(2):106–14.

77. Franchi J, Coutadeur MC, Marteau C, Mersel M, Kupferberg A. Depigmenting effects of calcium D-pantetheine-S-sulfonate on human melanocytes. Pigment Cell Res. 2000;13(3):165–71.

78. Li YH, Chen JZ, Wei HC, Wu Y, Liu M, Xu YY, et al. Efficacy and safety of intense pulsed light in treatment of melasma in Chinese patients. Dermatol Surg. 2008;34(5):693–700. discussion 700-1

79. Negishi K, Kushikata N, Tezuka Y, Takeuchi K, Miyamoto E, Wakamatsu S. Study of the incidence and nature of "very subtle epidermal melasma" in relation to intense pulsed light treatment. Dermatol Surg. 2004;30(6):881–6. discussion 6

80. Lee WR, Shen SC, Pai MH, Yang HH, Yuan CY, Fang JY. Fractional laser as a tool to enhance the skin permeation of 5-aminolevulinic acid with minimal skin disruption: a comparison with conventional erbium: Yag laser. J Control Release. 2010 Jul 14;145(2):124–33.

81. Rokhsar CK, Fitzpatrick RE. The treatment of melasma with fractional photothermolysis: a pilot study. Dermatol Surg. 2005;31(12):1645–50.

82. Kroon MW, Wind BS, Beek JF, van der Veen JP, Nieuweboer-Krobotová L, Bos JD, et al. Nonablative 1550-nm fractional laser therapy versus triple topical therapy for the treatment of melasma: a randomized controlled pilot study. J Am Acad Dermatol. 2011;64(3):516–23.

83. Kim JH, Kim H, Park HC, Kim IH. Subcellular selective photothermolysis of melanosomes in adult zebrafish skin following 1064-nm Q-switched Nd:YAG laser irradiation. J Invest Dermatol. 2010;130(9):2333–5.

84. Wattanakrai P, Mornchan R, Eimpunth S. Low-fluence Q-switched neodymium-doped yttrium aluminum garnet (1,064 nm) laser for the treatment of facial melasma in Asians. Dermatol Surg. 2010;36(1):76–87. https://doi.org/10.1111/j.1524-4725.2009.01383.x.

85. Passeron T, Fontas E, Kang HY, Bahadoran P, Lacour JP, Ortonne JP. Melasma treatment with pulsed-dye laser and triple combination cream: a prospective, randomized, single-blind, split-face study. Arch Dermatol. 2011;147(9):1106–8.

86. Lee HI, Lim YY, Kim BJ, Kim MN, Min HJ, Hwang JH, et al. Clinicopathologic efficacy of copper bromide plus/yellow laser (578 nm with 511 nm) for treatment of melasma in Asian patients. Dermatol Surg. 2010;36(6):885–93.

87. Ferrara N. Binding to the extracellular matrix and proteolytic processing: two key mechanisms regulating vascular endothelial growth factor action. Mol Biol Cell. 2010;21(5):687–90.

88. Bastaki M, Nelli EE, Dell'Era P, Rusnati M, Molinari-Tosatti MP, Parolini S, et al. Basic fibroblast growth factor-induced angiogenic phenotype in mouse endothelium. A study of aortic and microvascular endothelial cell lines. Arterioscler Thromb Vasc Biol. 1997;17(3):454–64.

Macular Pigmentation of Uncertain Etiology

13

Johannes F. Dayrit and Prasad Kumarasinghe

Understanding Macular Pigmentation of Uncertain Etiology

Ashy dermatosis (AD), erythema dyschromicum perstans (EDP), lichen planus pigmentosus (LPP), and idiopathic eruptive macular pigmentation (IEMP) manifest clinically as acquired macules and patches of hyperpigmentation. The etiology and pathogenesis of each disease remains an enigma, and presently there is no consensus on effective treatment. The clinical features overlap and racial variations may exist. And because these diseases share similarities in clinical presentation, the term "macular pigmentation of uncertain etiology" (MPUE) has been suggested as the proper nomenclature until the condition is accurately diagnosed. Although a global consensus on the definition of these entities is still lacking, more recent publications suggest that small and large macular pigmentation of

uncertain etiology (i.e., AD, EDP, and IEMP) should be considered as separate entities from those associated with lichen planus . While agreeing that ashy dermatosis, EDP, and LPP are forms of MPUE, AD with the classic presentation on the trunk, EDP with erythematous borders predominantly on the trunk, and LPP on the face and neck, these terms may still be used, especially by clinicians who are familiar with the classic types. For all other non-specific forms of small and large macules of pigmentation, the term MPUE or AMPUE (acquired macular pigmentation of uncertain etiology) can be used. A review of related literature differentiates IEMP from AD and EDP based on the self-limiting course of the disease. Lesions of IEMP usually disappear within a few months to a few years, in contradistinction to AD and EDP which persist for several years [1]. There is a pressing need to fully understand and properly define these skin conditions as patchy hyperpigmentation creates both cosmetic and psychological problems for the darker-skinned populations (Fitzpatrick skin types III and above).

J. F. Dayrit
Department of Dermatology, Research Institute for Tropical Medicine, Metro Manila, Philippines

Department of Internal Medicine, De La Salle Health Sciences Institute, Cavite, Philippines

P. Kumarasinghe (✉)
Department of Dermatology, Fiona Stanley Hospital and University of Western Australia, Perth, WA, Australia

Ashy Dermatosis

Ashy dermatosis was first described in 1957 by Oswaldo Ramirez in El Salvador, who reported 139 patients who abruptly developed

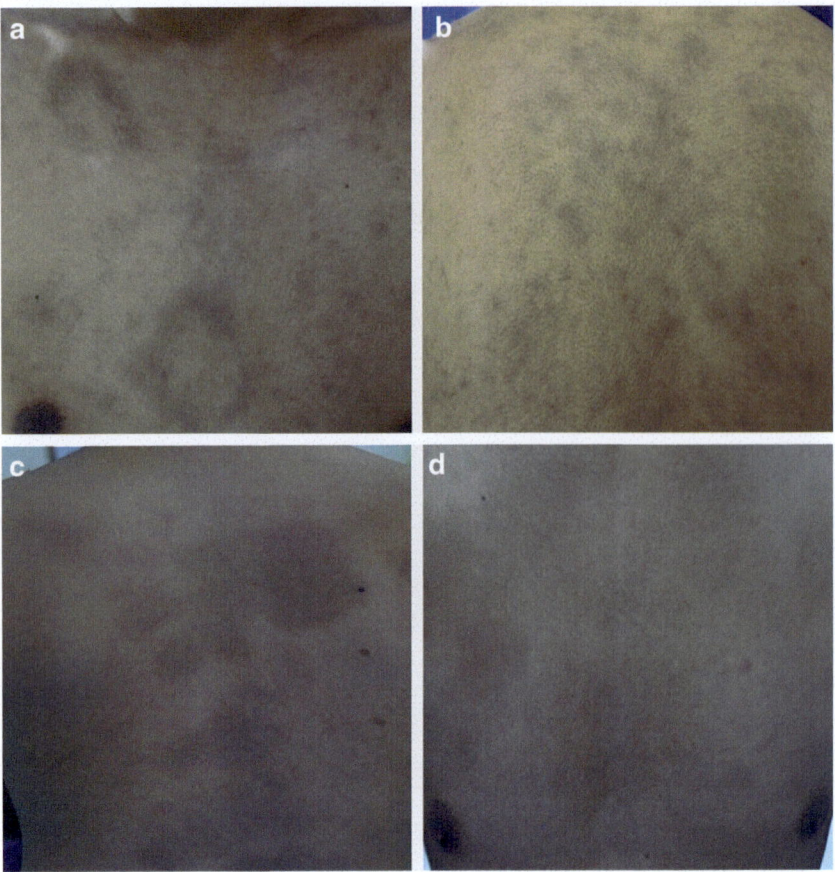

Fig. 13.1 Ashy dermatosis in two Filipino males (**a**) 17 years old and (**b**) 18 years old with ash-gray patches on the trunk for 12 (**a, b**) and 10 months (**c, d**), respectively. The size of the lesions ranged from 1 to 5 cm

ash-gray-colored macules (from 1 cm to very large patches), without any classical lesions of lichen planus (Fig. 13.1). Some of the cases showed transient non-elevated erythematous borders. From the original case series, majority of the subjects were young adults from Central America. The etiology of the disease was unknown, and no predisposing factors have been identified. The disease runs a chronic course and is refractory to any form of treatment. Pruritus or preceding papules and plaques are usually not present, and there is no nail nor mucosal involvement [2, 3].

The main histological features of AD based on the original study of Ramirez were hydropic or vacuolar alteration of the basal cell layer, dermal melanosis, and a perivascular infiltrate of lymphocytes, histiocytes, and melanin-laden macrophages (Fig. 13.2). Likewise, Weedon described the histopathology of AD as thinning of the epidermis with mild vacuolar alteration of the basal cell layer, marked melanin incontinence, and a lymphocytic infiltrate. These histological changes are reminiscent of what is called "burnt-out" appearance [4], used to describe post-inflammatory changes secondary to interface dermatitis such as in lichen planus, lupus erythematosus, erythema multiforme, and drug eruptions.

Erythema Dyschromicum Perstans

In 1961, Convit and colleagues reported five patients in Venezuela presenting with similar signs and symptoms described by Ramirez in

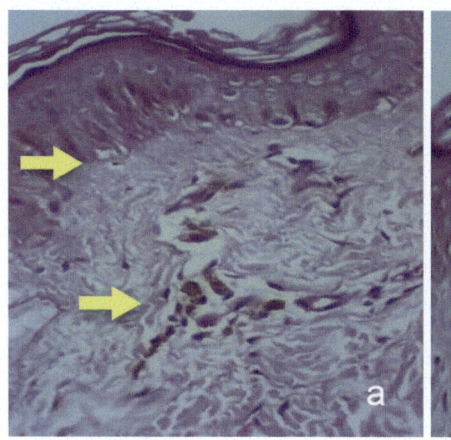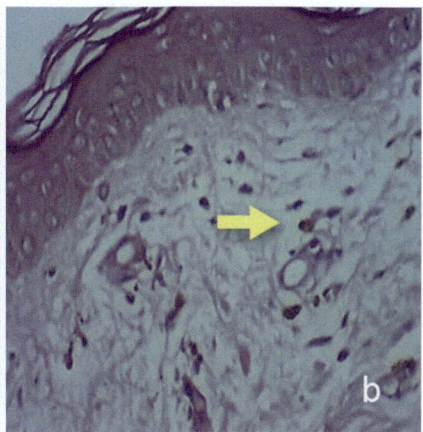

Fig. 13.2 Histopathological findings of established AD show (**a**, **b**) absence or subtle vacuolar change in the basal layer, prominent pigment incontinence in the papil-lary dermis, and a mild superficial perivascular lympho-cytic infiltrate. H&E X400 (**a**, **b**)

1957, but in addition having an elevated erythematous border in active lesions, which disappeared after several months. The macules sometimes become confluent to cover extensive areas of the body [5]. It is important to note that the patients described by Convit and colleagues resembled those of Ramirez, except for the presence of raised erythematous margins in the active part of the lesions, and to date, this is the only recognized significant difference between the so-called cases of AD and EDP (Fig. 13.3a–d).

The histologic findings of cases described in literature were consistent with a lichenoid tissue reaction pattern, and the term "erythema dyschromicum perstans" was proposed to name this skin condition. As an attempt to resolve conflicts in terminology, Weedon [4] proposed that the term EDP should be used in cases where lesions have or have previously had an erythematous border, while AD should be used for other cases where the "erythematous feature" is lacking. However some authors consider that ashy dermatosis and EDP are the same [3], and other authors believe that the two entities can only be considered different until an etiological basis for each has finally been established.

Histologically, EDP shows discrete areas of follicular hyperkeratosis, vacuolar alteration of the basal cell layer, pigment incontinence, and a sleeve-like perivascular infiltrate of lymphocytes

and macrophages filled with melanin-containing granules. The erythematous component of EDP lesions shows vacuolar alteration of the basal cell layer, presence of occasional colloid bodies, melanin-laden macrophages, and a perivascular infiltrate of lymphocytes and histiocytes (Fig. 13.4a–d). The infiltrate may be more pronounced in the upper portion of the dermis. However, in the ashy blue-gray macules and patches, melanin incontinence is a more prominent histological finding, while the vacuolar change in the basal cell layer and the lymphohistiocytic infiltrate in the dermis may only be mild or absent [6]. Similarly, Pinkus divided the histopathological findings of EDP into two phases: early and late. A lichenoid infiltrate of lymphocytes and vacuolar alteration of the basal cell layer predominate in the early phase. As the lesions mature, there is reduction in the density of the infiltrate leaving only residual vacuolar alteration of the basal cells. There is also significant melanin incontinence, and there is a tendency toward the loss of the rete ridge pattern in mature lesions [7].

Direct immunofluorescence examination of lesional skin shows numerous, small, intensely staining, epidermal and dermal, globular deposits of immunoglobulins, C3, and fibrinogen, corresponding to the colloid bodies seen on routine light microscopy. Electron microscopy findings

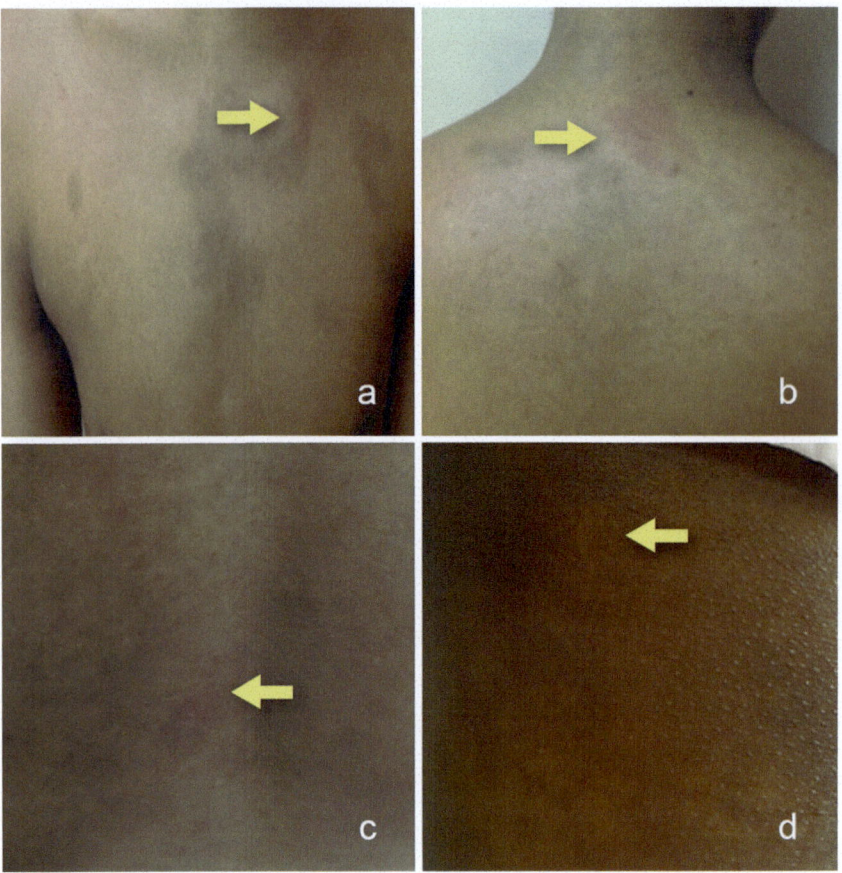

Fig. 13.3 Erythema dyschromicum perstans in four Filipinos (**a–d**) who presented clinically with ash-gray patches on the trunk with areas of elevated erythematous periphery

are non-specific and reflect the inflammatory nature of the condition [8].

To date, the cause of EDP is still unknown, and in the vast majority of cases, no ingestants, inhalants, or contactants have been implicated [8]. Pinkus [7] has postulated that unidentified set of environmental pollutants may be affecting certain predisposed individuals.

In general, treatment has been unsuccessful in either halting the progress of the condition or reversing the hyperpigmentation. Among the various modalities that have been tried are avoidance of sun exposure, use of sunscreens, chemical peels, broad-spectrum antibiotics, oral and topical corticosteroids, oral vitamin therapy, chloroquine, griseofulvin, and DMSO [8].

Lichen Planus Pigmentosus

Bhutani and colleagues [9] reported 40 cases in India with lesions similar to those described by Ramirez. The patients are young (20–45), and there is equal sex predilection. Men present a decade earlier than women (20 vs 34). The clinical and histological findings in 11 of the patients (27.5%) presented by Bhutani had an association with lichen planus; hence, they proposed to name the condition lichen planus pigmentosus. It is believed to be a macular variant of lichen planus, and more recent observations show that it usually starts on the face, neck, and ears (Fig. 13.5). Only a minority of cases of LPP have past or current evidence of typical lichen planus. It is sometimes associated with pruritus, and oral mucosal involvement is sometimes seen [10]. If pruritus is

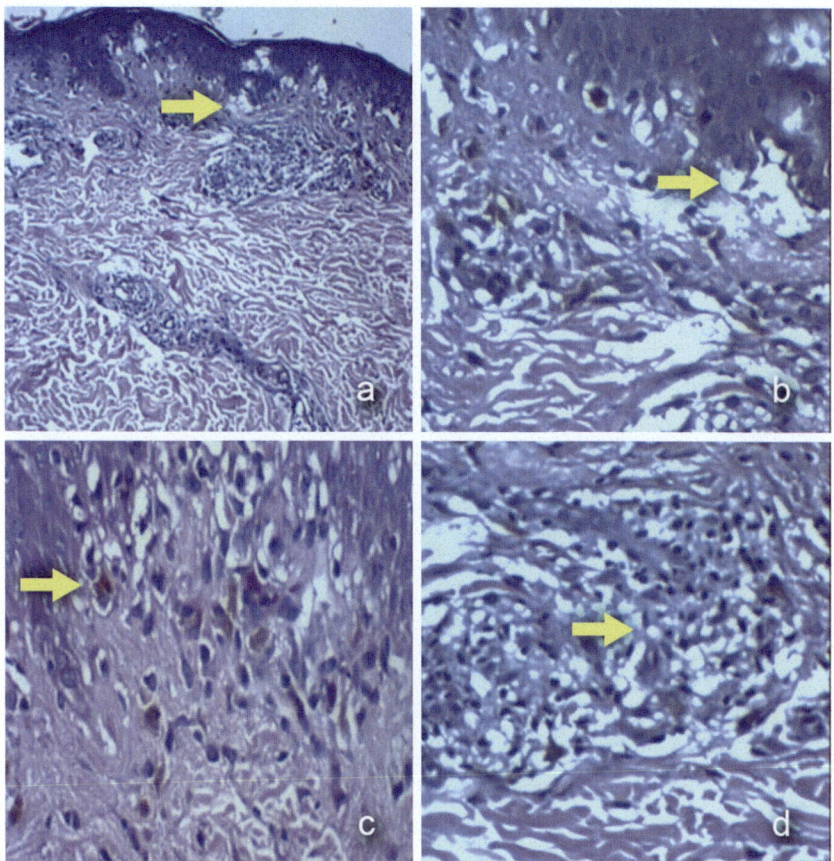

Fig. 13.4 Biopsy of erythematous part of an EDP lesion shows more pronounced vacuolar alteration of the basal cell layer, melanin-laden macrophages, and sleeve-like mononuclear perivascular infiltrate (**a, b**). A biopsy taken from the ash-gray patch shows milder vacuolar alteration and more prominent pigment incontinence (**c, d**) H&E ×100 (**a**), H&E ×400 (**b–d**)

a prominent feature in a patient presenting with ash-gray patches on the head and neck, other diagnoses such as post-inflammatory hyperpigmentation should be considered carefully.

Controversy exists regarding the relationship of AD, EDP, and LPP based on clinical and histopathological features. Pinkus [7, 11] included ashy dermatosis and atrophic lichen planus in the same section of his classification of "lichenoid tissue reaction patterns" because of their histological similarities. Novick and Phelps [8] suggested that EDP is a variant of lichen planus based on similarities in clinical presentation, histopathological, DIF, and electron microscopy findings. In the original study of Bhutani and colleagues, in 9 of the 40 patients they studied, the

typical clinical and histological lesions of EDP were accompanied, preceded, or followed by lesions of lichen planus.

On the other hand, Vega and colleagues in 1992 [12] reviewed 20 cases of AD and 11 cases of LPP and tried to distinguish these two entities despite similar histopathological findings. In the LPP patient group, the average age at onset was 46 years (range 9–68), and there was no sex predilection. The pattern of distribution was localized in six (54%) of cases and generalized in five cases (46%). The main areas affected in the localized form are the face ($n = 4$) and submammary, axillary, and inguinal folds ($n = 1$ each). There was slight variation in the morphology of the lesions in LPP and AD, such that the macules

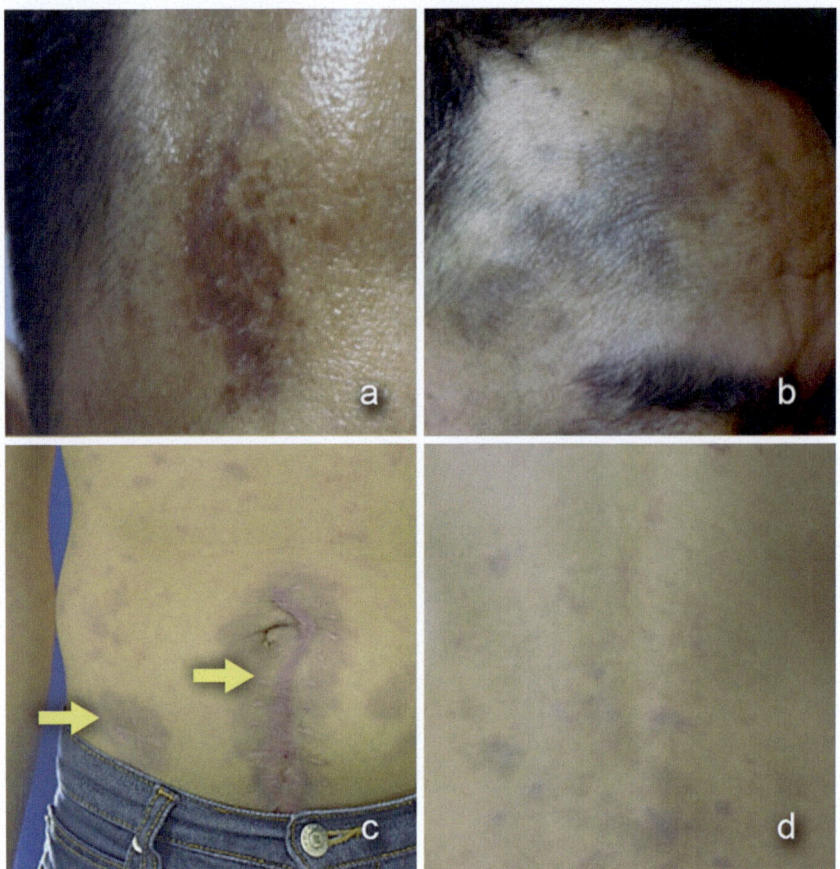

Fig. 13.5 Lichen planus pigmentosus in two Filipino males showing blackish-brown patches on the forehead (**a**, **b**). In another case of LPP in a 19-year-old male, Koebner phenomenon was observed on surgical scars on the abdomen (**c**) while lesions on the back showed ash-gray patches similar to AD and EDP (**d**)

in LPP were black-brown, irregularly shaped, and with ill-defined borders, and none of the subjects presented with the elevated, active red borders present in AD. While all the cases of AD were asymptomatic, seven (62%) of the individuals with LPP had pruritus [12].

Treatment in the LPP patients consisted mainly of topical steroids, keratolytics, and 10% aqueous solution of dimethyl sulfoxide; others received griseofulvin, prednisone (1 mg/kg), retinoids (etretinate), or chloroquine. Only one patient showed an almost complete resolution with topical steroids, while the rest did not show any changes [12]. More recently Muthu and colleagues [13] have shown improvement with low-dose (20 mg/day for 6 months) isotretinoin in early cases of LPP in Indian patients. Topical

tacrolimus has also been reported to be effective in LPP patients (53.8%) by some authors [14]. However, more studies are needed to assess the efficacy of these new and promising treatment modalities.

Vega and colleagues believed that ashy dermatosis predominates in type IV skin, and there are probably some undefined ecological and nutritional conditions involved that are not applicable to other races or countries in North America and Europe [12]. However, the nutritional deficiency theory is not tenable as migrants from South Asian ethnicities with affluent lifestyles living in the West also develop similar skin lesions despite a healthy diet.

The histopathological finding of LPP is characterized by an atrophic epidermis with vacuolar alteration of the basal layer; a scarce lymphohistiocytic or lichenoid infiltrate with incontinence of pigment and the presence of melanin-laden macrophages are seen in the dermis [12].

A biopsy of a raised lesion shows typical lichen planus pathology characterized by sawtoothing of the rete ridges, wedge-shaped hypergranulosis, vacuolar alteration of the basal layer, civatte bodies, and a lichenoid lymphocytic infiltrate. A biopsy of a macule, on the other hand, reveals a relatively flat epidermis with loss of the rete pattern, focal vacuolar change with occasional necrotic keratinocytes and civatte bodies, dermal melanophages, and lymphocytic infiltrate [11]. The lichenoid inflammatory infiltrate, which is often focal and peri-infundibular, is a helpful histological feature which may differentiate LPP from either EDP or AD (Fig. 13.6a–d). Direct immunofluorescence helps confirm the diagnosis of LPP showing the presence of IgM and IgG, complement, and fibrin (Fig. 13.6e), but these findings may also be observed in EDP [11].

In the study by Vega and colleagues, treatment of LPP included topical steroids, keratolytics, or 10% aqueous solution of dimethyl sulfoxide. The others tried griseofulvin, prednisone, etretinate, or chloroquine. Majority showed no response to treatment [12].

Idiopathic Eruptive Macular Pigmentation

In 1978, Degos and colleagues reported seven pediatric cases with pigmented macules, 5–25 mm in diameter, distributed over the neck, trunk, and limbs, and introduced the nomenclature idiopathic eruptive macular pigmentation [15]. Three of the cases were de novo eruptions

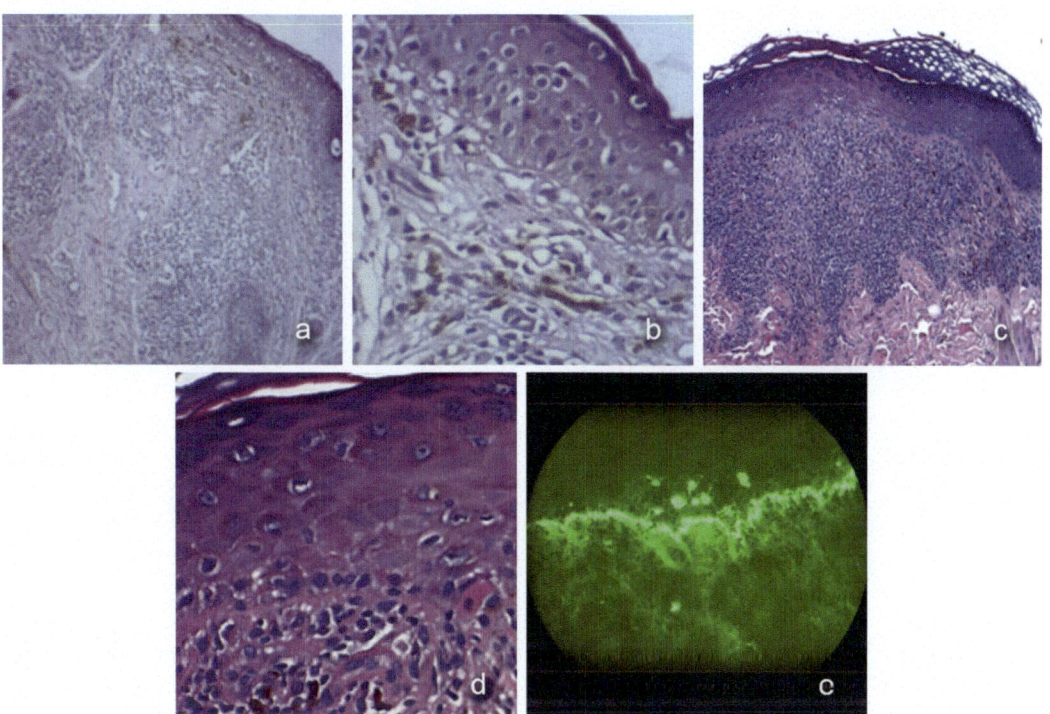

Fig. 13.6 Histopathology of lichen planus pigmentosus in the early stages (**a–c**) may show wedge-shaped hypergranulosis and vacuolar alteration of the basal cell layer. Colloid bodies and a dense lichenoid infiltrate of lymphocytes are seen in the dermis (**d**). Immunofluorescence shows deposition of C3, IgM colloid bodies, and fibrinogen at the DEJ (**e**)

presenting similar to ashy dermatosis. However, the lack of a palpable erythematous border and vacuolar degeneration of the basal cell layer distinguished these conditions from erythema dyschromicum perstans and lichen planus pigmentosus. Because of the widespread brown to gray macules on the neck, trunk, and extremities, a close differential diagnosis is urticaria pigmentosa (UP). However, in IEMP, Darier's sign is negative (absence of urticaria), and in UP, histopathology would show increased density of mast cells in the dermal papillae. Several reports followed which improved the definition of idiopathic eruptive macular eruption. In 1996, Sanz de Galdeano et al. outlined the basic criteria for diagnosing the condition [16]. (Fig. 13.7)

1. Eruption of brownish, nonconfluent, asymptomatic macules involving the trunk, neck, and proximal extremities in children and adolescents (Fig. 13.8)
2. Absence of preceding inflammatory lesions
3. No previous drug exposure
4. Basal cell layer hyperpigmentation of the epidermis and prominent dermal melanophages

without visible basal layer damage or lichenoid inflammatory infiltrate (Fig. 13.9)
5. Normal mast cell count

The clinical and histopathological features of IEMP were further studied by Jang and colleagues [17] in a series of ten cases among Asians. His subjects consisted of six male and four female children or young adults. The lesions appeared suddenly, persisted from 2 months to 5 years, and disappeared gradually in nine patients. In one patient the lesions did not disappear. Histopathological findings included increased pigmentation in the basal layer in an otherwise normal epidermis, melanin incontinence in the upper dermis, and a mild lymphocytic inflammatory infiltrate. A characteristic feature of IEMP is that the condition improves spontaneously without any treatment and typically regresses over a course of some months to a few years [16–18].

Joshi and colleagues later described nine cases from India similar to previously reported cases of IEMP but with the characteristic feature of velvety thickening of the patchy pigmented lesions with histopathological features of pigmented

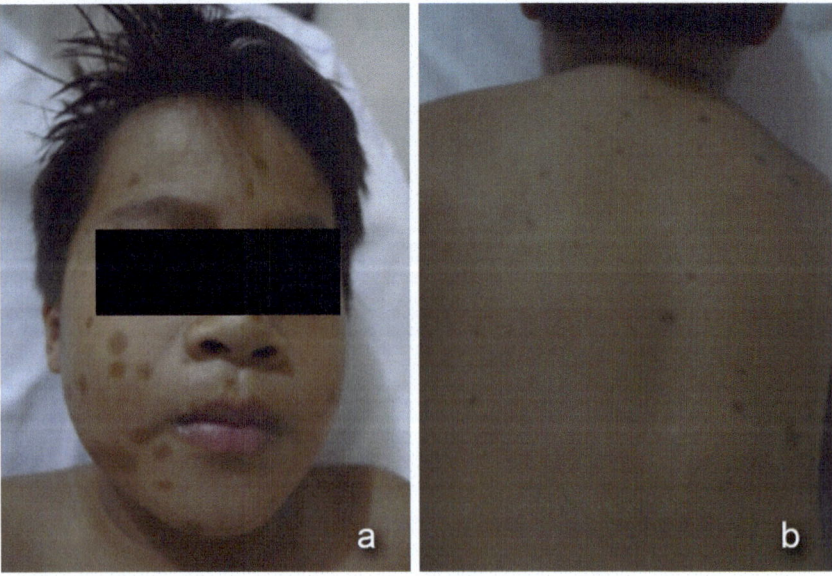

Fig. 13.7 (**a**, **b**) Idiopathic eruptive macular pigmentation in a 7-year-old Filipino boy showing widespread nonconfluent ash-gray macules

papillomatosis similar to acanthosis nigricans [19, 20]. The patient group consisted of seven male and seven female children, whose ages ranged from 6 to 14. The skin lesions were widespread, discrete, and <2 cm. Although the term "IEMP with papillomatosis" has been cited since and used by some other authors as well, it appears to be a paradox that plaque lesions are described as a variant of a macular skin pigmentary disorder (IEMP). Until further evidence is available, it is difficult to categorize IEMP with or without papillomatosis as an eruptive form of acanthosis nigricans [1, 21].

Riehl's Melanosis (Pigmented Contact Dermatitis)

In 1917, Riehl identified several patients with dark-brown to grayish-brown facial pigmentation on the face and neck, which he postulated to be due to nutritional deficiencies during the World War era [22] .Subsequently, different authors identified similar clinical findings that were linked to the use of certain oils, hydrocarbons, formaldehyde, aniline dyes, and Tinopal CH 3566 (optical whitener) from detergents. Some of these substances have been implicated and

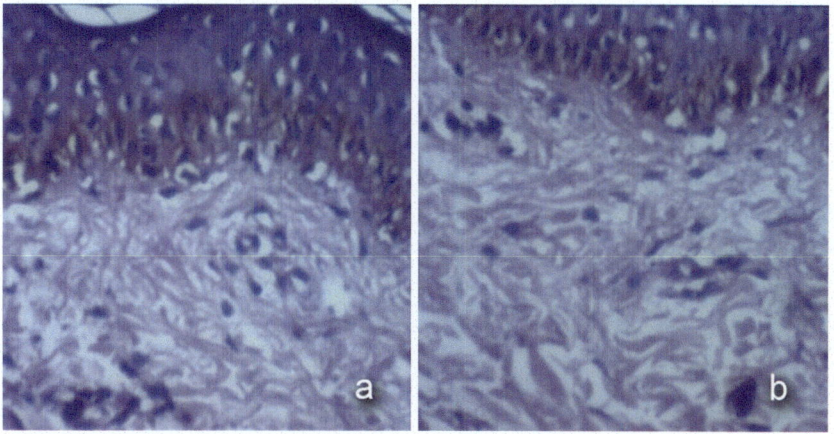

Fig. 13.8 (**a, b**) Histopathological findings of IEMP show prominent hyperpigmentation of the basal cell layer melanin-laden macrophages, and a mild lymphocytic infiltrate is present in the dermis

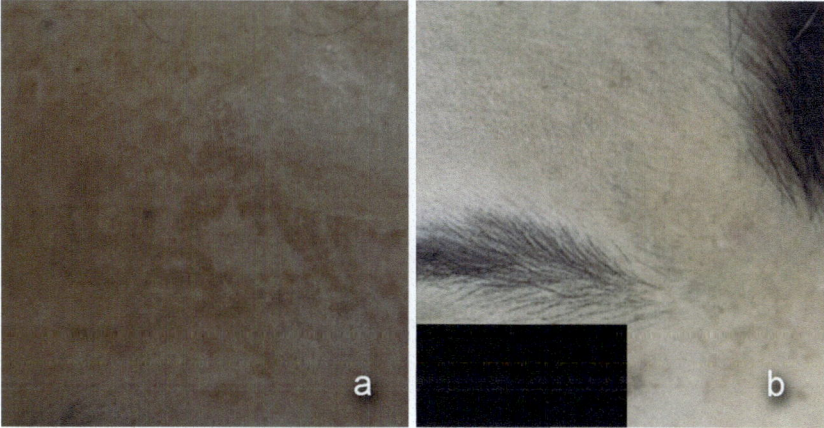

Fig. 13.9 (**a, b**) Riehl's melanosis type of pigmented contact dermatitis in two Filipino males presenting with brownish-gray reticular pigmentation on the bitemporal areas with positive patch tests to paraphenylenediamine and disperse blue dye

documented by patch testing in occupationally related pigmented contact dermatitis [23].

In Japan, the condition is believed to be associated with contact sensitivity to cosmetics or to a photocontact dermatitis resulting from fragrances, musk ambrette, lemon oil, and some bactericidal compounds hence the use of the term "pigmented cosmetic dermatitis" [24, 25]. Most patients presented with no preceding eczematous lesions [26, 27].

Clinically, Riehl's melanosis presents as non-pruritic brownish-gray pigmentation that develops rapidly over the face, more intense on the forehead and the temples. It often has a reticulated pattern (Fig. 13.10a). Although it commonly affects the face, other sun-exposed areas as well as the thighs or axilla can be affected if the textile dyes are implicated [26, 28, 30].

It is not uncommon to find cases with the clinical features of Riehl's melanosis in patients who have not been exposed to any toxins, dyes, or allergy-causing substances as described above. Therefore, clinicians need to critically evaluate the possible etiological factors that lead to this type of pigmentation. Furthermore, spurious associations and causality should be clarified.

Spongiosis and exocytosis of lymphocytes, which are diagnostic features of contact dermatitis, are not present in PCD. Histopathologic features of PCD include epidermal atrophy, vacuolar alteration of the basal cell layer, pigment incontinence, and a lymphocytic inflammatory infiltrate in the dermis. Periodic acid-Schiff stain shows a thickened basal layer (Fig. 13.10) [24, 29, 30]. Confocal microscopy shows basal cell layer liquefaction and pigment incontinence [29].

Patch testing, photo-patch, or repeated open application test (ROAT) is necessary to identify the allergens, and complete avoidance of the allergen often leads to improvement. Hypoallergenic soap and cosmetics and sun protection are essential management. Topical lightening products may be considered, but recently the use of intense-pulsed light therapy and Q-switched Nd:YAG lasers has shown more promising results [31–33].

Approach to the Diagnosis of Macular Pigmentation of Uncertain Etiology

Many types of skin diseases can cause transient, small macules of hyperpigmentation in dark-skinned races. Typical examples are lichen planus, drug eruptions, pityriasis rosea, secondary syphilis, allergic contact dermatitis, viral exanthem, and cutaneous mastocytosis. In AD, EDP,

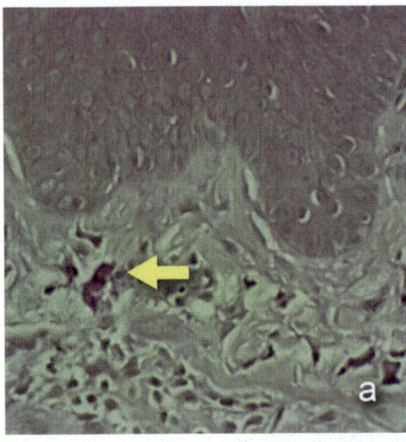 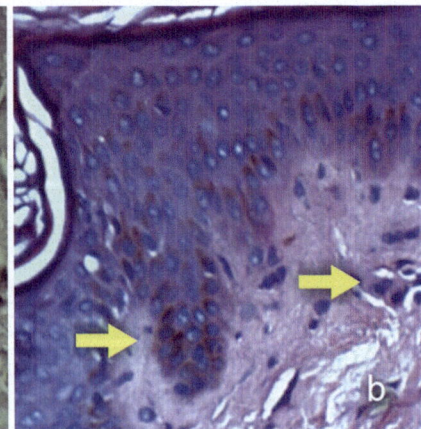

Fig. 13.10 Histopathology shows acanthosis, subtle vacuolar change and melanin-laden macrophages, and a sparse inflammatory infiltrate in the absence of spongiosis (**a**). Elongation of the rete ridges and prominent basal cell layer hyperpigmentation are also seen in another case of Riehl's melanosis (**b**). The presence of melanin-laden macrophages in the dermal papillae is a clue to the diagnosis.

and LPP, the patches are larger and are more persistent [1]. Subtle differences may be appreciated in dermoscopy. To date, there is no large study which evaluated the different dermoscopy patterns seen in AD and EDP. Pirmez and colleagues, however, identified 4 patterns of pigmentation in 37 cases of LPP with accompanying frontal fibrosing alopecia which include pseudonetwork, speckled blue-gray dots, dotted pattern, and blue-gray dots in circles. The changes observed in dermoscopy correlate with the presence and depth of melanin pigments in the dermis, interface dermatitis, and involvement of eccrine glands and hair follicles [34]. Pseudonetworks and gray dots are also prominent dermoscopy characteristics of Riehl's melanosis (Fig. 13.11d) [29]. Patch testing is mandatory to rule out post-inflammatory hyper-

pigmentation secondary to allergic contact dermatitis. Table 13.1 shows the clinical characteristics of AD, EDP, LPP, and IEMP.

The following algorithm facilitates categorizing various types of small and large macules of hyperpigmentation of uncertain etiology (Fig. 13.12). We strongly recommend carefully ruling out drug-induced hyperpigmentations and other etiologies before categorizing as LPP, EDP, AD, or IEMP. These other conditions include Addison's disease, hemochromatosis, ochronosis, argyria, pigmented mycosis fungoides, dermatomyositis, and vitamin B12 deficiency. Furthermore if a particular case of acquired macular pigmentation of uncertain etiology (AMPUE) does not fit in with the typical presentations of AD/EDP, LPP, or IEMP, it is better to label it as "macular pigmentation of uncertain etiology" or

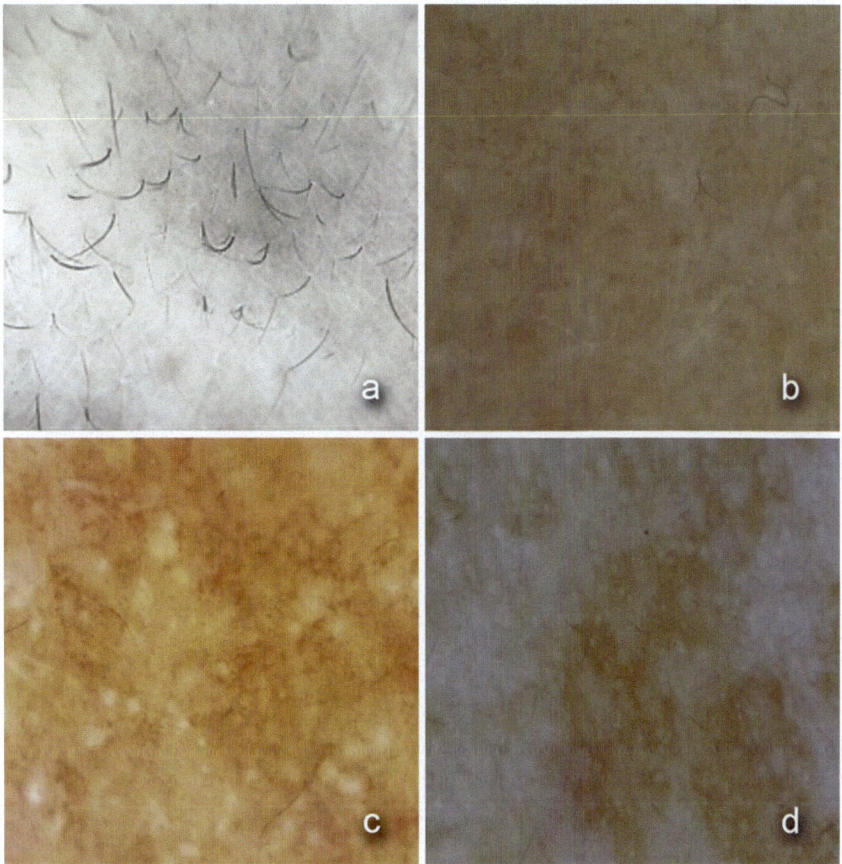

Fig. 13.11 Dermoscopy findings in (**a**) ashy dermatosis, (**b**) erythema dyschromicum perstans, (**c**) lichen planus pigmentosus, and (**d**) Riehl's melanosis which show thin reticular lines and blue-gray dots

Table 13.1 Clinical characteristics of ashy dermatosis, erythema dyschromicum perstans, lichen planus pigmentation, and idiopathic eruptive macular pigmentation.

	Ashy dermatosis	Erythema dyschromicum perstans	Lichen planus pigmentosus	Idiopathic eruptive macular pigmentation	Riehl's melanosis
Epidemiology	Adults Central and South America Dark skin (skin type IV and above), more in women	Adults Central and South America, occasionally Asia Skin type III and above	Adults and adolescents South Asian, south east Asian, African skin types IV and above	Children, adolescents skin types IV and above	Adults
Size	1 cm to very large patches	1 cm to large patches	0.5 cm to large confluent patches	0.5–2.5 cm	<0.5 cm very small macules
Color	Ash-colored, shades of gray, blue-gray hyperpigmented	Fresh lesions have erythematous borders, older lesions ash-colored, shades of gray, blue-gray hyperpigmented	Hyperpigmented dark brown to gray	Hyperpigmented, dark brown to gray	Brownish gray
Lesion	Macules	Macules	Macules	Macules	Macules
Palpable erythematous border	–	+ (active lesion) disappears after several months	–	–	–
Sites of predilection	Symmetrical face, neck, trunk, and upper extremities	Trunk, arms, neck, and face Spares palms, soles, scalp, nails, and mucous membranes	Face, neck, upper trunk, arms, axillae, groins	Neck, trunk, and limbs	Face (forehead temples, neck)
Pruritus	–	–	±	–	–
Associated conditions	–	–	Classic lichen planus ±		
Course	Chronic, insidious	Chronic	Chronic	Months–few years	Chronic

"acquired macular pigmentation of uncertain etiology" and investigate further and monitor for further developments [21].

Conclusion

Acquired macular pigmentation is a significant problem for many patients, more so among the dark-skinned races. A good history and a complete examination are essential to arrive at a rational diagnosis. Acquired macular pigmentation of uncertain etiology(AMPUE) has certain characteristic pigmentation patterns; they include ashy dermatosis, erythema dyschromicum perstans, lichen planus pigmentosus, idiopathic eruptive macular hypermelanosis, Riehl's melanosis, and idiopathic eruptive macular pigmentation. Ashy dermatosis and erythema dyschromicum perstans appear to be in the same spectrum, but EDP shows raised erythematous borders in the fresh lesions. These two conditions are considered synonymous by many. Histopathology alone cannot differentiate the four conditions. The subtle differences observed should be further studied in a large number of cases, supplemented by the use of special stains and immunofluorescence studies. All other cases of acquired macular pigmentation without a known aetiology, where the pattern of pigmentation is not characteristic, are best kept under the umbrella of AMPUE

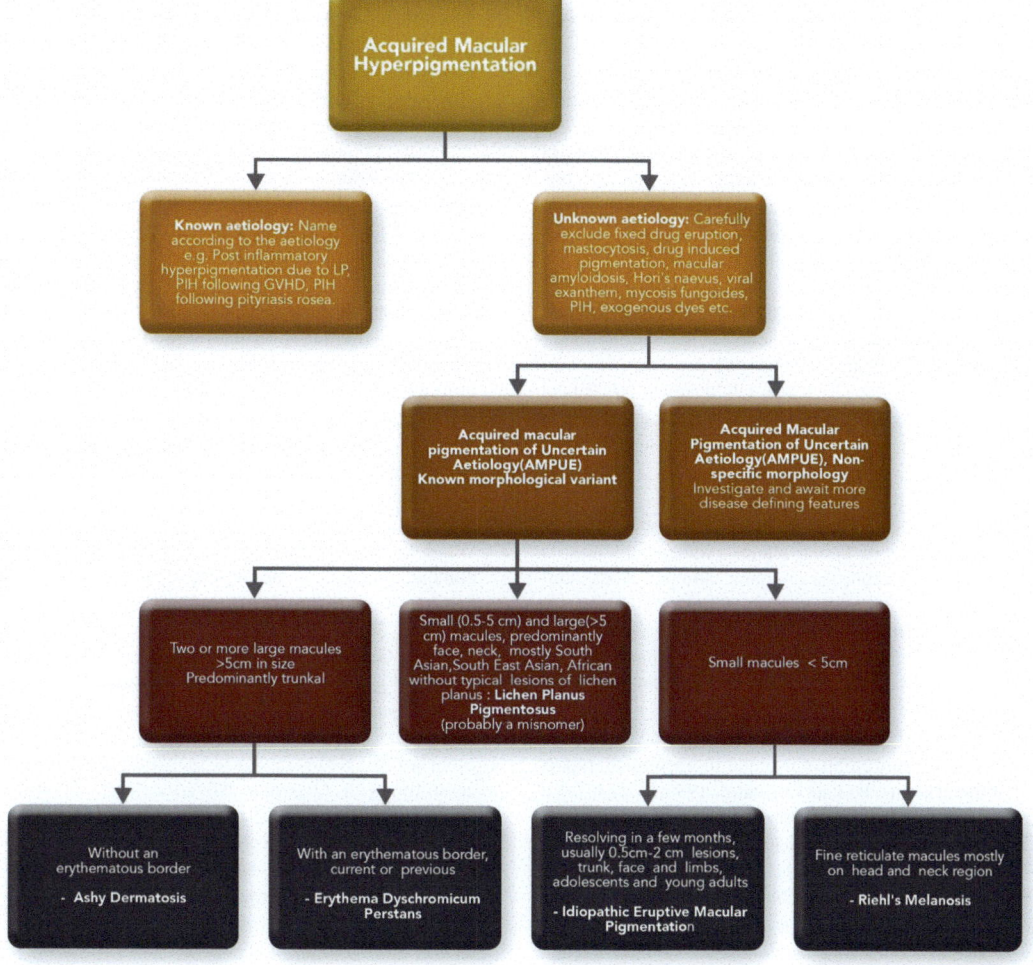

Fig. 13.12 Proposed algorithm for acquired macular hyperpigmentation (Modified from Chandran and Kumarasinghe [21])

until more disease-defining features develop or the etiology becomes clearer.

As the research into all forms of acquired macular pigmentation gains momentum, hopefully the etiology/etiologies will be uncovered, and more effective treatments will be found for this cosmetically undesirable disease condition.

References

1. Kumarasinghe SP. Understanding macular pigmentation of uncertain aetiology. Indian J Dermatol Venereol Leprol. 2015;81:581–3.

2. Ramirez CO. Los Cenicientos (1957) Problema Clinico. In: Report of the first central American congress of dermatology, San Salvador, December 5–8, 1957. San Salvador: Publisher; 1957. p. 122–30.

3. Ramirez CO. The ashy dermatosis (erythema dyschromicum perstans). Epidemiological study and report of 139 cases. Cutis. 1967;3:244–7.

4. Weedon D. Weedon's skin pathology. 2nd ed. London: Churchill Livingstone Elsevier; 2002. p. 37.

5. Convit J, Kerdel-Vegas F, Rodriguez G. Erythema dyschromicum perstans. A hitherto undescribed skin disease. J Invest Dermatol. 1961;36:457–62.

6. Sanchez NP, Pathak MA. Circumscribed dermal melanosis: classification, light, histochemical and electron microscopic studies on 3 patients with erythema dyschromicum perstans. Int J Dermatol. 1985;24:630.

7. Novick NL, Phelps R, Tom C. Erythema dyschromicum perstans. Int J Dermatol. 1985;24(10):630–3.

8. Pinkus H. Lichenoid tissue reactions. A speculative review of the clinical spectrum of epidermal basal cell damage with special reference to erythema dyschromicum perstans. Arch Dermatol. 1973;107:840–6.

9. Bhutani LK, Bedi TR, Pandhi RK. Lichen planus pigmentosus. Dermatologica. 1974;149:43–50.

10. Kanwar AJ, Dogra S, Handa S, Parsad D, Radotra BDA. Study of 124 Indian patients with lichen planus pigmentosus. Clin Exp Dermatol. 2003;28:481–5.

11. Knox JM, Dodge BG, Freeman RG. Erythema dyschromicum perstans. Arch Dermatol. 1968;97:262–72.

12. Vega ME, Waxtein L, Arenas R, Hodyo M, Dominguez-Soto L. Ashy dermatosis and lichen planus pigmentosus: a clinicopathologic study of 31 cases. Int J Dermatol. 1992;31:90–4.

13. Muthu SK, Narang T, Saikia UN, Kanwar AJ, Parsad D, Dogra S. Low-dose oral isotretinoin therapy in lichen planus pigmentosus: an open-label non-randomized prospective pilot study. Int J Dermatol. 2016;55(9):1048–54.

14. Al-Mutairi N, El-Khalawany M. Clinicopathological characteristics of lichen planus pigmentosus and its response to tacrolimus ointment: an open label, non-randomized, prospective study. J Eur Acad Dermatol Venereol. 2010;24(5):535–40.

15. Degos R, Civatte J, Belaich S. La pigmentation maculeuse éruptive idiopathique. Ann Dermatol Venereol. 1978;105:177–82.

16. de Galdeano CS, Leaute-Labreze C, Bioulac-Sage P, et al. Idiopathic eruptive macular pigmentation: report of five patients. Pediatr Dermatol. 1996;13:274–7.

17. Jang KA, Choi JH, Sung KJ, Moon KC, Koh JK. Idiopathic eruptive macular pigmentation: report of 10 cases. J Am Acad Dermatol. 2001;44(2):351–3.

18. Stinco G, Favot F, Scott CA, et al. Pigmentatio maculos eruptive idiopathica: a case report and review of related literature. Int J Dermatol. 2007;46:1267–70.

19. Joshi R. Idiopathic eruptive macular pigmentation with papillomatosis: report of nine cases. Indian J Dermatol Venereol Leprol. 2007;73:402–5.

20. Joshi R, Palwade PK. Idopathic eruptive macular pigmentation or acanthosis nigricans? Indian J Dermatol Venereol Leprol. 2010;76:591.

21. Chandran V, Kumarasinghe SP. Macular pigmentation of uncertain aetiology revisited: two case reports and a proposed algorithm for clinical classification. Australas J Dermatol. 2017;58(1):45–9.

22. Riehl G. Uber eine eigenartige melanose. Wien Klin Wochensschr. 1917;30:280–1.

23. Findlay GH. Some observations on the melanosis of Riehl. S Afr Med J. 1952 May 3;26(18):373–5.

24. Rorsman H. Riehl's melanosis. Int J Dermatol. 1982;21:75–80.

25. Nakayama H, Matsuo S, Hayakawa K, Takahashi K, Shigematsu T. Pigmented cosmetic dermatitis. Int J Dermatol. 1984;23:299–305.

26. Kozuka T, Tashiro M, Sano S, Fujimoto K, Nakamura Y, Hashimoto S, et al. Brilliant Lake red R as a cause of pigmented contact dermatitis. Contact Dermatitis. 1979;5:297.

27. Fujimoto K, Hashimoto S, Kozuka T, Tashiro M, Sano S. Occupational pigmented contact dermatitis from azo dyes. Contact Dermatitis. 1985;12:15–7.

28. Shenoi SD, Rao R. Pigmented contact dermatitis. Indian J Dermatol Venereol Leprol. 2007 Sep-Oct;73(5):285–7.

29. Wang L, Xu AE. Four views of Riehl's melanosis: clinical appearance, dermoscopy, confocal microscopy and histopathology. J Eur Acad Dermatol Venereol. 2014 Sep.;28(9):1199–206.

30. Serrano G, Pujol C, Cuadra J, Gallo S, Aliaga A. Riehl's melanosis: pigmented contact dermatitis caused by fragrances. J Am Acad Dermatol. 1989;5(2):1057–60.

31. Smucker JE, Kirby JS. Riehl melanosis treated successfully with Q-switch Nd:YAG laser. J Drugs Dermatol. 2014 Mar;13(3):356–8.

32. On HR, Hong WJ, Roh MR. Low-pulse energy Q-switched Nd:YAG laser treatment for hair-dye-induced Riehl's melanosis. J Cosmet Laser Ther. 2015 Jun.;17(3):135–8.

33. Chung BY, Kim JE, Ko JY, Chang SEA. Pilot study of a novel dual--pulsed 1064 nm Q-switched Nd: YAG laser to treat Riehl's melanosis. J Cosmet Laser Ther. 2014 Dec.;16(6):290–2.

34. Pirmez R, Duque-Estrada B, Donati A, Campos-do-Carmo G, Valente NS, Romiti R, et al. Clinical and dermoscopic features of lichen planus pigmentosus in 37 patients with frontal fibrosing alopecia. Br J Dermatol. 2016;175(6):1387–90.

Post-inflammatory Hyperpigmentation

14

Michelle Rodrigues and Ana Sofia Ayala-Cortés

Post-inflammatory Hyperpigmentation

Post-inflammatory hyperpigmentation (PIH), most commonly seen in those with skin of color, is a reactive hypermelanosis of the skin that occurs after inflammation. Excess melanin is deposited in the epidermis or dermis [1, 2]. A negative impact on quality of life has been extensively documented in the literature [3–5].

Cutaneous inflammation that promotes PIH may be endogenous or exogenous. The former originates from primary dermatoses, while exogenous inflammation arises from external insults to the skin such as trauma or physical injury [6].

PIH affects males and females equally but is more prevalent in darker skin phototypes (Fitzpatrick IV–VI) [3]. Several studies have demonstrated that all pigmentary disorders are more frequent in skin of color patients [7]. Halder et al. reported that for those with skin of color, pigmentary disorders were the third most common reason for presentation to a dermatologist, while it was the seventh most common reason for presentation for Caucasian patients [8]. In addition, in 2007, Alexis et al. reported that pigmentary disorders were the second most common skin problem in African American patients [9].

Pathogenesis

PIH results from cutaneous inflammation that promotes cytokine production. The inflammation releases and oxidizes arachidonic acid via peroxidase, cyclooxygenase, and 5-lipoxygenase into intermediates that form prostaglandins, leukotrienes, and thromboxanes [10]. The melanocyte-stimulating properties of these intermediates together with interleukin 1 and 6, tumor necrosis factor, epidermal growth factor, nitric oxide, and other reactive oxygen species are well known [2, 11, 12]. These cytokines may induce an excessive production of melanin or an irregular dispersion of it into the epidermis. If the inflammation damages the basement membrane zone, the melanin falls into the dermis and is eventually phagocytized by melanophages in the upper dermis. This process of phagocytosis can take many months to years to clear meaning that dermal PIH in particular may linger for many months or years [2, 13].

M. Rodrigues
Department of Dermatology, St. Vincent's Hospital, Fitzroy, VIC, Australia

A. S. Ayala Cortés (✉)
Dermatology Department, Hospital Universitario Dr. José Eleuterio González de la Universidad Autónoma de Nuevo León, Monterrey, NL, Mexico

P. Kumarasinghe (ed.), *Pigmentary Skin Disorders*, Updates in Clinical Dermatology,
https://doi.org/10.1007/978-3-319-70419-7_14

Etiology

Any dermatosis causing inflammation can cause PIH. The degree of inflammation and disruption of the basement membrane determines the extent, color, and location of the melanin. The pigment, for example, is darker and deeper in the dermis when the basement membrane is affected or with chronic or recurrent inflammation [1]. An increased number of epidermal melanocytes are noted in endogenous causes of PIH [14].

A large group of primary cutaneous diseases may result in PIH [12] including acne, atopic dermatitis, and connective tissue diseases [2]. PIH is one of the main complications of acne, which is evident after the erythema has faded [4]. However, conditions like lichen planus, erythema dyschromicum perstans, and Riehl's melanosis have distinct patterns and distributions of pigmentation, which result in corresponding distinct clinical and morphological patterns of PIH [6].

On the other hand, exogenous inflammation may also cause PIH. Physical injury, photosensitization, contact dermatitis, infections, infestations, and skin-directed therapies like chemical peels and laser are just some of the culprits. Further examples from the former group are ionizing and nonionizing radiation, mechanical trauma, freezing, and direct thermal injury. Other exogenous inflammation sources include drug reactions, including fixed drug and lichenoid drug eruptions [6, 15].

Cosmetic procedures are a common exogenous cause of exogenous PIH in those with skin of color and are becoming more frequent due to the increase in the number of cosmetic procedures being performed in this group of patients [16]. Mandy et al. reported an incidence of 28% of PIH in 25 patients treated with dermabrasion for acne scarring [17]. PIH is especially common after treatment with intense-pulsed light therapy (IPL) in skin of color patients [18] with between 3% and 28% of patients reporting PIH after IPL treatment for melasma [19, 20]. Q-switched lasers have also been implicated in the development of PIH with an incidence between 10% and 25% documented [21, 22]. Fractional CO2 laser, due to thermal damage to surrounding tissue, has been associated with an even higher incidence of PIH with 68–92% of Fitzpatrick skin type IV patients developing PIH 1 month after use [23, 24]. On average, PIH lasted 3.8 months. It should be noted that the cryogen spray used with some lasers can also cause thermal injury that results in transient PIH (Fig. 14.1).

Picosecond lasers, such as the alexandrite picosecond laser, were approved by the Food and Drug Administration (FDA) in 2012 for the treatment of pigmentation [25]. One retrospective study reported 6 out of 56 Fitzpatrick skin type IV–VI patients developed PIH after a 755 nm alexandrite picosecond laser treatment for acne and other scars, striae, and pigmented lesions. A spot size of 6 mm, fluence of $0.71/cm^2$, repetition rate of 5 Hz, and pulse width of 750–850 ps were used. Face treatments used 3000–7000 pulses with an average of 2–4 passes. In all cases PIH resolved after 2 weeks and 3 months [26]. A similar side-effect profile has not been seen in lighter skin types [27].

Certain dermatoses may increase the risk of PIH, like erythema multiforme and lichen planus [28], where the basement membrane is damaged and the pigments falls and is phagocyted by dermal melanophages, persisting there for years [29]. All the skin inflammatory reactions that disturb the dermoepidermal junction, including lichenoid dermatoses such as lichen planus, ashy dermatosis, fixed drug eruption, and erythema multiforme, cause melanin to drop into the

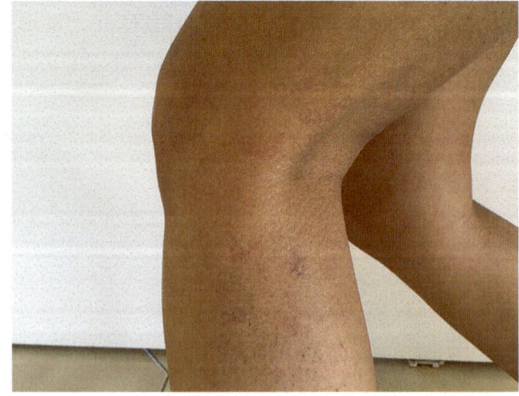

Fig. 14.1 PIH post-alexandrite laser with built-in cryogen spray for hair removal in skin phototype 4

dermis causing more sustained dermal pigmentation [30].

Clinical Manifestations

Asymptomatic macules or patches with varying intensity of pigmentation, from light brown to black, may be observed [31]. PIH is more common in patients with skin of color, though subtle pigmentation is also seen in those with lighter skin phototypes [1]. In epidermal PIH lesions are dark brown and accentuated by Wood's lamp examination, with well-circumscribed borders. Dermal PIH, on the contrary, presents with poorly circumscribed dark gray pigmentation and is not accentuated by Wood's lamp examination. The distribution, size, and shape of the lesions correspond to the location of the previous inflammatory dermatosis [32] (Figs. 14.2, 14.3 and 14.4).

Diagnosis

PIH is a clinical diagnosis. A history of a previous inflammatory dermatosis in the affected areas will clinch the diagnosis [31]. Occasionally, however, erythema and scale, especially in those with skin of color, may be so transient or mild that the prior inflammation is not recalled by the patient. In such cases, the distribution and configuration of the hyperpigmentation might be helpful for determining the previous inflammatory condition (Fig. 14.5) [1]. Wood's lamp examination and a skin biopsy may be necessary to determine the location of the melanin, which may help navigate management options. For quantification of the melanin, colorimetry or a narrow-band reflectance spectroscopy can be used but has limited availability [12].

Histopathology

Skin biopsy specimens of the hyperpigmented areas demonstrate accumulation of epidermal or dermal melanin [1]. In the epidermis the basal

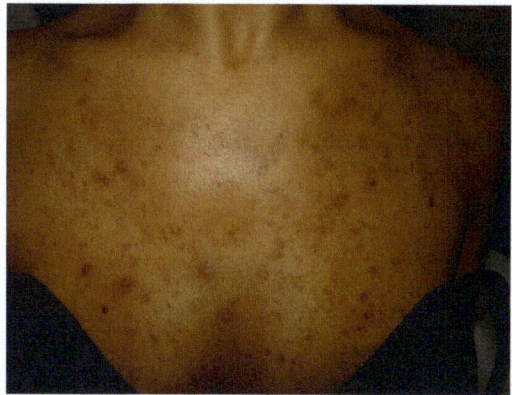

Fig. 14.2 PIH secondary to acne on the chest of a female of African descent

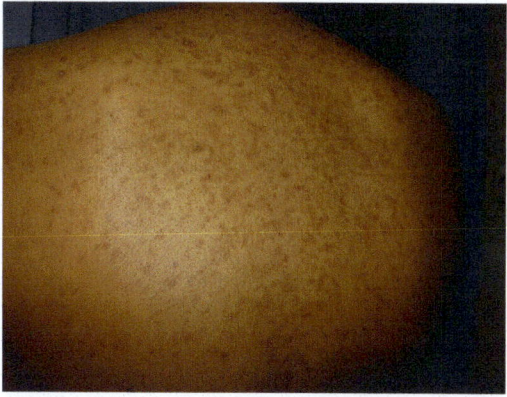

Fig. 14.3 PIH secondary to acne on the back of a female of African descent

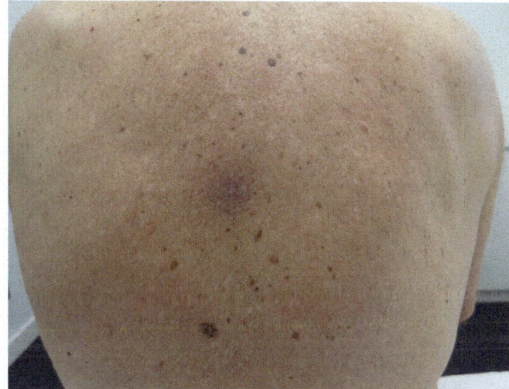

Fig. 14.4 PIH secondary to systemic lupus erythematosus on the back of an elderly Caucasian man

cells may be hyperpigmented, while the papillary dermis demonstrates variable numbers of mela-nophages [33] (Figs. 14.6 and 14.7).

Differential Diagnoses

Some of the dermatoses that need to be differentiated from PIH include melasma, erythema dyschromicum perstans, idiopathic eruptive macular pigmentation, lichen planus pigmentosus, acanthosis nigricans, macular amyloidosis, fixed drug eruption, and drug-induced pigmentation [34]. Tetracycline, clofazimine, antimalarial drugs, and hormones are some of the many culprits that cause drug-induced pigmentation that can mimic PIH clinically [31].

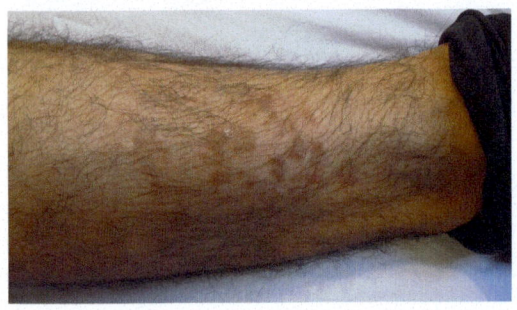

Fig. 14.5 PIH secondary to psoriasis on the leg of a Latin American male patient

Prevention

Preventing the offending dermatosis is not always possible so it is imperative to treat the cutaneous inflammation as early as possible in order to minimize the risk of PIH [31]. Once pigmentary changes are observed, management is challenging and protracted [32].

Given cosmetic procedures are a common source of PIH, it is important to identify high-risk patients (e.g., history of PIH, existing inflammatory dermatoses), to ensure adequate pre- and post-procedure care, and to choose appropriate treatment settings and regimens.

Sun avoidance, sun protection, and topical bleaching agents at least 2 weeks before and 6 weeks after procedures such as peels are critical [28, 35]. Several bleaching agents for prevention of PIH are described, including tretinoin, hydroquinone, alpha hydroxy acids, kojic acid, and azelaic acid [36].

Test areas before full laser treatments and superficial peels and intimate understanding of laser and peeling end points, lower laser fluences, epidermal cooling during treatment, and lengthening treatment intervals should be considered in high-risk individuals.

Given the inflammatory cascade promotes prostaglandin, leukotriene, and thromboxane activity, anti-inflammatory medications such as topical corticosteroids can theoretically reduce PIH. Twice-daily application for 2 days of 0.05%

Fig. 14.6 20× magnification of PIH secondary to systemic lupus erythematosus (SLE) (Picture courtesy of Dr. Andrew Ryan, pathologist)

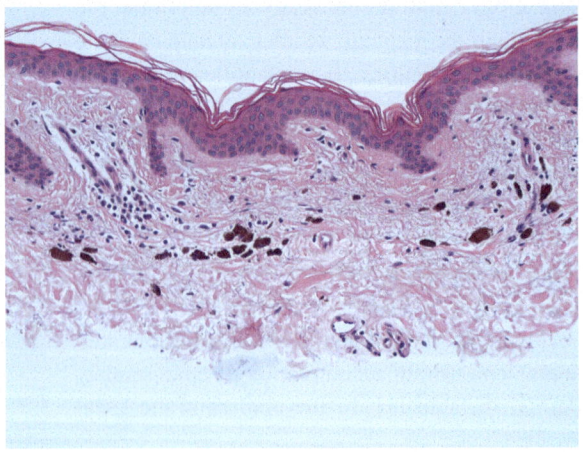

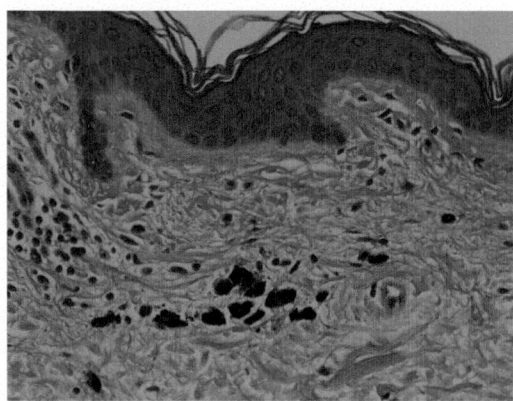

Fig. 14.7 40× magnification of PIH secondary to SLE (Picture courtesy of Dr. Andrew Ryan, pathologist)

clobetasol propionate ointment post-fractional CO_2 laser for acne scarring on the face significantly decreased the incidence of PIH [37]. Although controversial, prophylactic systemic prednisolone (10 mg for 3 days) has also been used to prevent PIH after a 10,600-nm carbon dioxide fractional laser for facial acne scars in Asian patients [38]. Recently Song et al. suggested that the "golden" time period to prevent PIH is at least 1 week after a Q-switched alexandrite laser treatment, advising the prophylactic application of topical corticosteroids at least for the first 7 days post-laser treatment. The study revealed that topical steroid post-irradiaton reduced the inflammatory cell infiltrate and degenerative epidermal change, with a removal of pigmentation and the majority of the melanocytes at day 7 [39].

Treatment

PIH may be challenging to treat, especially if it is dermal in origin. A plethora of topical creams, chemical peels, and lasers have been described as being helpful [31] (Table 14.1).

Waiting for spontaneous resolution may be appropriate for some patients. However, the impact on quality of life needs to be considered when formulating a management plan [12]. Additionally, the localization of the pigment needs to be considered in order to choose the best treatment and to provide realistic expectations [32] (Tables 14.2 and 14.3).

Table 14.1 Treatment modalities

Topical	Photoprotection
	Hydroquinone
	Mequinol
	Retinoids (tretinoin, adapalene, tazarotene)
	Azelaic acid
	Kojic acid
	Arbutin
	Niacinamide
	N-Acetylglucosamine
	Ascorbic acid
	Licorice extract
	Soy
	Combination therapy
Chemical peels	Glycolic acid
	Salicylic acid
Laser and light therapies	Intense-pulsed light
	Long-pulsed dye laser
	Q-switched Nd:Yttrium aluminum garnet laser
	Q-switched ruby laser
	Erbium-doped Fraxel SR 1500
	CO2 laser

Table 14.2 PIH treatment algorithm

First-line treatments	Photoprotection +
	Expectant treatment
	Or
	Hydroquinone 4%
Second-line treatments	Photoprotection +
	Combination therapy: Hydroquinone/retinoid/other depigmentation agents[a]
	Or
	Chemical peels[a]
	Or
	Laser/light therapy[a]

HQ hydroquinone
[a]see Table 14.1.

Cosmetic Camouflage

If mild or recalcitrant, cosmetic camouflage can be used [40]. In contrast to regular cosmetics, camouflage products are more durable (up to 16 h) and water-resistant [41]. Searching for one that is hypoallergenic, noncomedogenic, and

Table 14.3 Second-line treatments.

Depigmentation agents	*Tyrosinase inhibitors*
	  Hydroquinone
	  Mequinol
	  Retinoids
	  Azelaic acid
	  Kojic acid
	  Arbutin
	  N-Acetylglucosamine
	  Ascorbic acid
	Melanosome transfer inhibitors
	  Niacinamide
	  Soy
	Melanin disperser
	  Licorice extract

Chemical peels	Glycolic acid Salicylic acid
Laser and light therapies	Long-pulsed dye laser Q-switched Nd:yttrium aluminum garnet Q-switched ruby laser Intense-pulsed light Erbium-doped Fraxel

resistant to perspiration and with a good concealing ability is important [42].

Photoprotection

Sun avoidance and the use of sunscreen are important, even in skin of color patients. Patients must be advised to use a broad-spectrum sunscreen with a sun protection factor of at least 30 in addition to sun-protective hats and clothing. The sunscreen should be reapplied every 2 h if swimming or sweating or with intense sun exposure [2].

Hydroquinone (HQ)

HQ is currently the gold-standard treatment for PIH. This topical medication is a phenolic compound that inhibits tyrosinase and blocks the conversion of dihydroxyphenylalanine (DOPA) to melanin [43]. Additional mechanisms are inhibition of DNA and RNA synthesis, selective melanocyte cytotoxicity, melanosome degradation by phenol oxidases, and autoxidation forming oxygen radicals [2, 44]. Concentrations of 2% are

usually used initially, but the concentration may be titrated up to 10% depending on response and adverse cutaneous reactions [2]. HQ is most commonly used at night for 3–6 months or even longer in selected cases. Application with Q-tips may be helpful for small areas of PIH. An initial evaluation at 12 weeks is recommended, as most patients who will respond are likely to do so by this time [12, 44].

Controlled studies evaluating HQ for PIH are scarce with most studies using HQ in combination with other treatment modalities. Patients must be educated about potential side effects of HQ application. Possible side effects include contact dermatitis and hypopigmentation of the surrounding normal skin described as the "halo effect" [45]. Adjunctive treatment with a corticosteroid may reduce irritation [2]. Rarely, prolonged use of high concentration HQ (5–6%) has been associated with exogenous ochronosis [46, 47]. While the incidence of ochronosis in the United States is low, a high prevalence has reported in those of African descent in South Africa [2].

Mequinol

An alternative tyrosinase inhibitor is mequinol with which there is a lower incidence of cutaneous irritation. It is available at 2% concentration usually with 0.01% tretinoin [48]. Studies have shown no significant difference between this and 4% HQ over 12 weeks [49].

Retinoids

Retinoids are analogs of vitamin A [2] that remove melanin as epidermal turnover or skin desquamation occurs [50]. Topical options include tretinoin, adapalene, and tazarotene and are usually applied at night. Irritant dermatitis is a common and may itself lead to PIH in darker skin phototypes so patients should be counseled appropriately about this. Other side effects include erythema, burning, scaling, and dryness [3]. However, studies have shown a lower incidence of retinoid dermatitis with ada-palene [51].

Azelaic Acid

Isolated from *Malassezia furfur*, azelaic acid is a dicarboxylic acid that inhibits tyrosinase, DNA synthesis, and mitochondrial enzymes. It has cytotoxic and antiproliferative effects on abnormal melanocytes and results in cutaneous depigmentation [52]. Twice-daily application of 20% formula is most commonly used. Common side effects are pruritus, erythema, scaling, burning, and dryness [3]. Chan et al. reported a combination of azelaic acid, 4% hydroquinone, and a moderate-potency steroid twice daily 2 weeks preoperatively and 4 weeks postoperatively for lasers, light sources, and radiofrequency in Asian patients [18]. The incidence of steroid-induced rosacea and other steroid-induced side effects was not discussed in this study but should be considered.

Kojic Acid

Kojic acid is an aromatic acid tyrosinase inhibitor obtained as a fungal metabolite of certain species of *Acetobacter*, *Aspergillus*, and *Penicillium* [53]. One to four percent kojic acid is usually combined with other depigmentation agents to increase its efficacy. Side effects include allergic contact dermatitis, erythema, stinging, and mild exfoliation. Clinical studies for PIH have not been conducted; however, multiple studies demonstrate that kojic acid is efficient when combined with HQ or glycolic acid for melasma [3].

Arbutin

Arbutin is a beta-D-glucopyranoside of hydroquinone that inhibits melanosomal tyrosinase activity and, at a concentration of 3%, has been reported to be effective for the treatment of cuta-neous hyperpigmentation [54]. It is obtained from dried leaves of certain plants such as pear, blueberry, and cranberry. However, patients must be advised that a higher concentration may irritate and induce PIH [55]. There are currently no studies available assessing arbutin in the treatment of PIH.

Niacinamide

Niacinamide is the physiologically active amide of vitamin B3 (niacin) and has been reported to reduce skin hyperpigmentation. It works by inhibiting melanosome transfer from melanocytes to keratinocytes. Unlike most of the skin-lightening medications, it does not have an effect on tyrosinase activity or melanin synthesis [56]. While studies evaluating niacinamide for PIH are lacking, it has been studied for facial hyperpigmentation with good results. Few side effects such as mild cutaneous irritation have been reported [57].

N-Acetylglucosamine

N-Acetylglucosamine is a precursor to hyaluronic acid found in all human tissues and has been found to reduce melanin production in melanocytes in culture by inhibiting the glycosylation of tyrosinase [58]. A 2% concentration has been used to treat facial hyperpigmentation [58, 57].

Ascorbic Acid

Ascorbic acid (vitamin C) is a natural antioxidant that interferes with activity of tyrosinase and melanin synthesis. Furthermore it has a photoprotective effect, promotes collagen synthesis, and reduces dermal injury [2, 59]. Combination with other agents is usually the best approach [60]. A 5–10% concentration is recommended, with mild side effects such as skin irritation noted.

Botanicals

Components of licorice have been shown to inhibit tyrosinase activity. It is widely used in skin-lightening cosmeceuticals [61, 62]. Soybeans affect the transfer of melanosomes from melanocytes to keratinocytes, inducing subtle skin lightening [63, 64]. Further studies to demonstrate efficacy in PIH would be useful.

Combination Therapy

The classic combination treatment is the triple combination derived from the Kligman formula. It comprises HQ, tretinoin, and a corticosteroid. The original Kligman formula was described for the treatment of melasma, PIH, ephelides, and lentigines in 1975 and is formulated with HQ 5% + tretinoin 0.1% and dexamethasone 0.1%. The corticosteroid reduces irritation risk and may also inhibit melanin synthesis, while the tretinoin increases HQ penetration and treats hyperpigmentation [65].

Bauman et al., in a randomized, investigator-blinded study, reported on an 8-week treatment regimen with HQ 4% + tretinoin 0.05% + fluocinolone acetonide 0.01% vs. HQ 4% + tretinoin 0.05% vs. fluocinolone acetonide 0.01% + tretinoin 0.05% in patients with PIH post-acne. The best results were seen with the triple combination cream [12]. Two different studies in Asian patients with PIH revealed good results with tretinoin 0.05–0.1%, HQ 4–5%, and lactic acid 7% [66, 67].

PIH post-acne in skin of color patients has been successfully treated with combination of HQ 4% + glycolic acid 10% + vitamin E [68].

While various combination therapies have been used over time, the first-line treatment is still HQ 4% together with sun protection.

Chemical Peels

Chemical peels are considered second line for recalcitrant PIH. This potentially costly treatment modality must be used with caution due to the risk of worsening PIH, especially in those with skin of color or those that have an altered epidermal barrier function. Peels should be reserved for those who have not demonstrated good results after 3 months of topical treatment [69].

Superficial chemical peels should be used for skin of color patients [43]. Glycolic acid (20–70%) and salicylic acid (20–30%) peels are commonly used in combination with topical treatments such as HQ or tretinoin. While they demonstrate efficacy alone, they enhance the efficacy of topical therapy and are therefore a possible adjunct to topical therapy [32, 70–72].

Laser and Light Therapies

Laser and light therapies are also considered second-line treatment modalities for recalcitrant cases of PIH [12]. Some studies reveal improvement of PIH with lasers such as 595-nm long-pulsed dye laser, low-fluence 1064-nm Q-switched (QS) Nd:yttrium aluminum garnet (YAG) laser, and non-ablative and ablative lasers [69, 73]; contrastingly, others show PIH due to laser therapy. This is more common in those with skin of color.

Several studies have revealed improvement without significant side effects when 1064-nm Q-switched Nd-YAG laser is used for acne-induced PIH [4, 74, 75]. While intense-pulsed light (IPL) demonstrated efficacy in one study examining 25 Korean patients with PIH, results of other studies were not as positive [69, 76]. Fractional thermolysis and non-ablative 1550 fractional lasers have demonstrated variable results [77–80] and should only be considered in a select group of patients if all other treatment options have failed. Of course, test areas are recommended to ensure efficacy and minimize adverse effects.

Future Directions

Picosecond lasers, a recently developed laser modality, have recently been described for the treatment of pigmented lesions and pigmentation on the face and have been deemed safe in those with skin of color. They are able to deliver greater mechanical stress with less thermal damage than nanosecond lasers [26, 81, 82]. There are currently no studies demonstrating efficacy of picosecond lasers in PIH.

Tranexamic acid (TA) is an antiplasmin agent and has demonstrated efficacy for the treatment of melasma [83, 84]. More recently, it has been successfully used in one patient with PIH in combination with weekly low-fluence 1064-nm Q-switched Nd:YAG laser [85]. Further studies are required to assess its efficacy before this treatment can be recommended for PIH.

Other therapies have been described for hyperpigmentation but require well-constructed studies to assess their efficacy. These include coffeeberry extract, lignin peroxidase, undecylenoyl phenylalanine, topical methimazole, aloesin, dioic acid, and cysteamine cream [12, 86–91].

References

1. Ruiz-Maldonado R, Dela Luz Orozco-Covarrubias M. Postinflammatory hypopigmentation and hyperpigmentation. Semin Cutan Med Surg. 1997;16(1):36–43.
2. Davis EC, Callender VD. Postinflammatory hyperpigmentation: a review of the epidemiology, clinical features, and treatment options in skin of color. J Clin Aesthet Dermatol. 2010;3(7):20–31.
3. Callender VD, St.Surin-Lord S, Davis EC, Maclin M. Postinflammatory hyperpigmentation: etiologic and therapeutic considerations. Am J Clin Dermatol. 2011;12(2):87–99.
4. Zawar V, Agarwal M, Vasudevan B. Treatment of postinflammatory pigmentation due to acne with Q-switched neodymium-doped yttrium aluminum garnet in 78 Indian cases. J Cutan Aesthet Surg. 2015;8(4):222–6.
5. Abad-Casintahan F, Chow S, Goh C, Kubba R, Hayashi N, Noppakun N, et al. Frequency and characteristics of acne-related post-inflammatory hyperpigmentation. J Dermatol. 2016;43(7):826–8.
6. Epstein JH. Postinflammatory hyper-pigmentation. Clin Dermatol. 1989;7(2):55–65.
7. Halder RM, Nootheti PK, Lanka S, Asia S. Ethnic skin disorders overview. J Am Acad Dermatol. 2003;48(6):143–8.
8. Halder R, Grimes P, McLaurin C. Incidence of common dermatoses in a predominately black dermatologic practice. Cutis. 1983;32:388–90.
9. Alexis A, Sergay A, Taylor S. Common dermatologic disorders in skin of color: a comparative practice survey. Cutis. 2007;80:387–94.
10. Tomita Y, Maeda K, Tagami H. Melanocyte-stimulating properties of arachidonic metabolites: possible role in postinflammatory pigmentation. Pigment Cell Res. 1992;5:357–61.
11. Cardinali G, Kovacs D, Picardo M. Mechanisms underlying post-inflammatory hyperpigmentation: lessons from solar lentigo. Ann Dermatol Venereol. 2012;139(Suppl):S148–52. Available from: https://doi.org/10.1016/S0151-9638(12)70127-8.
12. Taylor S, Grimes P, Lim J, Im S, Lui H. Postinflammatory hyperpigmentation. J Cutan Med Surg [Internet]. 2009;13(4):183–91. Available from: http://cms.sagepub.com/lookup/doi/10.2310/7750.2009.08077
13. Youn SW. *In vivo* model for postinflammatory hyperpigmentation: a step forward. Br J Dermatol [Internet]. 2016;174(4):721–2. Available from: http://doi.wiley.com/10.1111/bjd.14333
14. Papa C, Kligman A. The behavior of melanocytes in inflammation. J Invest Dermatol. 1965;45:465–73.
15. Wintroub BU, Stern R. Cutaneous drug reactions: pathogenesis and clinical classification. J Am Acad Dermatol [Internet]. American Academy of Dermatology, Inc. 1985;13(2 Pt 1):167–79. Available from: https://doi.org/10.1016/S0190-9622(85)70156-9
16. Callender V. Acne in ethnic skin: special considerations for therapy. Dermatol Ther. 2004;17(2):184–95.
17. Mandy SH. Tretinoin in the preoperative and postoperative management of dermabrasion. J Am Acad Dermatol [Internet]. 1986;15(4):878–9. Available from: http://www.sciencedirect.com/science/article/pii/S0190962286702454
18. Chan HHL. Effective and safe use of lasers, light sources, and radiofrequency devices in the clinical management of Asian patients with selected dermatoses. Lasers Surg Med. 2005;37(3):179–85.
19. Li Y-H, Chen JZS, Wei H-C, Wu Y, Liu M, Xu Y-Y, et al. Efficacy and safety of intense pulsed light in treatment of melasma in Chinese patients. Dermatol Surg [Internet]. 2008;34(5):693–700–1. Available from: http://www.ncbi.nlm.nih.gov/pubmed/18318729.
20. Negishi K, Kushikata N, Tezuka Y, Takeuchi K, Miyamoto E, Wakamatsu S, et al. Study of the incidence and nature of "very subtle epidermal melasma" in relation to intense pulsed light treatment. Dermatologic Surg. 2004;30(6):881–6.
21. Chan H, Fung W, Ying S, Kono T. An in vivo trial comparing the use of different types of 532 nm Nd:YAG lasers in the treatment of facial lentigines in oriental patients. Dermatol Surg. 2000;26(8):743–9.
22. Murphy M, Huang M. Q-switched ruby laser treatment of benign pigmented lesions in Chinese skin. Ann Acad Med Singap. 1994;23(1):60–6.

23. Sriprachya-anunt S, Marchell N, Fitzpatrick R, Goldman M, Rostan E. Facial resurfacing in patients with Fitzpatrick skin type IV. Lasers Surg Med. 2002;30:86–92.

24. Shamsaldeen O, Peterson J, Goldman M. The adverse events of deep fractional CO(2): a retrospective study of 490 treatments in 374 patients. Lasers Surg Med. 2011;43(6):453–6.

25. Lee S, Lee M, Noh T, Choi K, Won C, Chang S, et al. Successful treatment of tattoos with a picosecond 755-nm alexandrite laser in Asian skin. Ann Dermatol. 2016;28(5):673–5.

26. Haimovic A, Brauer J, Cindy Y, Geronemus R. Safety of a picosecond laser with diffractive lens array (DLA) in the treatment of Fitzpatrick skin types IV to VI: a retrospective review. J Am Acad Dermatol. 2016;74(5):931–6.

27. DC W, Fletcher L, Guiha I, Goldman MP. Evaluation of the safety and efficacy of the picosecond alexandrite laser with specialized lens array for treatment of the photoaging décolletage. Lasers Surg Med. 2016;48(2):188–92.

28. Chan HHL, Manstein D, CS Y, Shek S, Kono T, Wei WI. The prevalence and risk factors of postinflammatory hyperpigmentation after fractional resurfacing in Asians. Lasers Surg Med. 2007;39(5):381–5.

29. Vashi NA, Kundu RV. Facial hyperpigmentation: causes and treatment. Br J Dermatol. 2013;169:41–56.

30. Tienthavorn T, Tresukosol P, Sudtikoonaseth P. Patch testing and histopathology in Thai patients with hyperpigmentation due to erythema dyschromicum perstans, Lichen planus pigmentosus, and pigmented contact dermatitis. Asian Pacific J Allergy Immunol. 2014;32(2):185–92.

31. Lacz NL, Vafaie J, Kihiczak NI, Schwartz RA. Postinflammatory hyperpigmentation: a common but troubling condition. Int J Dermatol. 2004;43(5):362–5.

32. Pandya AG, Guevara IL. Disorders of hyperpigmentation. Dermatology Clin. 2000;18(1):91–8.

33. Calonje J, Brenn T, Lazar A, McKee P. McKee's pathology of the skin: with clinical correlations. 4th ed. China: Elsevier/Saunders; 2012. p. 932–3.

34. Goldsmith L, Katz S, Gilchrest B, Paller A, Leffell D, Wolff K. Fitzpatrick's dermatology in general medicine. 8th ed. New York: McGraw-Hill; 2012. p. 804–25.

35. Wanitphakdeedecha R, Phuardchantuk R, Manuskiatti W. The use of sunscreen starting on the first day after ablative fractional skin resurfacing. J Eur Acad Dermatology Venereol. 2013:1522–8.

36. Goldman M. The use of hydroquinone with facial laser resurfacing. J Cutan Laser Ther. 2000;2(2):73–7.

37. Nutjira Cheyasa K, Manuskiatti W, Maneeprasopcho KP, Wanitpha Kdee Decha R. Topical corticosteroids minimise the risk of postinflammatory hyperpigmentation after ablative fractional Co2laser resurfacing in Asians. Acta Derm Venereol. 2015;95(2):201–5.

38. Cho S, Lee S, Kang J, Kim Y, Chung W, Oh S. The efficacy and safety of 10,600-nm carbon dioxide fractional laser for acne scars in Asian patients. Dermatol Surg. 2009;35(12):1955–61.

39. Song HS, Park JY, Kim SJ, Kang HY. In vivo time-sequential histological study focused on melanocytes: suggestion of golden time for intervention to prevent post-laser pigmentary changes. J Eur Acad Dermatology Venereol. 2016;30(2):306–10.

40. Holme S, Beattie P, Fleming C. Cosmetic camouflage advice improves quality of life. Br J Dermatol. 2002;147(5):946–9.

41. McMichael L. Skin camouflage. Br J Dermatol. 2012;344:d7921.

42. Nonni J. Medical makeup: the correction of hyperpigmentation disorders. Ann Dermatol Venereol. 2012;139(Suppl 4):S170–6. Available from: https://doi.org/10.1016/S0151-9638(12)70131-X.

43. Grimes P. Management of hyperpigmentation in darker racial ethnic groups. Semin Cutan Med Surg. 2009;28(2):77–85.

44. Rossi A, Perez M. Treatment of hyperpigmentation. Facial Plast Surg Clin North Am. 2011;19(2):313–24.

45. Badreshia-Bansal S, Draelos Z. Insight into skin lightening cosmeceuticals for women of color. J Drugs Dermatol. 2007;6(1):32–9.

46. Stratigos AJ, Katsambas AD. Optimal management of recalcitrant disorders of hyperpigmentation in dark-skinned patients. Am J Clin Dermatol. 2004;5(3):161–8.

47. Touart D, Sau P. Cutaneous deposition diseases. Part II. J Am Acad Dermatol. 1998;39(4 Pt 1):527–44.

48. Fleischer AJ, Schwartzel E, Colby S, Altman D. The combination of 2% 4-hydroxyanisole (Mequinol) and 0.01% tretinoin is effective in improving the appearance of solar lentigines and related hyperpigmented lesions in two double-blind multicenter clinical studies. J Am Acad Dermatol. 2000;42(3):459–67.

49. Taylor S, Callender V. A multicenter, 12-week, phase 3b trial: a combination solution of mequinol 2%/tretinoin 0.01% 60. vs hydroquinone 4% cream in the treatment of mild to moderate postinflammatory hyperpigmentation. J Am Acad Dermatol. 2006;54(Suppl):AB194.

50. Kang H, Valerio L, Bahadoran P, Ortonne J. The role of topical retinoids in the treatment of pigmentary disorders: an evidence-based review. Am J Clin Dermatol. 2009;10(4):251–60.

51. Jacyk W, Mpofu P. Adapalene gel 0.1% for topical treatment of acne vulgaris in African patients. Cutis. 2001;68(4 Suppl):48–54.

52. Nguyen Q, Bui T. Azelaic acid: pharmacokinetic and pharmacodynamic properties and its therapeutic role in hyperpigmentary disorders and acne. Int J Dermatol. 1995;34(2):75–84.

53. Shokeen D. Postinflammatory Hyperpigmentation in Patients With Skin of Color co co. 2016;97(January):9–11.

54. Maeda K, Fukuda M. Arbutin: mechanism of its depigmenting action in human melanocyte culture. J Pharmacol Exp Ther. 1996;276:765–9.

55. Zhu W, Gao J. The use of botanical extracts as topical skin-lightening agents for the improvement of skin pigmentation disorders. J Investig Dermatol Symp Proc [Internet]. Elsevier Masson SAS; 2008;13(1):20–4. Available from: https://doi.org/10.1038/jidsymp.2008.8.

56. Hakozaki T, Minwalla L, Zhuang J, Chhoa M, Matsubara A, Miyamoto K, et al. The effect of niacinamide on reducing cutaneous pigmentation and suppression of melanosome transfer. Br J Dermatol. 2002;147(1):20–31.

57. Kimball AB, Kaczvinsky JR, Li J, Robinson LR, Matts PJ, Berge CA, et al. Reduction in the appearance of facial hyperpigmentation after use of moisturizers with a combination of topical niacinamide and N-acetyl glucosamine: results of a randomized, double-blind, vehicle-controlled trial. Br J Dermatol. 2010;162(2):435–41.

58. Bissett D, Robinson L, Raleigh P, Miyamoto K, Hakozaki T, Li J, et al. Reduction in the appearance of facial hyperpigmentation by topical N-acetyl glucosamine. J Cosmet Dermatol. 2007;6(1):20–6.

59. Espinal-Perez LE, Moncada B, Castanedo-Cazares JP. A double-blind randomized trial of 5% ascorbic acid vs. 4% hydroquinone in melasma. Int J Dermatol. 2004;43(8):604–7.

60. Draelos Z. Skin lightening preparations and the hydroquinone controversy. Dermatol Ther. 2007;20:308–13.

61. Fu B, Li H, Wang X, Lee FSC, Cui S. Isolation and identification of flavonoids in licorice and a study of their inhibitory effects on tyrosinase. J Agric Food Chem. 2005;53(19):7408–14.

62. Yokota T, Nishio H, Kubota Y, Mizoguchi M. The inhibitory effect of glabridin from licorice extracts on melanogenesis and inflammation. Pigment Cell Res [Internet]. 1998;11(6):355–61. Available from: http://www.scopus.com/inward/record.url?eid=2-s2.0-0032239708&partnerID=40&md5=b1e30198618d92632c40359d552c332b

63. Paine C, Sharlow E, Liebel F, Eisinger M, Shapiro S, Seiberg M. An alternative approach to depigmentation by soybean extracts via inhibition of the PAR-2 pathway. J Invest Dermatol [Internet]. Elsevier Masson SAS; 2001;116(4):587–95. Available from: https://doi.org/10.1046/j.1523-1747.2001.01291.x.

64. Sah A, Stephens T, Kurtz E. Topical acne treatment improves postacne postinflammatory hyperpgmentation (PIH) in skin of color [poster]. J Am Acad Dermatol 2005;52(Suppl):P25.

65. Kligman A, Willis I. A new formula for depigmenting human skin. Arch Dermatol 1975;111(1):40–48.

66. Yoshimura K, Harii K, Aoyama T, Shibuya F, Iga T. A new bleaching protocol for hyperpigmented skin lesions with a high concentration of all-trans retinoic acid aqueous gel. Aesthet Plast Surg. 1999;23(4):285–91.

67. Yoshimura K, Harii K, Aoyama T, Iga T. Experience with a strong bleaching treatment for skin hyperpigmentation in Orientals. Plast Reconstr Surg. 2000;105(3):1097–108.

68. Cook-Bolden F. The efficacy and tolerability of a combination cream containing 4% hydroquinone in the treatment of post-inflammatory hyperpigmentation in skin types IV-VI. Cosmet Dermatol. 2004;17:149–55.

69. Eimpunth S, Wanitphadeedecha R, Manuskiatti W. A focused review on acne-induced and aesthetic procedure-related postinflammatory hyperpigmentation in Asians. J Eur Acad Dermatology Venereol. 2013;27(SUPPL. 1):7–18.

70. Burns R, Prevost-Blank P, Lawry M, Lawry T, Faria D, Fivenson D. Glycolic acid peels for postinflammatory hyperpigmentation in black patients. A comparative study. SODermatol Surg. 1997;23(3):171–4.

71. Grimes P. The safety and efficacy of salicylic acid chemical peels in darker racial-ethnic groups. Dermatol Surg. 1999;25(1):18.

72. Ahn H, Kim I. Whitening effect of salicylic acid peels in Asian patients. Dermatol Surg. 2006;32(3):372–5.

73. Vijay Z, Madhuri A, Biju V. Treatment of postinflammatory pigmentation due to acne with Q-switched neodymium-doped yttrium aluminum garnet in 78 Indian cases. J Cutan Aesthet Surg. 2015;8(4):222–6.

74. Kim S, Cho K. Treatment of facial postinflammatory hyperpigmentation with facial acne in Asian patients using a Q-switched neodymium-doped yttrium aluminum garnet laser. Dermatol Surg. 2010;36:1374–80.

75. Cho S, Park S, Kim J, Al E. Treatment of postinflammatory hyper- pigmentation using 1064-nm Q-switched Nd:YAG laser with low fluence: report of three cases. J Eur Acad Dermatol Venereol. 2009;23:12061207.

76. Park J, Kim J, Kim W. Treatment of persistent facial postinflammatory hyperpigmentation with novel pulse-in-pulse mode intense pulsed light. Dermatol Surg. 2016;42(2):218–24.

77. Katz T, Goldberg L, Firoz B, Friedman P. Fractional photothermolysis for the treatment of postinflammatory hyperpigmentation. Dermatol Surg. 2009;35:1844–8.

78. Rokhsar C, Ciocon D. Fractional photothermolysis for the treatment of postinflammatory hyperpigmentation after carbon dioxide laser resurfacing. Dermatol Surg. 2009;35:535–7.

79. Kroon M, Wind B, Meesters A, Wolkerstorfer A, Wietze van der Veen J, Bos J, et al. Non-ablative 1550 nm fractional laser therapy not effective for erythema dyschromicum perstans and postinflammatory hyperpigmentation: a pilot study. J Dermatolog Treat. 2012;23:339–44.

80. Oram Y, Akkaya AD. Refractory postinflammatory hyperpigmentation treated with fractional CO2 laser. J Clin Aesthet Dermatol. 2014;7(3):42–4.

81. Brauer J, Kazlouskaya V, Alabdulrazzaq H, Bae Y, Bernstein L, Anolik R, et al. Use of a picosecond pulse duration laser with specialized optic for treatment of facial acne scarring. JAMA Dermatol. 2015;151(3):278–84.

82. Forbat E, Al-Niaimi F. The use of picosecond lasers beyond tattoos. J Cosmet Laser Ther [Internet]. 2016;18(6):345–7. Available from: https://www.tandfonline.com/doi/full/10.1080/14764172.2016.1188209

83. Padhi T, Pradhan S. Oral tranexamic acid with fluocinolone-based triple combination cream versus fluocinolone-based triple combination cream alone in melasma: an open labeled randomized comparative trial. Indian J Dermatol. 2015;60(5):520.

84. Lee H, Thng T, Goh C. Oral tranexamic acid (TA) in the treatment of melasma: a retrospective analysis. J Am Acad Dermatol. 2016;75(2):385–92.

85. Lee YB, Park SM, Kim J-W, Yu DS. Combination treatment of low-fluence Q-switched Nd:YAG laser and oral tranexamic acid for post-inflammatory hyperpigmentation due to allergic contact dermatitis to henna hair dye. J Cosmet Laser Ther [Internet]. 2016;18(2):95–7. Available from: http://www.tandfonline.com/doi/full/10.3109/14764172.2015.1114634

86. Katoulis A, Alevizou A, Bozi E, Makris M, Zafeiraki A, Mantas N, et al. A randomized, double-blind, vehicle-controlled study of a preparation containing undecylenoyl phenylalanine 2% in the treatment of solar lentigines. Clin Exp Dermatol. 2010;35(5):473–6.

87. Kasraee B, Handjani F, Parhizgar A, Omrani G, Fallahi M, Amini M, et al. Topical methimazole as a new treatment for postinflammatory hyperpigmentation: report of the first case. Dermatology. 2005;211(4):360–2.

88. Choi S, Lee S, Kim J, Chung M, Park Y. Aloesin inhibits hyperpigmentation induced by UV radiation. Clin Exp Dermatol. 2002;27(6):513–5.

89. Tirado-Sánchez A, Santamaría-Román A, Ponce-Olivera R. Efficacy of dioic acid compared with hydroquinone in the treatment of melasma. Int J Dermatol. 2009;48(8):893–5.

90. Draelos Z. A split-face evaluation of a novel pigment-lightening agent compared with no treatment and hydroquinone. J Am Acad Dermatol. 2015;72:105.

91. Mansouri P, Farshi S, Hashemi Z, Kasraee B. Evaluation of the efficacy of cysteamine 5% cream in the treatment of epidermal melasma: a randomized double-blind placebo-controlled trial. Br J Dermatol. 2015;173(1):209–17.

Lasers in Pigmentary Skin Disorders

15

Melissa A. Levoska, Tasneem F. Mohammad, and Iltefat H. Hamzavi

Introduction

Pigmentary disorders are characterized by either hypo- or hyperpigmentation and contribute to a significant portion of visits to the dermatology clinic. Many of these conditions are associated with negative impacts on quality of life [1]. Laser-based therapies have been used to treat multiple pigmentary disorders, including lentigines, nevus of Ota, melasma, post-inflammatory hyperpigmentation (PIH), drug-induced hyperpigmentation, vitiligo, and idiopathic guttate hypomelanosis (IGH). In this chapter, we review the use of lasers in the management of several common pigmentary disorders.

Laser Basics

The acronym LASER stands for light amplification by stimulated emission of radiation. Over the last half-century, advances in laser technology and a greater understanding of their mechanism of action have expanded their utility in dermatology. Today, lasers are the primary treatment modality for various pigmentary and scarring

M. A. Levoska • T. F. Mohammad • I. H. Hamzavi (✉)
Department of Dermatology, Henry Ford Hospital,
Detroit, MI, USA
e-mail: mlevoska@med.wayne.edu; ihamzavi1@hfhs.org

disorders [2]. Other applications include improving topical drug delivery and hair removal [2, 3].

Along with wavelength and pulse duration, fluence and irradiance are important concepts to understand (see Fig. 15.1). Fluence, or dose, is the energy distributed per unit area and is measured in J/cm^2. This value can be calculated by multiplying the device irradiance by the exposure time. Irradiance, or fluence rate, refers to the rate of energy delivered per unit area and is calculated using the laser's power output and the beam's cross-sectional area. The irradiance of a laser can be increased exponentially by using a smaller spot size, which essentially decreases the diameter of the beam. The higher the irradiance, the less time is required to administer a desired dose.

Several factors must be taken into account when choosing a laser to treat pigmentary abnormalities. First, the wavelength of the laser must be such that it will penetrate the skin to an appropriate depth. Secondly, the wavelength must match the absorption spectra of the specific chromophore, which is typically melanin in the case of pigmentary disorders. This ensures that firing of the laser will cause appropriate absorption of photons by the chromophore, leading to the desired thermal or photobiologic event. In addition, the absorption spectra of other chromophores must be taken into account to ensure that there is minimal targeting of these structures. The pulse duration of the laser is important as shorter pulses target smaller structures than longer pulse

© Springer International Publishing AG, part of Springer Nature 2018
P. Kumarasinghe (ed.), *Pigmentary Skin Disorders*, Updates in Clinical Dermatology,
https://doi.org/10.1007/978-3-319-70419-7_15

$$\text{FLUENCE} \;=\; \frac{\text{Laser Pulse Energy (Joules)}}{\text{Spot Cross-Sectional Area (cm}^2\text{)}} \;=\; \begin{matrix} \text{Irradiance (Watts/cm}^2\text{)} \\ \times \\ \text{Exposure time (seconds)} \end{matrix}$$

$$\text{POWER} \;=\; \frac{\text{Laser Pulse Energy (Joules)}}{\text{Pulse Duration (seconds)}}$$

$$\text{IRRADIANCE} \;=\; \frac{\text{POWER (Watts)}}{\text{Spot Cross-Sectional Area (cm}^2\text{)}}$$

Fig. 15.1 Important formulas for laser therapy

Table 15.1 Clinical applications of various lasers and light therapies

Type of laser	Wavelength	Pigmentary disorder	Other clinical applications
EL	308 nm	Vitiligo [4]	Psoriasis [5]
CuBr	510 or 578 nm	Melasma [6]	Vascular lesions, telangiectasias [7]
QSRL	694 nm	Nevus of Ota [8], solar lentigines [9, 10], drug-induced hyperpigmentation [11–13]	Tattoos [14, 15]
QSAL	755 nm	Nevus of Ota [16–18], solar lentigines [19–21], melasma [22, 23], drug-induced hyperpigmentation [24–28]	Tattoos [15]
Nd:YAG QS, frequency-doubled	532 nm	Vitiligo [29], solar lentigines [30–32], minocycline-induced hyperpigmentation [33]	Tattoos [15]
Nd:YAG, QS	1064 nm	PIH [34–36]	Tattoos [15]
long-pulsed	1064 nm	–	Hair removal [37], viral warts [38], ablative resurfacing [39]
IPL	515–1200 nm	Solar lentigines [40]	Wrinkles [41]
FCO$_2$	10,600 nm	Vitiligo [42–46], refractory melasma [22, 47, 48], IGH [49, 50]	Drug delivery [51]

Abbreviations: *EL* XeCl excimer laser, *CuBr* copper bromide (quasi-continuous wave) laser, *QSRL* Q-switched ruby laser, *QSAL* Q-switched alexandrite, *Nd:YAG* neodymium yttrium-aluminum-garnet, *QS* Q-switched, *IPL* intense pulsed light, *FCO₂* fractional carbon dioxide, *MKTP* melanocyte-keratinocyte transfer procedure, *IGH* idiopathic guttate hypomelanosis.

durations. Larger spot sizes typically allow deeper penetration into the skin, and the fluence must be adjusted based on skin thickness and the patient's skin type.

Table 15.1 includes an overview of lasers and their clinical utility. We will focus our attention on discussing the xenon chloride excimer (EL), fractional carbon dioxide (FCO$_2$), Q-switched ruby (QSRL), Q-switched alexandrite (QSAL), and neodymium yttrium-aluminum-garnet (QS Nd:YAG) lasers.

Laser Safety and Procedures

Lasers are relatively safe, but there are a few potential hazards including fires and ocular injuries. Lasers can be put into standby mode to help prevent accidental laser firing [52], and proper eye protection (based on the wavelength of the laser used) can minimize ocular risk. Providers can refer to the article by Tanzi et al. for more information on laser safety [52]. Epidermal cooling is also important to prevent nonselective thermal damage and minimize pain. This can be done by using ice packs, fans, cold air blowers, or a cooling tip on the laser device [53].

Xenon Chloride Excimer Laser

The xenon chloride excimer laser emits monochromatic, coherent light at a wavelength of 308 nm. Originally studied in psoriasis patients, monochromatic excimer light (MEL) was found to upregulate apoptotic markers and be cytotoxic to T cells in the epidermis and dermis [54]. Light emitted at a wavelength of 308 nm requires lower doses to damage DNA in human lymphocytes than light emitted at longer wavelengths [55]. Subsequently, EL requires a smaller apoptotic dose (defined as the amount of energy necessary to incite apoptosis of 50% of T cells) than narrowband ultraviolet B (NB-UVB) phototherapy (95 mJ/cm^2 vs. 320 mJ/cm^2, respectively). Furthermore, EL induces apoptosis of a greater percentage of T cells in vitro than NB-UVB [56], which correlates with clinical findings.

Use in Disorders of Hypopigmentation

Vitiligo
EL is used to induce repigmentation for the treatment of hypopigmentary disorders, most notably for the treatment of localized vitiligo [4, 57]. Like NB-UVB, the target chromophore and mechanism of action of the excimer laser are not well understood but may involve a combination of immunomodulatory effects and alterations in melanocyte production by stimulating the proliferation of inactive melanocytes in the hair follicle [58, 59]. In contrast to other photo(chemo)therapies for vitiligo, the laser can be directed to treat the affected area, effectively sparing uninvolved skin from undesirable hyperpigmentation and photodamage [59, 60].

Treatment Outcomes
Several studies have shown that EL is effective at inducing repigmentation in stable localized and generalized vitiligo [61–67]. Spencer et al. found that 13 of 23 (56.5%) patches achieved at least partial repigmentation after 2–4 weeks of treatment [61]. Ostovari et al. found similar results, with 50% of lesions achieving some degree of repigmentation. It is important to note that the repigmentation produced was often a darker color than the patient's natural skin color but eventually blended to match the true color, especially after 6 months of laser treatment [65]. After 1 year, lesions that had a poor initial response were more likely to lose pigment than lesions that had initially achieved greater than 50% repigmentation [63]. After a 2-year follow-up period, pigmentation remained, demonstrating the therapy's potentially long-lasting effects [64].

Factors Impacting Treatment Outcomes
Location of the vitiligo patches can affect treatment outcomes. Lesions located in "UV-sensitive" areas such as the face, neck, and trunk are more responsive to treatment with EL than lesions in "UV-resistant" areas such as the knees, elbows, ankles, and feet. In particular, facial lesions seem to have the best response [57, 62, 64, 65, 68]. This may be due to the relatively high follicular density of the responsive areas compared to resistant areas [69, 70].

Skin type and disease duration also play a role in repigmentation. Patients with Fitzpatrick skin phototypes (SPT) III–VI have a better response to EL than those with lighter skin [61, 64]. EL is also more effective at inducing repigmentation early in a patient's disease course, as disease duration is negatively associated with repigmentation [65, 68].

While increasing the frequency of treatment sessions results in faster repigmentation, the total number of sessions, rather than treatment frequency, has a greater impact on the degree of repigmentation. Typically, sessions are performed two to three times per week, and the treatment course should be greater than 12 weeks to ensure good cosmetic results [71]. Adjuvant therapies, such as topical corticosteroids or calcineurin inhibitors, are often used in conjunction with EL to maximize treatment outcomes (Table 15.2).

Irradiance and fluence of the laser are additional factors that need to be considered. Basic science experiments on melanoblasts have shown that irradiance is more important than fluence in inducing repigmentation with the excimer laser, with higher irradiances inducing greater pigmentation than lower irradiances [86].

Advantages

There are several advantages to utilizing EL over traditional NB-UVB therapies. EL can stimulate repigmentation in a faster amount of time, with one study showing similar outcomes within 10 weeks of laser therapy compared to 12 weeks of NB-UVB [61, 63, 87].

There is conflicting data regarding the repigmentation response between EL and NB-UVB. In a direct comparison of NB-UVB and EL in patients with generalized vitiligo who had failed prior treatment regimens, EL produced a significantly better repigmentation response as assessed by investigators after the tenth treatment session [67]. In contrast, a more recent study found no difference in repigmentation between the two treatment modalities when compared using a more objective image analysis system to measure therapy outcomes.

Of note, a lower cumulative UV dose was necessary to induce repigmentation with EL than NB-UVB phototherapy [88]. As there is a potential concern for UV-induced carcinogenesis, the combination of fewer treatment sessions and targeted treatment reduces the amount of UV exposure [61, 64, 73].

Furthermore, EL's articulated arm makes it advantageous in areas that can be difficult to reach like skin folds [60]. EL has also proven to be effective for patients who failed to respond to other therapies, including prior phototherapy, suggesting that it may have a superior ability to activate melanocytes [61, 63, 66, 67].

Studies have also compared EL to the excimer lamp. EL has a smaller spot size than the lamp so it is more accessible and easy to use for small lesions [89]. While there is no significant difference in repigmentation response between the laser and lamp [89], the lamp is associated with more severe, persistent erythema than the laser [90].

Limitations

The excimer laser has several limitations. Most studies reported minimal side effects with two sessions per week [66]. However, Hofer et al. reported a higher number of side effects, including blistering and burning, when compared to narrow and broadband UVB therapy, which they attributed to unintentional overlapping laser exposures and the addition of an extra treatment session (three sessions per week) [63, 87]. The spot size diameter of the laser ranges from 14 to 30 mm, which limits its use to lesions that cover less than 20% body surface area. One study found that patient satisfaction was greater with NB-UVB rather than EL treatment, which should be considered when choosing a therapy [88]. EL's purchase price and maintenance over time may also limit its use [60].

Summary of Excimer Laser

EL is an effective therapy for vitiligo, especially in UV-sensitive areas like the face [59]. In UV-resistant areas, it may be more effective to use a combination of laser and topical immunomodulators [57]. While EL produces a more rapid treatment response than NB-UVB, it can take longer to achieve a more noticeable cosmetic improvement. In addition, lesions in UV-resistant areas may require more sessions [63]. When choosing a treatment method, patient satisfaction and preferences should also be taken into account [88]. Due to its lower cumulative UV dosage, EL should be considered in children and those with a long history of UV exposure [88].

Table 15.2 Combination treatment trials with excimer laser for vitiligo.

Treatment modality	Study sample	Treatment regimen	Treatment outcomes
Corticosteroids			
EL vs. EL + topical hydrocortisone 17-butyrate cream [72]	UV-sensitive areas (face and neck)	EL alone: 2/week for 24 sessions Combination therapy: EL as above. Topical cream twice daily for 3 weeks followed by cream-free week, repeated over three treatment periods	EL alone: ≥75% repigmentation in 16.6% of patients Combination therapy: ≥75% repigmentation in 42.8% of patients
Topical calcineurin inhibitors			
EL vs. EL + 0.1% tacrolimus [57]	UV-resistant areas UV-sensitive areas	EL alone: 2/week for 24 sessions Combination therapy: EL as above. Tacrolimus ointment 2/day	EL alone: ≥75% repigmentation in 0% of lesions Combination therapy: ≥75% repigmentation in 60% of lesions EL alone: ≥75% repigmentation in 77% of lesions Combination therapy: ≥75% repigmentation in 57% of lesions
EL + placebo cream vs. EL + 0.1% tacrolimus [73]	Chronic symmetric vitiligo	EL at maximum of 3/week for maximum of 24 sessions Tacrolimus or placebo cream twice daily	EL alone: 75% repigmentation in 20% of lesions Combination therapy: 75% repigmentation in 50% of lesions
EL vs. topical 0.1% tacrolimus ointment vs. EL + topical tacrolimus [74]	Nonsegmental vitiligo	EL alone: 2/week for >6 months Topical alone: topical tacrolimus 2/week Combination therapy: both as above	First 6 months, repigmentation greater in combination therapy group After 6 months, repigmentation equivalent between groups
Triple combination therapies			
EL + topical tacrolimus + corticosteroids [75]	Segmental vitiligo	Various time frames (retrospective study)	≥75% repigmentation in 50.3% of patients
EL + topical tacrolimus + oral prednisolone [76]	Segmental and localized vitiligo	EL 2/week for 24 sessions 0.1% topical tacrolimus 2/day Oral prednisolone (0.3 mg/kg/day) for 4–8 weeks	≥75% repigmentation in 64.3% of patients
Vitamin D3 analogs			
EL vs. EL + topical calcipotriol [77]	Bilateral symmetrical vitiligo	EL alone: 3/week for 24 sessions on both sides of body Combination therapy: EL as above. Calcipotriol on lesions on one side of body 2/day	No significant difference in repigmentation between the treatment sides
EL vs. EL + topical tacalcitol vs. topical tacalcitol [78]	Nonsegmental vitiligo	EL alone: 2/week for 32 sessions Topical alone: topical tacalcitol nightly Combination therapy: both as above	EL and combination group showed significantly better repigmentation than topical alone No significant difference between EL and combination group

(continued)

Table 15.2 (continued)

Treatment modality	Study sample	Treatment regimen	Treatment outcomes
308-nm MEL + vehicle vs. MEL + tacalcitol [79]	–	MEL alone: MEL once weekly for 12 sessions + vehicle 2/day Combination therapy: MEL as above. Topical tacalcitol 2/day	MEL alone: 75% repigmentation in 5.7% of patients Combination therapy: 75% repigmentation in 25.7% of patients. Combo more effective at repigmentation than MEL alone [79, 80].
NB-UVB +EL [81]	–	NB-UVB 2/week until no change in lesions size followed by EL 2/week	≥75% repigmentation in 12.5% of patients, more on the face and neck
Surgical therapies			
EL + split thickness skin grafting [82]	Focal or segmental vitiligo	Split thickness skin grafting followed by EL 2/week for 32 sessions	All patients achieved "excellent" repigmentation at 1-year follow-up
NB-UVB or EL + mini-punch grafting [83]	Segmental vitiligo	Mini-punch grafting followed by either NB-UVB or EL	≥75% repigmentation in 69.2% of patients
MKTP vs. MKTP + EL vs. EL vs. no treatment [84]	Stable vitiligo	MKTP alone Combination therapy: MKTP followed by EL 2 weeks after grafting 2–3/week for 24 sessions EL alone: EL as above	MKTP alone: ≥ 65% repigmentation in 11% of patches Combination therapy: ≥65% repigmentation in 40% of patches EL alone: ≥65% repigmentation in 0% of patches
Topical antioxidants			
MEL alone vs. MEL + topical antioxidant [85]	Localized stable vitiligo	MEL alone: 2/week for 24 sessions Combination therapy: MEL as above. Topical antioxidant hydrogel applied daily	MEL alone: 0% of lesions achieved >75% repigmentation Combination therapy: 20% of lesions achieved >75% pigmentation

Abbreviations: *EL* excimer laser, *UV* ultraviolet, *MEL* monochromatic excimer light, *NB-UVB* narrow-band ultraviolet B, *MKTP* melanocyte-keratinocyte transplantation procedure

Fractional Carbon Dioxide Laser

The fractional carbon dioxide laser emits light at a wavelength of 10,600 nm. It is considered a "tissue-selective" laser, as its target chromophore is water, which is distributed equally in tissue. In contrast to other lasers, it is not "pigment-selective" and can damage cells that do not contain melanin [91].

Ablative CO_2 lasers were first used in the early 1990s for skin rejuvenation, and while they can be used to treat photodamaged skin, they can cause significant side effects [92]. Fractional photothermolysis (FP) was subsequently developed in response [91]. First described by Manstein et al., FP involves the creation of small necrotic wound columns, or microscopic treatment zones (MTZs), in the epidermis and dermis with sparing of the surrounding tissue, which allows for more rapid reepithelization and healing [92, 93]. In addition, there is a lower risk of scarring, permitting its use in areas prone to scar formation, including the neck and chest. Compared to other resurfacing lasers like the erbium-doped: yttrium-aluminum-garnet (Er:YAG), FCO_2 ablates only part of the epidermis, which decreases healing and recovery time, [42, 47] and the lack of open wounds decreases the risk of infection [48].

FCO_2 is thought to trigger the release of various melanocyte growth factors involved in wound healing secondary to cutaneous injury [42]. In addition, the MTZs created by FCO_2 can also improve drug absorption [51].

Use in Disorders of Hypopigmentation

Vitiligo

In vitiligo, the FCO_2 laser has been used mainly in combination with other treatment modalities. Shin et al. found that half-body FCO_2 laser therapy followed by NB-UVB phototherapy was more effective at inducing pigmentation than half-body NB-UVB therapy alone in patients with recalcitrant vitiligo [42]. Another study compared FCO_2 therapy followed by 2 h of sunlight exposure, to sunlight exposure alone, finding that the combination treatment was more effective. Lesion location impacted outcomes, with those on the face, legs, and neck showing better responses; lesions on bony prominences had worse outcomes [43]. Other studies have looked at triple combination therapy with NB-UVB, topical corticosteroids, and FCO_2, which have shown favorable results, particularly for lesions located on the extremities [44] and hands [45]. FCO_2 can be used to improve drug delivery of topical medications, such as corticosteroids as well [51].

The FCO_2 laser can also be used in surgical procedures for disorders of hypopigmentation in order to prepare the recipient site for melanocyte transplantation. Advantages of using FCO_2 over the more traditional dermabrasion include an even plane of epithelial denudation, operator ease, decreased risk of scarring, and decreased risk of peripheral hypopigmentation [46].

Idiopathic Guttate Hypomelanosis (IGH)

IGH is a leucoderma of unknown etiology that tends to occur in UV-exposed areas, most commonly involving the distal aspects of the arms and legs. It also occurs in areas exposed to repeated trauma [94]. Shin et al. speculate that FCO_2 may function by ablating the epidermis, effectively removing dysfunctional melanocytes [49].

In a pilot study, 40 patients were treated in one treatment session with the 10,600-nm FCO_2 laser. At a 2-month follow-up visit, 42.5% of patients experienced >75% improvement in pigmentation. None of the patients had recurrence after 1 year. Notable side effects included pain during treatment and post treatment erythema, with two patients experiencing long-lasting erythema of 2-month duration. Four patients experienced PIH [49].

In a larger study of 200 patients, similar findings were obtained, with 47.9% of patients achieving >75% improvement, further demonstrating its utility in IGH [50].

Use in Disorders of Hyperpigmentation

Melasma

Fractional lasers may be particularly useful in dermal melasma, as the creation of MTZs can penetrate deeper into the skin, without creating open wounds [47].

Treatment

The FCO_2 laser was proposed to be a new alternative with fewer side effects; however results thus far have not been as promising. While the ultrapulse CO_2 laser was shown to be effective in treating melasma, it was associated with PIH and a relatively long healing time [22, 48]. Laser settings should be based on the type of melasma and the SPT of the patient. For epidermal melasma, lower energies can be used. In patients with SPT I or II, higher energies may be necessary for mixed or dermal melasma. The recommendations regarding the treatment of darker skin types are more varied, as caution must be used with this population due to the risk of PIH [95].

Summary of Fractional Lasers

In refractory vitiligo, FCO_2 is useful in combination with other treatment modalities, specifically in treatment-resistant areas. To our knowledge, no studies have been done evaluating FCO_2 as monotherapy. The addition of FCO_2 to NB-UVB phototherapy can lead to a quicker response and reduce the number of phototherapy sessions to achieve repigmentation [45]. It can be also used for recipient site preparation in vitiligo surgery. In melasma, FCO_2 should only be considered in refractory cases and used with caution in darker skin types [47].

Q-Switched Ruby Laser

Q-switched lasers produce high-energy beams with extremely short pulse durations in the nanosecond range, which is less than the thermal relaxation time of melanosomes. As such, the Q-switched ruby laser (QSRL) directly targets melanosomes in the epidermis and dermis [96] without visibly damaging other organelles lacking melanin [97]. Therefore, skin thickening and epidermal changes are not seen.

Use in Disorders of Hypopigmentation

Vitiligo

The QSRL can be used to depigment patients with widespread vitiligo involving most of their total body surface area [98, 99]. Compared to bleaching creams, the QSRL has several advantages including a faster treatment response, shorter treatment times, and fewer adverse effects [100–102]. However, QSRL is typically used to treat smaller, discrete areas, whereas bleaching creams may have greater utility for larger surface areas.

A larger retrospective study found that 48% of patients treated with QSRL had >75% depigmentation of the treated pigmented area after a follow-up of just over a year. Patients with active disease had better outcomes than patients with stable disease, likely due to activation of the autoreactive T-cell response, which attacks the remaining melanocytes [102].

A study evaluating both QSRL and the topical depigmenting agent 4-methoxyphenol (4-MP) in patients with vitiligo universalis found that 69% of patients experienced total depigmentation following QSRL treatment. However, 44% of these responders relapsed after 2 months to 1.5 years later, particularly in sun-exposed areas. The repigmentation

tended to appear in a perifollicular distribution. Patients treated with QSRL achieved quicker results; depigmentation was observed in a week to 2 weeks compared to 4–12 months for patients treated with 4-MP [99].

Of note, in patients undergoing depigmentation treatment, strict photoprotection should be stressed to prevent repigmentation. Patients who decide to undergo treatment with QSRL should be advised that multiple treatments may be necessary to achieve complete depigmentation of the treated area.

Disorders of Hyperpigmentation

Nevus of Ota
Nevi of Ota are formed from intradermal melanocytes and are usually located in the distribution of the first and second branches of the trigeminal nerve (see Fig. 15.2). The QSRL emits light at a wavelength of 694 nm, which is long enough to be effective at targeting and destroying atypical melanocytes in the dermis while preserving epidermal melanocytes [8, 103]. This explains why red light lasers, such as the QSRL, are better for treatment of dermal pigmentation than green light lasers [104].

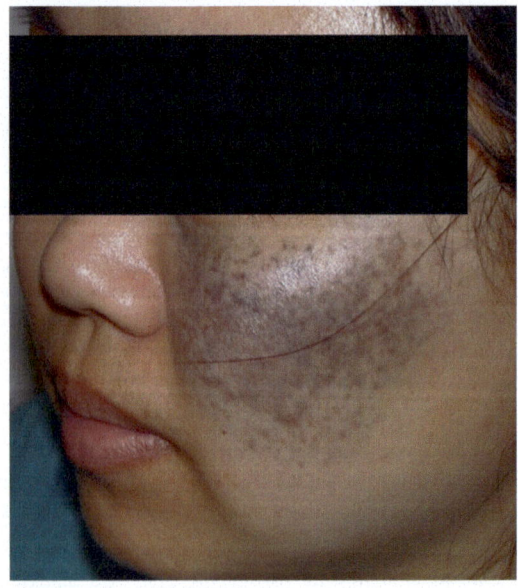

Fig. 15.2 Left cheek with nevus of Ota at baseline

Treatment Outcomes

Several studies have evaluated the efficacy of QSRL in the treatment of nevi of Ota. Of 35 Japanese patients who had four to five treatments with QSRL, 94.3% had an excellent response (≥70% lightening of the skin) [105]. Lowe et al. found that 85% of patients experienced >50% improvement in pigmentation after four laser treatment sessions, while 56.4% of patients with nevus of Ota showed greater than 75% clearance following a mean number of 5.5 laser treatments [106].

Factors Affecting Treatment Outcomes

Lesion color affects the number of treatments that are necessary to achieve clearance, with brown lesions requiring the least number of sessions followed by brown-violet. Blue-green and blue-violet lesions need the greatest number of treatments for successful clearance, which may be due to the increased number of dermal melanocytes observed in blue and green color variations [107]. This variation in color is secondary to the Tyndall effect, where the presence of melanin deeper in the dermis has a bluish appearance due to the scattering of light.

Limitations

Side effects of the QSRL included punctate erosions limited to the area of the lesion and transient PIH after the initial treatment [105, 106]. Lowe et al. reported transient hyperpigmentation and hypopigmentation in some patients that resolved in 3 months [103]. In the first large study evaluating complications of QSRL treatment, hypopigmentation was the most common side effect and was observed in 16.8% of patients, which was greater than other laser therapies [16, 106]. Higher fluences are associated with a greater risk of hypopigmentation, and subsequent studies have used lower fluences to avoid this complication [106]. Scarring and textural changes were not reported [103, 105].

QSRL Compared to Other Treatment Modalities

A few studies have compared QSRL to other Q-switched lasers to assess its efficacy. Tse et al. performed a bisected lesion study, using QSRL and the 1064-nm QS Nd:YAG to treat nevi of Ota. Lesion halves treated with QSRL had 57% mean clearance compared to 42% mean clearance in the lesion halves treated with the 1064-nm QS Nd: YAG [30]. Fewer treatment sessions were required to achieve >75% clearance when QSRL was used as opposed to QSAL or QS Nd:YAG [106].

Melasma

Treatment Outcomes

Multiple studies have shown that the QSRL is not an effective treatment for melasma, particularly for dermal and mixed melasma [30, 96, 108] and that hyperpigmentation may occur after treatment [96, 109]. In addition, recurrence is common following therapy [108, 110].

Conversely, new studies have shown positive outcomes with a new fractional QSRL that was developed to help decrease healing time and reduce adverse events [111]. Hilton et al. showed that fractional QSRL significantly reduced the Melasma Area and Severity Index (MASI) score by 72.3% at time intervals of 4 and 6 weeks after treatment in Caucasian patients with epidermal or mixed melasma [112]. Jang et al. studied Korean women (skin types III–IV) with dermal or mixed melasma treated with fractional QSRL and found a significant decrease in mean MASI score of 30%. Hypopigmentation or PIH was not observed in this set of patients, which may be due to their use of lower energy fluences than previous studies. Studies with longer follow-up periods are needed to evaluate long-term results beyond the 4-month period used in this study [113].

Post-inflammatory Hyperpigmentation

PIH can occur after a cutaneous insult triggers an inflammatory response. To prevent the development or worsening of PIH, the inciting inflammatory condition must be treated [47]. Treatment of existing PIH can be difficult. Taylor and Anderson did not find QSRL to be an effective treatment for PIH. In three out of four patients with PIH secondary to various causes, including lichen planus, thermal burns, and morphea, there was worsening of hyperpigmentation following QSRL therapy, which was dose-independent. Other patients developed hypopigmented and hyperpigmented patches [96]. Kopera et al. studied eight patients and found similar results; one patient experienced lesion darkening and only one patient achieved subjectively good results [109]. In a study of patients who developed hyperpigmentation following sclerotherapy, Tafazzoli et al. found that QSRL was effective at lightening lesions, possibly due to its ability to target hemosiderin [114]. In a case report, QSRL improved the appearance of PIH secondary to hemosiderin deposition in one patient by 77%. More research needs to be done to evaluate whether these results can be replicated [30].

Solar Lentigines

Treatment Outcomes
The target chromophore in solar lentigines is melanin, making QSRL a reasonable treatment option. However, there is concern about the risk of PIH and hypopigmentation, particularly in patients with darker skin types. To address this concern, a study was conducted of Iranian patients with SPT II to IV. All patients treated with the QSRL achieved complete resolution of their lesions after two sessions, demonstrating its efficacy in patients with slightly darker skin types [9]. Tse et al. found that QSRL resulted in 66% mean percent clearing in patients with solar lentigines [30]. QSRL has also been compared to various other treatment modalities for lentigines (Table 15.3).

Limitations
Post-procedural PIH was more common in darker skin types, but these pigmentary changes tended to resolve after 6 months, and the difference in pigmentary changes between light and dark skin types was not statistically significant [9]. While pain associated with treatment may be a limiting factor [10], adequate epidermal cooling can help alleviate some of the discomfort associated with the procedure.

Drug-Induced Hyperpigmentation
Many medications are associated with skin discoloration, including psychotropic drugs such as imipramine and chlorpromazine. It is thought that these medications may react with sunlight to produce free radicals and activate tyrosinase. The increased melanin then traps the free radicals, producing hyperpigmentation [118]. Imipramine-induced hyperpigmentation occurs in photosensitive areas, such as the face and arms. Changes in iris color have been reported as well [119]. A literature review reported that it could take years of treatment with imipramine before patients experience hyperpigmentation, ranging from 1 to 22 years [120]. Even after stopping these medications, the discoloration may persist.

Several other drugs have also been found to induce hyperpigmentation including amiodarone, heavy metals, and anti-malarial drugs [120, 121]. Minocycline, a tetracycline antibiotic, induces hyperpigmentation that appears to histologically reflect either melanin or hemosiderin, which explains why QSRL may be an effective treatment option [11]. There are several types of minocycline-induced hyperpigmentation. Type I is usually blue-black in color and involves areas prone to scarring, whereas type II is blue-gray and occurs in areas of normal skin on the extremities. Type III is a brown color with darker discoloration of UV-exposed areas [24, 33].

Treatment Outcomes
QSRL has been shown to effectively treat discoloration caused by several different medications including amiodarone and minocycline [11, 12]. In a case report, a patient with minocycline-induced facial hyperpigmentation was treated with the QSRL and the 1064-nm QS Nd:YAG laser. The spot treated with the QSRL had improved pigmentation both clinically and histologically, while the spot treated with the QS Nd:YAG showed only minimal histologic improvement and no clinical improvement. Additionally, the QSRL treatment did not cause any side effects, such as crusting or textural changes [11]. Another study of four patients with hyperpigmentation on either the face, lips, or legs were treated with QSRL 1 month after discon-

Table 15.3 Comparing QSRL to other treatment modalities for solar lentigines

Treatment modality	Study sample	Treatment regimen	Treatment outcomes
QSRL vs. TCT (hydroquinone 5%, tretinoin 0.03%, and dexamethasone 0.03%) [115]	Symmetric lentigines on bilateral dorsal hands	1 session at baseline on right hand, possible second session if necessary after 4 weeks TCT once daily on left hand for 7 weeks	After treatment and at 3-month follow-up, significantly improved clearing with QSRL based on physician and patient rating
QSRL vs. fractional CO_2 laser [10]	Symmetric lentigines on bilateral dorsal hands	3 monthly sessions with QSRL for one hand and fractional CO_2 for the other	At 2-month and 4-month follow-up, significantly improved clearing with QSRL than with FCO_2 based on physician rating
QSRL vs. frequency-doubled, 532-nm QS Nd:YAG [116]	Facial lentigines >8 mm in size	Patients randomized into one of four groups Groups 1 and 2 were treated with QSRL Groups 3 and 4 treated with frequency-doubled 532-nm QS Nd:YAG Groups 1 and 3 treated with "aggressive" irradiation Groups 2 and 4 treated with "mild" irradiation	Percentage of lesions achieving excellent clearance: 43.3% in group 1, 62.6% in group 2, 52.2% in group 3, 62.7% in group 4 No difference in lesion clearing between the different types of lasers and between higher and lower irradiances Higher incidence of PIH in groups 1 and 3
QSRL vs. 595-nm LPDL [117]	Facial lentigines	Each patient was treated with 1 session of QSRL and 1 session of LPDL	Significant difference in clearing with LPDL than with QSRL QSRL: 70.3% lesion clearing LPDL: 83.3% lesion clearing Erythema and hyperpigmentation more common with QSRL

Abbreviations: *QSRL* Q-switched ruby laser, *TCT* triple combination therapy, *QS Nd:YAG* quality-switched neodymium yttrium-aluminum-garnet, *PIH* post-inflammatory hyperpigmentation, *LPDL* long-pulsed dye laser

tinuing minocycline, and all patients experienced complete resolution without any scarring or hypopigmentation [13].

Summary for QSRL

QSRL is frequently regarded as the gold standard treatment for nevi of Ota [8, 30] as they are very responsive to laser therapy and recurrence is unusual [104]. This is particularly true in skin types I–IV, whereas in skin type V there is a higher risk of depigmentation. Since the laser is absorbed by melanin, patients with darker skin are at risk for pigmentary abnormalities, so it should be used with caution in these patients [52].

For solar lentigines, QSRL may be more effective than topical treatments. There is not enough evidence to support QSRL's use in the treatment of PIH and melasma. The new fractionated QSRL may be considered in patients with melasma, but more studies are necessary to evaluate its efficacy. With regard to drug-induced hyperpigmentation, QSRL is an effective option.

Q-Switched Alexandrite Laser

The Q-switched alexandrite laser (QSAL) has a longer wavelength of 755 nm, compared to the QSRL at 694 nm. Therefore, it can penetrate deeper into the dermis than the QSRL, making it more advantageous in destroying dermal melanin [122]. It also has a longer pulse duration of 50–100 ns, compared to the pulse duration of the QSRL of 25–40 ns [123].

Disorders of Hypopigmentation

Vitiligo

There is a single case reported in the literature of a patient with refractory vitiligo (including prior QSRL therapy) who was treated with QSAL for ten treatment sessions and had an excellent response, demonstrating its potential effectiveness as a depigmentation therapy [124]. Larger studies are needed to confirm these findings in patients with vitiligo.

Disorders of Hyperpigmentation

Nevus of Ota

Treatment Outcomes

In a study evaluating the efficacy of the QSAL for treatment of nevi of Ota, all 48 patients achieved >75% improvement in pigmentation after undergoing a varying number of treatment sessions that ranged from 3 to 11 [17]. Another study found that the QSAL required about four to five treatments to achieve ≥50% improvement in pigmentation [16]. In a small study of seven patients, five achieved complete clearance after four to six treatment sessions [18].

Factors Affecting Treatment Outcomes

Lesions with melanocyte depths of <1 mm had good to excellent pigment removal, although complete clearance is not always possible [125].

Complications

Use of the QSAL is associated with a higher incidence of hypopigmentation compared to other lasers, which can be temporary or persist for several years [16, 17].

Hyperpigmentation can also occur secondary to PIH, especially in skin types IV and V [125]. Tissue swelling and pain may also occur after treatment [122]. Again, these symptoms can be reduced by epidermal cooling before, during, and after treatment. Pain after treatment is more severe after QSAL treatment than the 1064-nm QS Nd:YAG, but this resolved after 1 week and long-term discomfort was less common with the QSAL [122].

Combination Trials

Combined use of the QSAL and the QS Nd:YAG resulted in improved clearance compared to either laser alone. However, the QSAL had a greater estimated probability of clearance with fewer treatment sessions than the QS Nd:YAG [16]. There is also slightly less pain and swelling associated with the QSAL compared to the QS Nd:YAG [122].

Solar Lentigines

In a study using the QSAL for treatment of solar lentigines, 76% of lesions responded to initial treatment. Hypopigmentation was the only side effect observed [19, 20]. Factors that affect treatment outcomes include the intensity of lesional pigment and fluence settings used [126, 127]. Lighter lesions do not respond as well to laser treatment as darker lesions [126]. As such, pretreatment with cryotherapy, which can induce lesion darkening, followed by treatment with the alexandrite laser may be an option [126].

A split-face study of 17 patients with solar lentigines was performed comparing the QSAL to intense pulsed light (IPL) therapy. Both treatments improved scoring of pigmentation, although hyperpigmentation was found more frequently in patients treated with the QSAL [21].

Melasma

A few studies have analyzed the combination of pulsed CO_2 laser and QSAL in the treatment of melasma, which utilizes both ablative and nonablative lasers. The pulsed CO_2 laser can destroy abnormal melanocytes in the epidermis, while the QSAL acts in the dermis [22].

A split-face study in six Thai patients compared QSAL monotherapy to a combined treatment with QSAL and ultrapulse CO_2 laser. A significant reduction in MASI score was observed on the side receiving combination treatment (five of six patients). Although three patients had a decrease in MASI score on the side treated with QSAL alone, it was not statistically significant, and one patient had worsening of the MASI score. Patients with darker skin were more likely to develop hyperpigmentation [47, 128].

Other studies have resulted in more encouraging outcomes. A study comparing pulsed CO_2 monotherapy to combination treatment with CO_2 and QSAL in patients with skin types IV–VI found that all patients had complete resolution. Two patients developed peripheral hyperpigmentation, but both were in the CO_2 laser monotherapy group [22]. In a split-face study comparing QSAL and the 1064-nm Nd:YAG in 16 patients with SPT I–IV with mixed-type facial melasma, both treatment groups experienced a significant improvement in pigmentation that was maintained at a 6-month follow-up visit. There was no significant difference in objective or subjective improvement between the two groups [23].

Drug-Induced Hyperpigmentation

In a case report of one patient who developed facial discoloration following treatment with minocycline (type III minocycline-induced hyperpigmentation), the 1064-nm QS Nd:YAG, QSAL, and QSRL were compared. After two treatment sessions, the QSAL resulted in a 50% improvement in pigmentation with minimal adverse effects. The QSRL resulted in 90% improvement, but was more painful. The QS Nd:YAG did not improve pigmentation. After two additional treatments with the QSAL, the patient experienced complete resolution. The authors concluded that QSAL was the most appropriate of the three lasers for treatment since it was effective with fewer side effects [24]. Another case report also found the QSAL with a fluence of 6 J/cm² to be effective in treating hyperpigmentation on the legs, with maintenance of results at 3-year follow-up [25]. A case series of six patients with type II and type III hyperpigmentation reported resolution after three to five treatment sessions [26].

Another case report described a patient who developed facial hyperpigmentation after taking desipramine and perphenazine that was persistent despite discontinuing the medications and undergoing chemical peels. She was treated with three 755-nm QSAL treatments and experienced complete resolution. Other patients with hyperpigmentation secondary to psychotropic medications also experienced lesional lightening with QSAL [27, 28].

Summary for QS Alexandrite Laser

For the treatment of melasma and Nevi of Ota, combination therapies may be more effective at inducing clearance than QSAL therapy alone. QSAL can successfully treat solar lentigines, although there is increased risk of hyperpigmentation. QSAL can effectively treat minocycline and psychotropic drug-induced hyperpigmentation as well.

Compared to other lasers, QSAL has a longer wavelength and pulse duration, with minimal risk of hypopigmentation, PIH, scarring, and tissue splatter. In addition, there is a lower incidence of transient hypopigmentation with QSAL compared to QSRL [41, 52].

Neodymium Yttrium-Aluminum-Garnet Laser

The Nd:YAG laser comes in several forms including continuous wave, quasi-continuous, frequency-doubled, and Q-switched. The Q-switched Nd:YAG laser functions at a wavelength of either 532 or 1064 nm. By using a potassium diphosphate crystal, the frequency-doubled laser emits light at a shorter wavelength of 532 nm, producing green light with a pulse duration of about 30 ns [52]. The 532-nm laser's target chromophore is melanin, and it is commonly used to treat epidermal pigmentation [52, 123, 129]. However, hemoglobin also absorbs at 532 nm, which poses the risk of vascular damage and subsequent erythema and PIH. The 1064-nm laser can more effectively treat dermal pigmentation due to its longer wavelength and has a lower risk of PIH [41]. Clinical end points of treatment should be tailored to the pigmentary skin disorder [130] (see Fig. 15.3).

Disorders of Hypopigmentation

Vitiligo

Only two studies have evaluated the use of Nd:YAG in vitiligo. In one study, the Dermalase frequency-doubled, Q-switched Nd:YAG was utilized at both the 532-nm and 1064-nm wavelengths for three monthly sessions but was unsuccessful at inducing repigmentation [131]. Another study found that the frequency-doubled, 532-nm Q-switched Nd:YAG was effective for depigmentation therapy [29]. In our experience, the 532-nm QS Nd:YAG is an effective method in removing pigment recalcitrant to topical agents in patients who desire depigmentation (see Figs. 15.4 and 15.5).

Disorders of Hyperpigmentation

Solar Lentigines

Few studies have evaluated the effectiveness of Nd:YAG lasers for the treatment of solar lentigines. Studies assessing the 532-nm Nd:YAG laser found that patients had improvement in pigmentation that was long-lasting. Higher energy

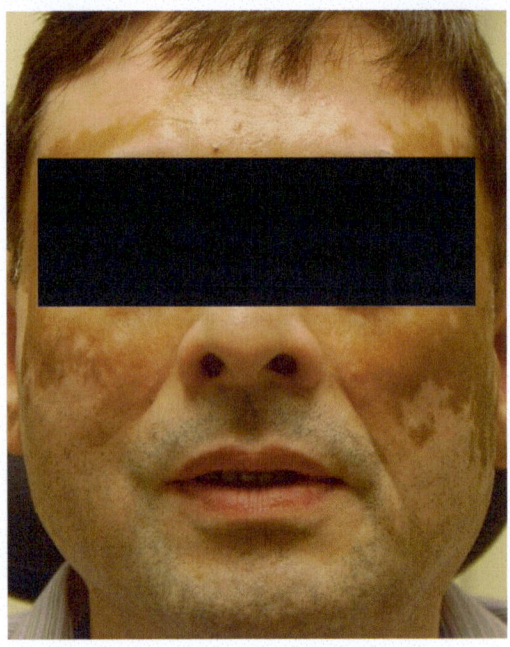

Fig. 15.4 Vitiligo patient with resistant facial pigmentation refractory to topical depigmenting agents at baseline

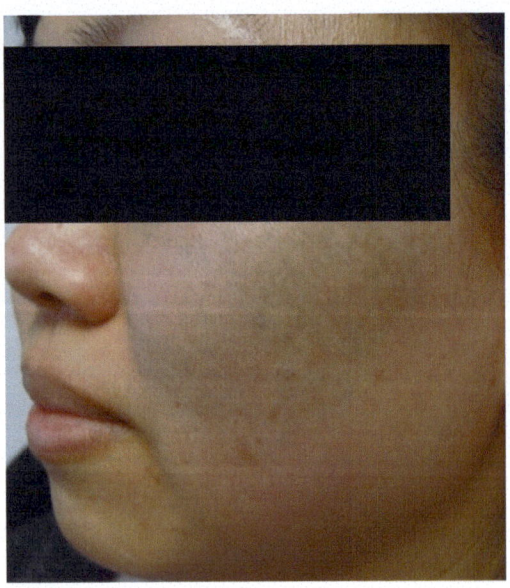

Fig. 15.3 Left cheek with nevus of Ota after four monthly sessions of treatment with the 1064-nm Q-switched Nd:YAG

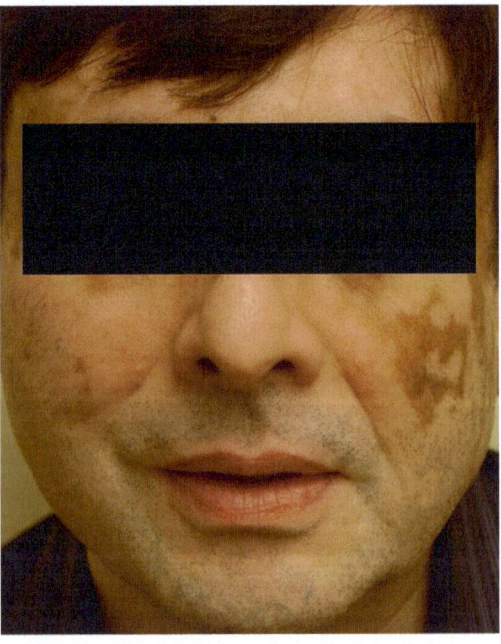

Fig. 15.5 Vitiligo patient with resistant facial pigmentation refractory to topical depigmenting agents 4 months after one treatment session with the 532-nm Q-switched Nd:YAG

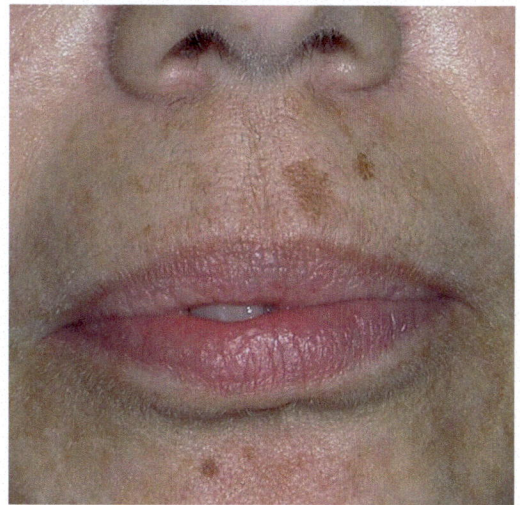

Fig. 15.6 Lentigines on the upper cutaneous lip at baseline

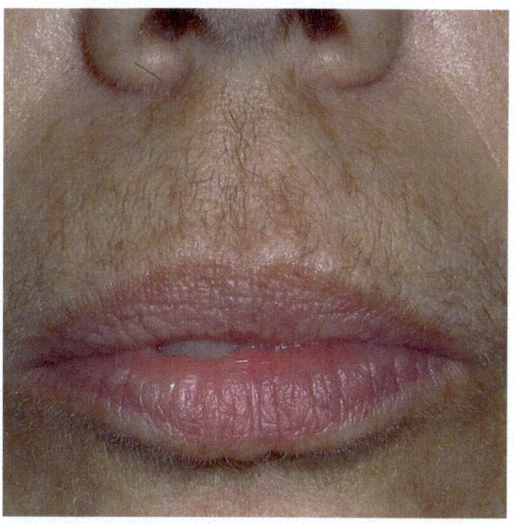

Fig. 15.7 Lentigines on the upper cutaneous lip 2 months after one session of treatment with the 532-nm Q-switched Nd:YAG

fluences are associated with greater lesional lightening, but have increased side effects, such as PIH [30–32] (see Figs. 15.6 and 15.7).

Comparisons to Other Treatment Modalities

In a study comparing the 532-nm Q-switched Nd:YAG to FCO$_2$, lesions treated with the Nd:YAG laser had a better response than FCO$_2$ alone. However, the 532-nm Nd:YAG had a higher pain score and slower healing time compared to the FCO$_2$ laser [132]. The 532-nm QS Nd:YAG was also compared to a new 660-nm QS Nd:YAG laser in Korean women with skin types III–IV as a treatment for facial lentigines. Of the seven patients who completed the study, both treatments produced significant improvements in pigmentation, with no statistically significant differences in treatment outcomes between the two modalities [133].

In a study comparing the 532-nm QS Nd:YAG, a krypton laser, a 532-nm diode-pumped vanadate laser, and liquid nitrogen (LN$_2$), laser therapy was more effective in lightening solar lentigines on the hands than LN$_2$. Notably, the 532-nm Nd:YAG laser was the most effective at clearing lentigines with fewer side effects than the other two lasers [134].

Another study compared the Versapulse 532-nm QS Nd:YAG, the Versapulse long-pulsed 532-nm Nd:YAG, and a conventional 532-nm QS Nd:YAG laser among Chinese patients. The Versapulse QS 532-nm laser was associated with the highest risk of hyperpigmentation and erythema, whereas the long-pulsed laser was the most effective at improving clearance of lentigines, with the lowest risk of hyperpigmentation. The risk of hyperpigmentation was independent of the type of SPT [135].

The frequency-doubled 532-nm Nd:YAG laser was also compared to 35% trichloroacetic acid (TCA) as a treatment for facial lentigines in patients with SPT III and IV. After one treatment, a greater number of lentigines (65%) treated with the laser had improved pigmentation compared to those treated with TCA. Although statistically significant, the difference between the two treatments was small [136].

Limitations

Complications associated with use of the frequency-doubled, 532-nm QS Nd:YAG include erythema, hypopigmentation, hyperpigmentation, and textural changes, primarily when using higher fluences of 4 or 5 J/cm^2, which usually improve with time [31, 32, 136].

Melasma

Both the 532-nm and 1064-nm Nd:YAG lasers have been studied in patients with melasma.

The longer wavelength of light with the 1064-nm laser allows it to travel deeper into the dermis, making it a better option for dermal and mixed melasma, especially in SPT III and IV. As the 532-nm laser emits green light, it is more effective for epidermal melasma [47]. Patients with melasma have increased vascularity and VEGF expression, and the QS Nd:YAG laser's efficacy in these patients may involve its ability to stimulate the formation of collagen within the papillary dermis and cause damage to the dermal vasculature [47, 137, 138].

Different clinical end points should be used depending on the type of melasma. For epidermal melasma, the laser should be passed along the area until whitening of the skin or hair is observed (see Fig. 15.8). For dermal or mixed melasma, the laser should be passed until the lesion darkens or there is perilesional erythema [130].

Treatment Outcomes

Early studies with the Nd:YAG laser for melasma used high fluences that caused complications. Recently, the concept of "laser toning" has been used to treat melasma. This technique involves using multiple passes of the QS Nd:YAG laser with a large spot size and low fluence (1.6–3.5 J/cm²). Polnikorn was the first to report laser toning, using weekly treatments of the 1064-nm QS Nd:YAG laser for 8–10 weeks, and found it to be successful on two patients with PIH and refractory melasma. Following laser treatment,

patients had a greater than 80% decrease in epidermal and dermal hyperpigmentation [130, 139]. Another study using a low-fluence 1064-nm QS Nd:YAG laser found significant improvement in pigmentation in patients with mixed-type facial melasma [23].

Cho et al. also used larger spot sizes and lower fluences in Korean patients with SPT IV and facial melasma with an average number of seven sessions. Twenty-eight percent (7/25) of these patients showed >75% total improvement, and 72% of patients were very satisfied or satisfied with the results [34]. Zhou et al. found that the mean melanin index using mexametry decreased by 35.8% after nine laser treatments with the 1064-nm QS Nd:YAG laser with fluences of 2.5–3.4 J/cm² and a 61.3% decrease in the mean MASI score. Patients with more severe melasma at baseline had worse outcomes after treatment [140].

Other studies have not been as promising, with low efficacy or recurrence of pigmentation after initial improvement and a higher incidence of adverse events [30, 141, 142].

Complications

Several studies have noted complications with this technique including hypopigmentation, punctate leukoderma, and more generalized depigmentation [34, 47, 141, 143, 144]. Leukotrichia can also occur, particularly with the 532-nm and 1064-nm Q-switched lasers at threshold and suprathreshold doses [145]. It is thought that hyperpigmentation may be due to the repeated passes of the laser with a greater cumulative laser dosage [144, 146].

To avoid these complications, using low-fluence settings with fewer passes may reduce the risk of hypo- and hyperpigmentation [142, 147–149]. This is especially important in patients with darker skin types, as they are more prone to developing pigmentary abnormalities [144]. To treat any resulting hypopigmentation, the excimer laser may be used to promote repigmentation [150]. Pain during and after the procedure is another complication that can often be managed by epidermal cooling devices.

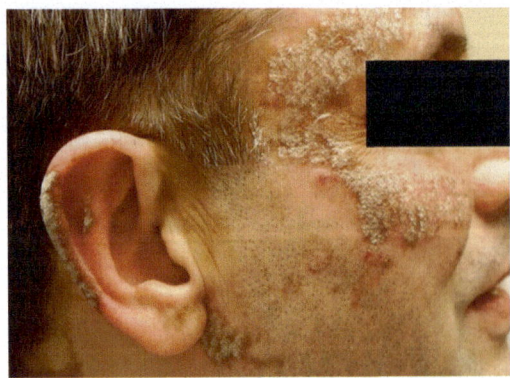

Fig. 15.8 Tissue whitening after laser firing is the biologic end point to achieve depigmentation

Long-Term Outcomes

Recurrence of melasma is common and long-term outcomes appear to be poor [140, 144]. To prevent this, it is important to avoid any exogenous inciting or exacerbating factors (oral contraceptive pills, sun exposure, etc.) and initiate maintenance therapy with topical bleaching agents (e.g., 7% alpha arbutin, etc.) and broad-spectrum sunscreens [130, 140].

Combination Therapies

Hydroquinone (HQ) is one of the most common topical lightening agents used for the treatment of melasma. Wattankrai et al. performed a split-face study of 22 patients with facial dermal or mixed melasma comparing topical 2% HQ alone vs. topical 2% HQ and 1064-nm QS Nd:YAG. Patients were told to apply the cream 2 weeks before beginning laser treatment. After seven treatment sessions, the side treated with laser had 92.5% improvement in pigmentation compared to the side treated with the HQ alone, which had 19.7% improvement in pigmentation. However, the side treated with combination therapy had increased side effects, and the improvement was transitory, with recurrence in all patients irrespective of treatment side [144].

Triple combination (TC) cream, which consists of HQ, a retinoid, and a steroid, is often prescribed as a first-line therapy for the treatment of melasma [151]. When used as pretreatment prior to laser therapy, it may improve treatment outcomes by decreasing melanin production prior to treatment and decreasing the risk of PIH. TC cream may also be used after laser therapy for maintenance [147].

The QS Nd:YAG has been studied in combination with other procedural therapies. The combination of microdermabrasion, low-fluence 1064-nm QS Nd: YAG (1.6–2 J/cm²), and a topical regimen between laser treatment sessions (sunscreen, hydroquinone, and either tretinoin or L-ascorbic acid) was evaluated in patients with refractory mixed-type melasma. Eighty-one percent had greater than 75% improvement after 1 month of treatment [152].

QS Nd:YAG laser has also been combined with IPL in the treatment of refractory melasma. IPL has a wavelength of 540 nm, effectively targeting melanin in the epidermis, while the 1064-nm laser's longer wavelength can target the dermis [153, 154]. Cunha et al. studied six patients with refractory melasma who received one laser treatment followed by IPL at each session. Patients applied a topical treatment that included Kligman's formula between their laser treatments. Combination therapy resulted in a statistically significant decrease in pigmentation compared to baseline [153]. Other studies have also shown improvement in melasma using the combination of Nd:YAG and IPL [148, 149]. The combination of low-fluence QS Nd:YAG and long-pulsed Nd:YAG laser (dual toning) in patients may also be effective in improving melasma [155].

Post-inflammatory Hyperpigmentation

With regard to clinical end points used for the treatment of post-inflammatory hyperpigmentation, the laser should be passed until lightening of the lesion is observed [130].

Relatively few studies have evaluated the effectiveness of the QS Nd:YAG laser for the treatment of PIH, but these have produced good results. In one patient with PIH and dermal melasma, ten weekly treatments with the 1064-nm QS Nd:YAG laser with a fluence of 3.4 J/cm² resulted in greater than 80% improvement in pigmentation without recurrence after 1 year [34]. Another study found that the 1064-nm QS Nd:YAG laser effectively treated PIH secondary to acne [35]. We also had a positive outcome with this laser in a patient with PIH refractory to prior medical management [36] (see Figs. 15.9 and 15.10). It is recommended to use sunscreen and a tyrosinase inhibitor, such as hydroquinone or alpha arbutin, after treatment for maintenance [130]. Use of the 532-nm QS Nd:YAG is less common for PIH, possibly because oxyhemoglobin absorbs light emitted from the 532-nm laser, which can lead to bruising and the potential development of additional PIH [47, 110]. However, one patient treated with this laser achieved good lightening of PIH [30].

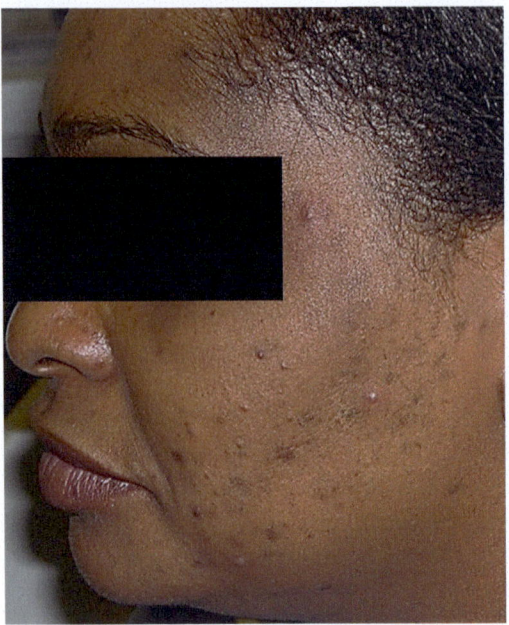

Fig. 15.9 Left cheek with post-inflammatory hyperpigmentation secondary to acne at baseline

Drug-Induced Hyperpigmentation

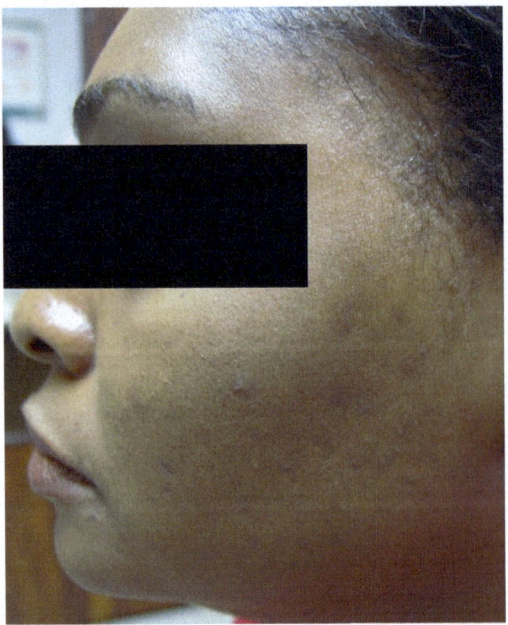

Fig. 15.10 Left cheek with post-inflammatory hyperpigmentation secondary to acne after four monthly sessions of treatment with the 1064-nm Q-switched Nd:YAG

Few studies have evaluated the effectiveness of the Nd:YAG lasers for drug-induced hyperpigmentation. One case report of a patient taking imipramine for 10 years did not find the Nd:YAG laser to be effective. However, the wavelength of the laser used in this patient was not reported [119].

There is mixed consensus of the utility of the Nd:YAG laser for minocycline-induced hyperpigmentation. One case report describes a patient who took minocycline for 6 years and developed type I facial blue-black pigmentation that did not resolve after discontinuing the medication or applying a topical hydroquinone cream. Two test sites were used to compare the different wavelengths of the QS Nd:YAG laser. One site was treated with the 1064-nm wavelength, while the other site was treated with the 532-nm wavelength. Eight weeks after one treatment session, there was complete resolution at the site treated with the 532-nm wavelength, while there was no change in pigmentation at the site treated with the 1064-nm wavelength laser. The authors speculated that the target chromophore in type I minocycline-induced hyperpigmentation may be iron, which the 532-nm laser effectively targets [33]. Another case report of type I minocycline-induced hyperpigmentation also did not find the 1064-nm QS Nd:YAG to clinically improve pigmentation [11].

In contrast, a woman with facial hyperpigmentation secondary to long-term use of minocycline was treated with the 1064-nm QS Nd:YAG laser for nine treatment sessions and experienced complete resolution [156]. In our experience, we have had good outcomes with the QS Nd:YAG without causing hypopigmentation, but additional treatment sessions were necessary.

Summary of Nd:YAG Lasers

The Nd:YAG is primarily used to treat disorders of hyperpigmentation including solar lentigines, PIH, and melasma. The long-pulsed 532-nm Nd:YAG is particularly useful for solar lentigines and also has some utility in PIH. The longer wavelength 1064-nm QS Nd:YAG is more useful for treating dermal pigmentation.

The management of melasma is complicated. Laser toning is controversial with mixed results, but the use of combination treatment with IPL and dual toning appears promising. When laser toning is performed, lower fluences should be used to avoid unwanted side effects. To avoid hypopigmentation and other complications, the number of treatment sessions and their frequency should be limited (less than once per week with a maximum of seven sessions) [47].

In the limited studies of minocycline-induced hyperpigmentation, the frequency-doubled 532-nm QS Nd:YAG laser may be effective, but the utility of the 1064-nm laser is unclear.

Summary and Future Directions

Lasers have been used with variable success to treat a variety of pigmentary disorders. EL can effectively treat vitiligo in UV-sensitive areas, with increased efficacy when used in combination with other treatments. FCO_2 is used for recipient site preparation in vitiligo surgery and for treatment of IGH. QSRL is the most effective in treating nevi of Ota and solar lentigines; it also can effectively treat hyperpigmentation induced by various drugs. The 1064-nm QS Nd:YAG may be useful for PIH, while the long-pulsed 532-nm Nd:YAG improves solar lentigines and the 532-nm QS Nd:YAG can treat minocycline-induced hyperpigmentation.

PIH and melasma can be the most difficult pigmentary disorders to treat. Laser treatment for melasma remains controversial and reserved for refractory cases, since lasers can cause inflammation and hyperpigmentation [104]. Treatment should be based on the melasma type, as epidermal melasma responds well to topical treatment. For patients who fail to respond to TC cream, laser therapy should be considered in combination with topical therapies [47, 147]. PIH is generally considered to be refractory to laser therapy [123]. While the limited studies performed have shown that the 1064-nm QS Nd:YAG may be a reasonable option, additional studies with larger sample sizes are needed. The long-pulsed Nd:YAG may be another alternative [157].

Several adverse events are possible with laser treatment and include hyperpigmentation, hypopigmentation, textural changes, scar formation, erythema, pain, and infection. Caution is advised when using lasers in darker skin types, particularly SPT IV to VI patients with melasma [158], and all patients should practice photoprotection to help prevent recurrence. However, maintenance therapy involving additional laser treatments or topical lightening agents may be necessary.

The clinical application of lasers in the field of dermatology is ever-changing and will continue to progress as more research is performed on the latest laser models along with greater understanding of the pathophysiology of skin conditions. Fractional lasers are still relatively new and need to be further studied. Most of the studies conducted are small, so larger randomized controlled and multi-armed combination trials are needed. The development of new lasers and techniques will undoubtedly improve their utility as well as improve outcomes for patients.

References

1. Taylor A, Pawaskar M, Taylor SL, Balkrishnan R, Feldman SR. Prevalence of pigmentary disorders and their impact on quality of life: a prospective cohort study. J Cosmet Dermatol. 2008;7(3):164–8.
2. Fabi SG, Metelitsa AI. Future directions in cutaneous laser surgery. Dermatol Clin. 2014;32(1):61–9.
3. Gomez C, Costela A, Garcia-Moreno I, Llanes F, Teijon JM, Blanco MD. Skin laser treatments enhancing transdermal delivery of ALA. J Pharm Sci. 2011;100(1):223–31.
4. Baltas E, Csoma Z, Ignacz F, Dobozy A, Kemeny L. Treatment of vitiligo with the 308-nm xenon chloride excimer laser. Arch Dermatol. 2002;138(12):1619–20.
5. Asawanonda P, Anderson RR, Chang Y, Taylor CR. 308-nm excimer laser for the treatment of psoriasis: a dose-response study. Arch Dermatol. 2000;136(5):619–24.
6. Lee HI, Lim YY, Kim BJ, Kim MN, Min HJ, Hwang JH, et al. Clinicopathologic efficacy of copper bromide plus/yellow laser (578 nm with 511 nm) for treatment of melasma in Asian patients. Dermatol Surg. 2010;36(6):885–93.
7. McCoy S, Hanna M, Anderson P, McLennan G, Repacholi M. An evaluation of the copper-bromide laser for treating telangiectasia. Dermatol Surg. 1996;22(6):551–7.

8. Goldberg DJ, Nychay SG. Q-switched ruby laser treatment of nevus of Ota. J Dermatol Surg Oncol. 1992;18(9):817–21.

9. Sadighha A, Saatee S, Muhaghegh-Zahed G. Efficacy and adverse effects of Q-switched ruby laser on solar lentigines: a prospective study of 91 patients with Fitzpatrick skin type II, III, and IV. Dermatol Surg. 2008;34(11):1465–8.

10. Schoenewolf NL, Hafner J, Dummer R, Bogdan Allemann I. Laser treatment of solar lentigines on dorsum of hands: QS Ruby laser versus ablative CO2 fractional laser - a randomized controlled trial. Eur J Dermatol. 2015;25(2):122–6.

11. Tsao H, Busam K, Barnhill RL, Dover JS. Treatment of minocycline-induced hyperpigmentation with the Q-switched ruby laser. Arch Dermatol. 1996;132(10):1250–1.

12. Wiper A, Roberts DH, Schmitt M. Amiodarone-induced skin pigmentation: Q-switched laser therapy, an effective treatment option. Heart. 2007;93(1):15.

13. Collins P, Cotterill JA. Minocycline-induced pigmentation resolves after treatment with the Q-switched ruby laser. Br J Dermatol. 1996;135(2):317–9.

14. Raulin C, Schonermark MP, Greve B, Werner S. Q-switched ruby laser treatment of tattoos and benign pigmented skin lesions: a critical review. Ann Plast Surg. 1998;41(5):555–65.

15. Choudhary S, Elsaie ML, Leiva A, Nouri K. Lasers for tattoo removal: a review. Lasers Med Sci. 2010;25(5):619–27.

16. Chan HH, Leung RS, Ying SY, Lai CF, Kono T, Chua JK, et al. A retrospective analysis of complications in the treatment of nevus of Ota with the Q-switched alexandrite and Q-switched Nd:YAG lasers. Dermatol Surg. 2000;26(11):1000–6.

17. Sami L, Changzheng H, Yan L. Factors affecting response, number of laser sessions and complications in nevus of Ota treated by Q-switched alexandrite laser: a retrospective study. G Ital Dermatol Venereol. 2016;107(2):160–8.

18. Alster TS, Williams CM. Treatment of nevus of Ota by the Q-switched alexandrite laser. Dermatol Surg. 1995;21(7):592–6.

19. Ortonne JP, Pandya AG, Lui H, Hexsel D. Treatment of solar lentigines. J Am Acad Dermatol. 2006;54(5 Suppl 2):S262–71.

20. Rosenbach A, Lee SJ, Johr RH. Treatment of medium-brown solar lentigines using an alexandrite laser designed for hair reduction. Arch Dermatol. 2002;138(4):547–8.

21. Wang CC, Sue YM, Yang CH, Chen CK. A Comparison of Q-switched alexandrite laser and intense pulsed light for the treatment of freckles and lentigines in Asian persons: a randomized, physician-blinded, split-face comparative trial. J Am Acad Dermatol. 2006;54(5):804–10.

22. Nouri K, Bowes L, Chartier T, Romagosa R, Spencer J. Combination treatment of melasma with pulsed CO2 laser followed by Q-switched alexandrite laser: a pilot study. Dermatol Surg. 1999;25(6):494–7.

23. Fabi SG, Friedmann DP, Niwa Massaki AB, Goldman MP. A Randomized, split-face clinical trial of low-fluence Q-switched neodymium-doped yttrium aluminum garnet (1,064 nm) laser versus low-fluence Q-switched alexandrite laser (755 nm) for the treatment of facial melasma. Lasers Surg Med. 2014;46(7):531–7.

24. Nisar MS, Iyer K, Brodell RT, Lloyd JR, Shin TM, Ahmad A. Minocycline-induced hyperpigmentation: comparison of 3 Q-switched lasers to reverse its effects. Clin Cosmet Investig Dermatol. 2013;6:159–62.

25. Green D, Friedman KJ. Treatment of minocycline-induced cutaneous pigmentation with the Q-switched alexandrite laser and a review of the literature. J Am Acad Dermatol. 2001;44(2 Suppl):342–7.

26. Alster TS, Gupta SN. Minocycline-induced hyperpigmentation treated with a 755-nm Q-switched alexandrite laser. Dermatol Surg. 2004;30(9):1201–4.

27. Wee SA, Dover JS. Effective treatment of psychotropic drug-induced facial hyperpigmentation with a 755-nm Q-switched alexandrite laser. Dermatol Surg. 2008;34(11):1609–12.

28. Atkin DH, Fitzpatrick RE. Laser treatment of imipramine-induced hyperpigmentation. J Am Acad Dermatol. 2000;43(1 Pt 1):77–80.

29. Majid I, Imran S. Depigmentation therapy with Q-switched Nd: YAG laser in universal vitiligo. J Cutan Aesthet Surg. 2013;6(2):93–6.

30. Tse Y, Levine VJ, McClain SA, Ashinoff R. The removal of cutaneous pigmented lesions with the Q-switched ruby laser and the Q-switched neodymium: yttrium-aluminum-garnet laser. A comparative study. J Dermatol Surg Oncol. 1994;20(12):795–800.

31. Rashid T, Hussain I, Haider M, Haroon TS. Laser therapy of freckles and lentigines with quasi-continuous, frequency-doubled, Nd:YAG (532 nm) laser in Fitzpatrick skin type IV: a 24-month follow-up. J Cosmet Laser Ther. 2002;4(3–4):81–5.

32. Kilmer SL, Wheeland RG, Goldberg DJ, Anderson RR. Treatment of epidermal pigmented lesions with the frequency-doubled Q-switched Nd:YAG laser. A controlled, single-impact, dose-response, multicenter trial. Arch Dermatol. 1994;130(12):1515–9.

33. Wilde JL, English JC 3rd, Finley EM. Minocycline-induced hyperpigmentation. Treatment with the neodymium:YAG laser. Arch Dermatol. 1997;133(11):1344–6.

34. Cho SB, Kim JS, Kim MJ. Melasma treatment in Korean women using a 1064-nm Q-switched Nd:YAG laser with low pulse energy. Clin Exp Dermatol. 2009;34(8):e847–50.

35. Kim S, Cho KH. Treatment of facial postinflammatory hyperpigmentation with facial acne in Asian patients using a Q-switched neodymium-doped yttrium aluminum garnet laser. Dermatol Surg. 2010;36(9):1374–80.

36. Parker J, Hamzavi I, editors. Q-switched Nd: YAG 1064-nm laser for the treatment of acne-Induced postinflammatory hyperpigmentation. Journal of the

American Academy of Dermatology; 2009: Mosby-Elsevier 360 Park Avenue South, New York, NY 10010–1710 USA.

37. Chan CS, Dover JS. Nd:YAG laser hair removal in Fitzpatrick skin types IV to VI. J Drugs Dermatol. 2013;12(3):366–7.

38. Shin, Y.S., et al., A comparative study of pulsed dye laser versus long pulsed Nd:YAG laser treatment in recalcitrant viral warts. J Dermatolog Treat, 2017. 28(5): p. 411–416.

39. Alshami MA. New application of the long-pulsed Nd-YAG laser as an ablative resurfacing tool for skin rejuvenation: a 7-year study. J Cosmet Dermatol. 2013;12(3):170–8.

40. Bjerring P, Christiansen K. Intense pulsed light source for treatment of small melanocytic nevi and solar lentigines. J Cutan Laser Ther. 2000;2(4):177–81.

41. Jones CE, Nouri K. Laser treatment for pigmented lesions: a review. J Cosmet Dermatol. 2006;5(1):9–13.

42. Shin J, Lee JS, Hann SK, Oh SH. Combination treatment by 10 600 nm ablative fractional carbon dioxide laser and narrowband ultraviolet B in refractory nonsegmental vitiligo: a prospective, randomized half-body comparative study. Br J Dermatol. 2012;166(3):658–61.

43. Helou J, Maatouk I, Obeid G, Moutran R, Stephan F, Tomb R. Fractional laser for vitiligo treated by 10,600 nm ablative fractional carbon dioxide laser followed by sun exposure. Lasers Surg Med. 2014;46(6):443–8.

44. Li L, Wu Y, Li L, Sun Y, Qiu L, Gao XH, et al. Triple combination treatment with fractional CO2 laser plus topical betamethasone solution and narrowband ultraviolet B for refractory vitiligo: a prospective, randomized half-body, comparative study. Dermatol Ther. 2015;28(3):131–4.

45. Vachiramon V, Chaiyabutr C, Rattanaumpawan P, Kanokrungsee S. Effects of a preceding fractional carbon dioxide laser on the outcome of combined local narrowband ultraviolet B and topical steroids in patients with vitiligo in difficult-to-treat areas. Lasers Surg Med. 2016;48(2):197–202.

46. Silpa-Archa N, Griffith JL, Williams MS, Lim HW, Hamzavi IH. Prospective comparison of recipient-site preparation with fractional carbon dioxide laser vs. dermabrasion and recipient-site dressing composition in melanocyte-keratinocyte transplantation procedure in vitiligo: a preliminary study. Br J Dermatol. 2016;174(4):895–7.

47. Arora P, Sarkar R, Garg VK, Arya L. Lasers for treatment of melasma and post-inflammatory hyperpigmentation. J Cutan Aesthet Surg. 2012;5(2):93–103.

48. Rokhsar CK, Fitzpatrick RE. The treatment of melasma with fractional photothermolysis: a pilot study. Dermatol Surg. 2005;31(12):1645–50.

49. Shin J, Kim M, Park SH, SH O. The effect of fractional carbon dioxide lasers on idiopathic guttate

hypomelanosis: a preliminary study. J Eur Acad Dermatol Venereol. 2013;27(2):e243–6.

50. Goldust M, Mohebbipour A, Mirmohammadi R. Treatment of idiopathic guttate hypomelanosis with fractional carbon dioxide lasers. J Cosmet Laser Ther. 2013. https://doi.org/10.3109/14764172.2013.803369.

51. Sklar LR, Burnett CT, Waibel JS, Moy RL, Ozog DM. Laser assisted drug delivery: a review of an evolving technology. Lasers Surg Med. 2014;46(4):249–62.

52. Tanzi EL, Lupton JR, Alster TS. Lasers in dermatology: four decades of progress. J Am Acad Dermatol. 2003;49(1):1–31. quiz -4

53. Hamzavi I, Lui H. The principles and medical applications of lasers and intense-pulsed light in dermatology. In: Lim HW, Honigsmann H, Hawk JLM, editors. Photodermatology. Basic and clinical dermatology. Boca Raton: CRC Press; 2007. p. 389–400.

54. Bianchi B, Campolmi P, Mavilia L, Danesi A, Rossi R, Cappugi P. Monochromatic excimer light (308 nm): an immunohistochemical study of cutaneous T cells and apoptosis-related molecules in psoriasis. J Eur Acad Dermatol Venereol. 2003;17(4):408–13.

55. de With A, Greulich KO. Wavelength dependence of laser-induced DNA damage in lymphocytes observed by single-cell gel electrophoresis. J Photochem Photobiol B. 1995;30(1):71–6.

56. Novak Z, Bonis B, Baltas E, Ocsovszki I, Ignacz F, Dobozy A, et al. Xenon chloride ultraviolet B laser is more effective in treating psoriasis and in inducing T cell apoptosis than narrow-band ultraviolet B. J Photochem Photobiol B. 2002;67(1):32–8.

57. Passeron T, Ostovari N, Zakaria W, Fontas E, Larrouy JC, Lacour JP, et al. Topical tacrolimus and the 308-nm excimer laser: a synergistic combination for the treatment of vitiligo. Arch Dermatol. 2004;140(9):1065–9.

58. Yu HS. Melanocyte destruction and repigmentation in vitiligo: a model for nerve cell damage and regrowth. J Biomed Sci. 2002;9(6 Pt 2):564–73.

59. Bordere AC, Lambert J, van Geel N. Current and emerging therapy for the management of vitiligo. Clin Cosmet Investig Dermatol. 2009;2:15–25.

60. Passeron T, Ortonne JP. Use of the 308-nm excimer laser for psoriasis and vitiligo. Clin Dermatol. 2006;24(1):33–42.

61. Spencer JM, Nossa R, Ajmeri J. Treatment of vitiligo with the 308-nm excimer laser: a pilot study. J Am Acad Dermatol. 2002;46(5):727–31.

62. Ostovari N, Passeron T, Zakaria W, Fontas E, Larouy JC, Blot JF, et al. Treatment of vitiligo by 308-nm excimer laser: an evaluation of variables affecting treatment response. Lasers Surg Med. 2004;35(2):152–6.

63. Hofer A, Hassan AS, Legat FJ, Kerl H, Wolf P. The efficacy of excimer laser (308 nm) for vitiligo at different body sites. J Eur Acad Dermatol Venereol. 2006;20(5):558–64.

64. Hadi S, Tinio P, Al-Ghaithi K, Al-Qari H, Al-Helalat M, Lebwohl M, et al. Treatment of vitiligo using the 308-nm excimer laser. Photomed Laser Surg. 2006;24(3):354–7.

65. Zhang XY, He YL, Dong J, JZ X, Wang J. Clinical efficacy of a 308 nm excimer laser in the treatment of vitiligo. Photodermatol Photoimmunol Photomed. 2010;26(3):138–42.

66. Taneja A, Trehan M, Taylor CR. 308-nm excimer laser for the treatment of localized vitiligo. Int J Dermatol. 2003;42(8):658–62.

67. Hong SB, Park HH, Lee MH. Short-term effects of 308-nm xenon-chloride excimer laser and narrow-band ultraviolet B in the treatment of vitiligo: a comparative study. J Korean Med Sci. 2005;20(2):273–8.

68. Do JE, Shin JY, Kim D-Y, Hann S-K, Oh SH. The effect of 308 nm excimer laser on segmental vitiligo: a retrospective study of 80 patients with segmental vitiligo. Photodermatol Photoimmunol Photomed. 2011;27(3):147–51.

69. Alhowaish AK, Dietrich N, Onder M, Fritz K. Effectiveness of a 308-nm excimer laser in treatment of vitiligo: a review. Lasers Med Sci. 2013;28(3):1035–41.

70. Greve B, Raulin C, Fischer E. Excimer laser treatment of vitiligo – critical retrospective assessment of own results and literature overview. J Dtsch Dermatol Ges. 2006;4(1):32–40.

71. Hofer A, Hassan AS, Legat FJ, Kerl H, Wolf P. Optimal weekly frequency of 308-nm excimer laser treatment in vitiligo patients. Br J Dermatol. 2005;152(5):981–5.

72. Sassi F, Cazzaniga S, Tessari G, Chatenoud L, Reseghetti A, Marchesi L, et al. Randomized controlled trial comparing the effectiveness of 308-nm excimer laser alone or in combination with topical hydrocortisone 17-butyrate cream in the treatment of vitiligo of the face and neck. Br J Dermatol. 2008;159(5):1186–91.

73. Kawalek AZ, Spencer JM, Phelps RG. Combined excimer laser and topical tacrolimus for the treatment of vitiligo: a pilot study. Dermatol Surg. 2004;30(2 Pt 1):130–5.

74. Park OJ, Park GH, Choi JR, Jung HJ, ES O, Choi JH, et al. A combination of excimer laser treatment and topical tacrolimus is more effective in treating vitiligo than either therapy alone for the initial 6 months, but not thereafter. Clin Exp Dermatol. 2016;41(3):236–41.

75. Bae JM, Yoo HJ, Kim H, Lee JH, Kim GM. Combination therapy with 308-nm excimer laser, topical tacrolimus, and short-term systemic corticosteroids for segmental vitiligo: a retrospective study of 159 patients. J Am Acad Dermatol. 2015;73(1):76–82.

76. Jang YH, Jung SE, Shin J, Kang HY. Triple combination of systemic corticosteroids, excimer laser, and topical tacrolimus in the treatment of recently developed localized vitiligo. Ann Dermatol. 2015;27(1):104–7.

77. Goldinger SM, Dummer R, Schmid P, Burg G, Seifert B, Lauchli S. Combination of 308-nm xenon chloride excimer laser and topical calcipotriol in vitiligo. J Eur Acad Dermatol Venereol. 2007;21(4):504–8.

78. SH O, Kim T, Jee H, Do JE, Lee JH. Combination treatment of non-segmental vitiligo with a 308-nm xenon chloride excimer laser and topical high-concentration tacalcitol: a prospective, single-blinded, paired, comparative study. J Am Acad Dermatol. 2011;65(2):428–30.

79. Lu-yan T, Wen-wen F, Lei-hong X, Yi J, Zhi-zhong Z. Topical tacalcitol and 308-nm monochromatic excimer light: a synergistic combination for the treatment of vitiligo. Photodermatol Photoimmunol Photomed. 2006;22(6):310–4.

80. Bae JM, Hong BY, Lee JH, Lee JH, Kim GM. The efficacy of 308-nm excimer laser/light (EL) and topical agent combination therapy versus EL monotherapy for vitiligo: a systematic review and meta-analysis of randomized controlled trials (RCTs). J Am Acad Dermatol. 2016;74(5):907–15.

81. Shin S, Hann SK, Combination OSH. Treatment with excimer laser and narrowband UVB light in vitiligo patients. Photodermatol Photoimmunol Photomed. 2016;32(1):28–33.

82. Al-Mutairi N, Manchanda Y, Al-Doukhi A, Al-Haddad A. Long-term results of split-skin grafting in combination with excimer laser for stable vitiligo. Dermatol Surg. 2010;36(4):499–505.

83. Tsuchiyama K, Watabe A, Sadayasu A, Onodera N, Kimura Y, Aiba S. Successful treatment of segmental vitiligo in children with the combination of 1-mm minigrafts and phototherapy. Dermatology. 2016;232(2):237–41.

84. Ebadi A, Rad MM, Nazari S, Fesharaki RJ, Ghalamkarpour F, Younespour S. The additive effect of excimer laser on non-cultured melanocyte-keratinocyte transplantation for the treatment of vitiligo: a clinical trial in an Iranian population. J Eur Acad Dermatol Venereol. 2015;29(4):745–51.

85. Soliman M, Samy NA, Abo Eittah M, Hegazy M. Comparative study between excimer light and topical antioxidant versus excimer light alone for treatment of vitiligo. J Cosmet Laser Ther. 2016;18(1):7–11.

86. Lan CC, HS Y, JH L, CS W, Lai HC. Irradiance, but not fluence, plays a crucial role in UVB-induced immature pigment cell development: new insights for efficient UVB phototherapy. Pigment Cell Melanoma Res. 2013;26(3):367–76.

87. Njoo MD, Spuls PI, Bos JD, Westerhof W, Bossuyt PM. Nonsurgical repigmentation therapies in vitiligo. Meta-analysis of the literature. Arch Dermatol. 1998;134(12):1532–40.

88. Linthorst Homan MW, Spuls PI, Nieuweboer-Krobotova L, de Korte J, Sprangers MA, Bos JD, et al. A randomized comparison of excimer laser versus narrow-band ultraviolet B phototherapy after punch grafting in stable vitiligo patients. J Eur Acad Dermatol Venereol. 2012;26(6):690–5.

89. Sun Y, Wu Y, Xiao B, Li L, Li L, Chen HD, et al. Treatment of 308-nm excimer laser on vitiligo: a systemic review of randomized controlled trials. J Dermatolog Treat. 2015;26(4):347–53.

90. Le Duff F, Fontas E, Giacchero D, Sillard L, Lacour JP, Ortonne JP, et al. 308-nm excimer lamp vs. 308-nm excimer laser for treating vitiligo: a randomized study. Br J Dermatol. 2010;163(1):188–92.

91. Omi T, Numano K. The role of the CO2 laser and fractional CO2 laser in dermatology. Laser Ther. 2014;23(1):49–60.

92. Geronemus RG. Fractional photothermolysis: current and future applications. Lasers Surg Med. 2006;38(3):169–76.

93. Manstein D, Herron GS, Sink RK, Tanner H, Anderson RR. Fractional photothermolysis: a new concept for cutaneous remodeling using microscopic patterns of thermal injury. Lasers Surg Med. 2004;34(5):426–38.

94. Shin MK, Jeong KH, IH O, Choe BK, Lee MH. Clinical features of idiopathic guttate hypomelanosis in 646 subjects and association with other aspects of photoaging. Int J Dermatol. 2011;50(7):798–805.

95. Sherling M, Friedman PM, Adrian R, Burns AJ, Conn H, Fitzpatrick R, et al. Consensus recommendations on the use of an erbium-doped 1,550-nm fractionated laser and its applications in dermatologic laser surgery. Dermatol Surg. 2010;36(4):461–9.

96. Taylor CR, Anderson RR. Ineffective treatment of refractory melasma and postinflammatory hyperpigmentation by Q-switched ruby laser. J Dermatol Surg Oncol. 1994;20(9):592–7.

97. Polla LL, Margolis RJ, Dover JS, Whitaker D, Murphy GF, Jacques SL, et al. Melanosomes are a primary target of Q-switched ruby laser irradiation in guinea pig skin. J Invest Dermatol. 1987;89(3):281–6.

98. Taneja A. Treatment of vitiligo. J Dermatolog Treat. 2002;13(1):19–25.

99. Njoo MD, Vodegel RM, Westerhof W. Depigmentation therapy in vitiligo universalis with topical 4-methoxyphenol and the Q-switched ruby laser. J Am Acad Dermatol. 2000;42(5 Pt 1): 760–9.

100. AlGhamdi KM, Kumar A. Depigmentation therapies for normal skin in vitiligo universalis. J Eur Acad Dermatol Venereol. 2011;25(7):749–57.

101. Kim YJ, Chung BS, Choi KC. Depigmentation therapy with Q-switched ruby laser after tanning in vitiligo universalis. Dermatol Surg. 2001;27(11): 969–70.

102. Komen L, Zweitbrock L, Burger SJ, van der Veen JP, de Rie MA, Wolkerstorfer A. Q-switched laser depigmentation in vitiligo, most effective in active disease. Br J Dermatol. 2013;169(6):1246–51.

103. Lowe NJ, Wieder JM, Sawcer D, Burrows P, Chalet M. Nevus of Ota: treatment with high energy fluences of the Q-switched ruby laser. J Am Acad Dermatol. 1993;29(6):997–1001.

104. Goldberg DJ. Laser treatment of pigmented lesions. Dermatol Clin. 1997;15(3):397–407.

105. Watanabe S, Takahashi H. Treatment of nevus of Ota with the Q-switched ruby laser. N Engl J Med. 1994;331(26):1745–50.

106. Kono T, Nozaki M, Chan HH, Mikashima Y. A Retrospective study looking at the long-term complications of Q-switched ruby laser in the treatment of nevus of Ota. Lasers Surg Med. 2001;29(2):156–9.

107. Ueda S, Isoda M, Imayama S. Response of naevus of Ota to Q-switched ruby laser treatment according to lesion colour. Br J Dermatol. 2000;142(1):77–83.

108. Goldberg DJ. Benign pigmented lesions of the skin. Treatment with the Q-switched ruby laser. J Dermatol Surg Oncol. 1993;19(4):376–9.

109. Kopera D, Hohenleutner U. Ruby laser treatment of melasma and postinflammatory hyperpigmentation. Dermatol Surg. 1995;21(11):994.

110. Stratigos AJ, Dover JS, Arndt KA. Laser treatment of pigmented lesions--2000: how far have we gone? Arch Dermatol. 2000;136(7):915–21.

111. Niwa Massaki AB, Eimpunth S, Fabi SG, Guiha I, Groff W, Fitzpatrick R. Treatment of melasma with the 1,927-nm fractional thulium fiber laser: a retrospective analysis of 20 cases with long-term follow-up. Lasers Surg Med. 2013;45(2):95–101.

112. Hilton S, Heise H, Buhren BA, Schrumpf H, Bolke E, Gerber PA. Treatment of melasma in Caucasian patients using a novel 694-nm Q-switched ruby fractional laser. Eur J Med Res. 2013;18:43.

113. Jang WS, Lee CK, Kim BJ, Kim MN. Efficacy of 694-nm Q-switched ruby fractional laser treatment of melasma in female Korean patients. Dermatol Surg. 2011;37(8):1133–40.

114. Tafazzoli A, Rostan EF, Goldman MP. Q-switched ruby laser treatment for postsclerotherapy hyperpigmentation. Dermatol Surg. 2000;26(7):653–6.

115. Imhof L, Dummer R, Dreier J, Kolm I, Barysch MJA. Prospective trial comparing Q-switched ruby laser and a triple combination skin-lightening cream in the treatment of solar lentigines. Dermatol Surg. 2016;42(7):853–7.

116. Negishi K, Akita H, Tanaka S, Yokoyama Y, Wakamatsu S, Matsunaga K. Comparative study of treatment efficacy and the incidence of post-inflammatory hyperpigmentation with different degrees of irradiation using two different quality-switched lasers for removing solar lentigines on Asian skin. J Eur Acad Dermatol Venereol. 2013;27(3):307–12.

117. Kono T, Manstein D, Chan HH, Nozaki M, Anderson RR. Q-switched ruby versus long-pulsed dye laser delivered with compression for treatment of facial lentigines in Asians. Lasers Surg Med. 2006;38(2):94–7.

118. Sicari MC, Lebwohl M, Baral J, Wexler P, Gordon RE, Phelps RG. Photoinduced dermal pigmentation in patients taking tricyclic antidepressants: histology, electron microscopy, and energy dispersive spectroscopy. J Am Acad Dermatol. 1999;40 (2 Pt 2):290–3.

119. Ming ME, Bhawan J, Stefanato CM, McCalmont TH, Cohen LM. Imipramine-induced hyperpigmentation: four cases and a review of the literature. J Am Acad Dermatol. 1999;40(2 Pt 1):159–66.

120. Metelitsa AI, Nguyen GK, Lin AN. Imipramine-induced facial pigmentation: case report and literature review. J Cutan Med Surg. 2005;9(6):341–5.

121. Dereure O. Drug-induced skin pigmentation. Epidemiology, diagnosis and treatment. Am J Clin Dermatol. 2001;2(4):253–62.

122. Chan HHL, King WWK, Chan ESY, Mok CO, Ho WS, Van Krevel C, et al. vivo trial comparing patients' tolerance of Q-switched Alexandrite (QS Alex) and Q-switched neodymium:yttrium-aluminum-garnet (QS Nd:YAG) lasers in the treatment of nevus of Ota. Lasers Surg Med. 1999;24(1):24–8.

123. Bukvic Mokos Z, Lipozencic J, Ceovic R, Stulhofer Buzina D, Kostovic K. Laser therapy of pigmented lesions: pro and contra. Acta Dermatovenerol Croat. 2010;18(3):185–9.

124. Rao J, Fitzpatrick RE. Use of the Q-switched 755-nm alexandrite laser to treat recalcitrant pigment after depigmentation therapy for vitiligo. Dermatol Surg. 2004;30(7):1043–5.

125. Kang W, Lee E, Choi GS. Treatment of Ota's nevus by Q-switched alexandrite laser : therapeutic outcome in relation to clinical and histopathological findings. Eur J Dermatol. 1999;9(8):639–43.

126. Vano-Galvan S, Matarredona JA, Harto A, Escudero A, Pascual JC, Jaen P. Treatment of light-coloured solar lentigines with cryotherapy plus alexandrite laser. J Eur Acad Dermatol Venereol. 2009;23(7):850–2.

127. Trafeli JP, Kwan JM, Meehan KJ, Domankevitz Y, Gilbert S, Malomo K, et al. Use of a long-pulse alexandrite laser in the treatment of superficial pigmented lesions. Dermatol Surg. 2007;33(12):1477–82.

128. Angsuwarangsee S, Polnikorn N. Combined ultrapulse CO2 laser and Q-switched alexandrite laser compared with Q-switched alexandrite laser alone for refractory melasma: split-face design. Dermatol Surg. 2003;29(1):59–64.

129. Spicer MS, Goldberg DJ. Lasers in dermatology. J Am Acad Dermatol. 1996;34(1):1–25. quiz 6-8

130. Polnikorn N. Treatment of refractory dermal melasma with the MedLite C6 Q-switched Nd:YAG laser: two case reports. J Cosmet Laser Ther. 2008;10(3):167–73.

131. Lanigan SW. Failure of Q-switched Nd/YAG laser to repigment vitiligo. Clin Exp Dermatol. 1996;21(3):245–6.

132. Vachiramon V, Panmanee W, Techapichetvanich T, Chanprapaph K. Comparison of Q-switched Nd:YAG laser and fractional carbon dioxide laser for the treatment of solar lentigines in Asians. Lasers Surg Med. 2016;48(4):354–9.

133. Noh TK, Chung BY, Yeo UC, Chang S, Lee MW, Chang SE. Q-switched 660-nm versus 532-nm Nd:YAG laser for the treatment for facial lentigines in Asian patients: a prospective, randomized, double-blinded, split-face comparison pilot study. Dermatol Surg. 2015;41(12):1389–95.

134. Todd MM, Rallis TM, Gerwels JW, Hata TR. A Comparison of 3 lasers and liquid nitrogen in the treatment of solar lentigines: a randomized, controlled, comparative trial. Arch Dermatol. 2000;136(7):841–6.

135. Chan HH, Fung WK, Ying SY, Kono T. An in vivo trial comparing the use of different types of 532 nm Nd:YAG lasers in the treatment of facial lentigines in oriental patients. Dermatol Surg. 2000;26(8):743–9.

136. Li YT, Yang KC. Comparison of the frequency-doubled Q-switched Nd:YAG laser and 35% trichloroacetic acid for the treatment of face lentigines. Dermatol Surg. 1999;25(3):202–4.

137. Schmults CD, Phelps R, Goldberg DJ. Nonablative facial remodeling: erythema reduction and histologic evidence of new collagen formation using a 300-microsecond 1064-nm Nd:YAG laser. Arch Dermatol. 2004;140(11):1373–6.

138. Kim EH, Kim YC, Lee ES, Kang HY. The vascular characteristics of melasma. J Dermatol Sci. 2007;46(2):111–6.

139. Rodrigues M, Pandya AG. Melasma: clinical diagnosis and management options. Australas J Dermatol. 2015;56(3):151–63.

140. Zhou X, Gold MH, Lu Z, Li Y. Efficacy and safety of Q-switched 1,064-nm neodymium-doped yttrium aluminum garnet laser treatment of melasma. Dermatol Surg. 2011;37(7):962–70.

141. Chan NP, Ho SG, Shek SY, Yeung CK, Chan HHA. Case series of facial depigmentation associated with low fluence Q-switched 1,064 nm Nd:YAG laser for skin rejuvenation and melasma. Lasers Surg Med. 2010;42(8):712–9.

142. Hofbauer Parra CA, Careta MF, Valente NY, de Sanches Osorio NE, Torezan LA. Clinical and histopathologic assessment of facial melasma after low-fluence Q-switched neodymium-doped yttrium aluminium garnet laser. Dermatol Surg. 2016;42(4):507–12.

143. Kim MJ, Kim JS, Cho SB. Punctate leucoderma after melasma treatment using 1064-nm Q-switched Nd:YAG laser with low pulse energy. J Eur Acad Dermatol Venereol. 2009;23(8):960–2.

144. Wattanakrai P, Mornchan R, Eimpunth S. Low-fluence Q-switched neodymium-doped yttrium aluminum garnet (1,064 nm) laser for the treatment of facial melasma in Asians. Dermatol Surg. 2010;36(1):76–87.

145. Anderson RR, Margolis RJ, Watenabe S, Flotte T, Hruza GJ, Dover JS. Selective photothermolysis of cutaneous pigmentation by Q-switched Nd: YAG laser pulses at 1064, 532, and 355 nm. J Invest Dermatol. 1989;93(1):28–32.

146. Choi M, Choi JW, Lee SY, Choi SY, Park HJ, Park KC, et al. Low-dose 1064-nm Q-switched Nd:YAG laser for the treatment of melasma. J Dermatolog Treat. 2010;21(4):224–8.

147. Jeong SY, Shin JB, Yeo UC, Kim WS, Kim IH. Low-fluence Q-switched neodymium-doped yttrium aluminum garnet laser for melasma with pre- or post-treatment triple combination cream. Dermatol Surg. 2010;36(6):909–18.

148. Na SY, Cho S, Lee JH. Intense pulsed light and low-fluence Q-switched Nd:YAG laser treatment in melasma patients. Ann Dermatol. 2012;24(3):267–73.

149. Yun WJ, Moon HR, Lee MW, Choi JH, Chang SE. Combination treatment of low-fluence 1,064-nm Q-switched Nd:YAG laser with novel intense pulse light in Korean melasma patients: a prospective, randomized, controlled trial. Dermatol Surg. 2014;40(8):842–50.

150. Kim HS, Jung HD, Kim HO, Lee JY, Park YM. Punctate leucoderma after low-fluence 1,064-nm quality-switched neodymium-doped yttrium aluminum garnet laser therapy successfully managed using a 308-nm excimer laser. Dermatol Surg. 2012;38(5):821–3.

151. Torok HM. A Comprehensive review of the long-term and short-term treatment of melasma with a triple combination cream. Am J Clin Dermatol. 2006;7(4):223–30.

152. Kauvar AN. Successful treatment of melasma using a combination of microdermabrasion and Q-switched Nd:YAG lasers. Lasers Surg Med. 2012;44(2):117–24.

153. Cunha PR, Pinto CA, Mattos CB, Cabrini DP, Tolosa JL. New insight in the treatment of refractory melasma: laser Q-switched Nd: YAG non-ablative fractionated followed by intense pulsed light. Dermatol Ther. 2015;28(5):296–9.

154. Ball Arefiev KL, Hantash BM. Advances in the treatment of melasma: a review of the recent literature. Dermatol Surg. 2012;38(7 Pt 1):971–84.

155. Choi CP, Yim SM, Seo SH, Ahn HH, Kye YC, Choi JE. Retreatment using a dual mode of low-fluence Q-switched and long-pulse Nd:YAG laser in patients with melasma aggravation after previous therapy. J Cosmet Laser Ther. 2015;17(3):129–34.

156. Greve, B., M.P. Schonermark, and C. Raulin, Minocycline-induced hyperpigmentation: treatment with the Qswitched Nd:YAG laser. Lasers Surg Med, 1998. 22(4): p. 223–7.

157. Agbai ONHI, Jagdeo J. Laser treatments for post-inflammatory hyperpigmentation: a systematic review. JAMA Dermatol. (Accepted).

158. Sheth VM, Pandya AG. Melasma: a comprehensive update: part II. J Am Acad Dermatol. 2011;65(4):699–714. quiz 5

Phototherapy in Pigmentary Disorders

16

Thiam Seng Colin Theng
and Eugene Sern-Ting Tan

Introduction

Phototherapy has its origins since 3000 BC
when the Egyptians applied the extracts of the
Ammi majus Linnaeus plant found along the
banks of Nile to treat vitiligo. This was the
start of photochemotherapy. It was only in
1948 that el Mofty first used purified
8-methoxypsoralen for the treatment of vitiligo. Since then, PUVA, both topical and oral,
has been the mainstay of treatment for vitiligo
for many years.

Over the years, with advances in technology,
newer phototherapy modalities like the NBUVB
and excimer laser and lamp have been introduced. These treatments have in recent years
increasingly become the preferred treatment
modality, due to their ease of administration and
lesser side effects. In this chapter, we will be
looking at phototherapy, in particular PUVA,
NBUVB and excimer laser and lamp for the
treatment of pigmentary disorders, with a focus
on vitiligo, which is the most common pigmentary problem treated with phototherapy.

PUVA

PUVA is a form of photochemotherapy that
involves the activation of a photosensitizer by UVA
light (320–400 nm) irradiation. The most commonly used photosensitizer is 8-methoxypsoralen
(8-MOP). Other photosensitizers that are used
include 4,5,8-trimethylpsoralen (trioxsalen, TMP),
which is a synthetic drug, and 5-methoxypsoralen
(5-MOP), both of which have less phototoxic side
effects than 8-MOP. PUVA treatment has proven to
be effective particularly in vitiligo and psoriasis.

Mechanism of Action of PUVA

Psoralen intercalates between the DNA base pairs
and, when activated by UVA, forms cross links
with the DNA, resulting in its anti-angiogenic,
anti-proliferative and immunosuppressive effects
[1]. How PUVA therapy works in vitiligo repigmentation is still uncertain; however, psoralens
are known to stimulate melanogenesis. When psoralens bind to DNA in the melanocytes, it stimulates the proliferation of the melanocytes and
increases the melanosome number and transfer to
keratinocytes [2]. Hepatocyte growth factor and

T. S. Colin Theng (✉)
The Skin Specialists & Medical Clinic, Mount
Alvernia Medical D, Singapore, Singapore
e-mail: colintheng@theskinspecialists.com.sg

E. S. Tan
Department of Dermatology, National Skin Centre,
Singapore, Singapore
e-mail: eugenetan@nsc.com.sg

© Springer International Publishing AG, part of Springer Nature 2018
P. Kumarasinghe (ed.), *Pigmentary Skin Disorders*, Updates in Clinical Dermatology,
https://doi.org/10.1007/978-3-319-70419-7_16

basic fibroblast growth factors have also been shown to be increased by PUVA treatment and may play a role in the regrowth and migration of follicular melanocytes in the basal layer of the skin [3].

Administration of PUVA

In systemic PUVA treatment, the 8-MOP is taken orally at a dose of 0.6 mg/kg body weight. This is usually taken 2 h before the irradiation, and this timing should be kept consistent to ensure consistent levels of the psoralen in the skin. The meal taken should also be consistent as the amount and type of food can also affect the absorption of the psoralen. During the day of the treatment, the patients are advised to avoid sun exposure for the next 12–24 h as the patient may still be photosensitive to sunlight. Protective eyewear should also be worn on the day of the treatment. Treatments are usually given two to three times a week, with at least a day's interval between treatments. It is important to realize that the peak erythema in PUVA occurs 48–96 h later, and consecutive-day treatments may increase the risk of burns [4].

Oral psoralen can cause nausea in some individuals. Other photosensitizers like 5-MOP and TMP, though less commonly used, are less erythemogenic compared with 8-MOP and cause less gastrointestinal side effects. The genital area is often shielded during treatment as the risk of photocarcinogenesis is believed to be higher here with PUVA therapy.

Efficacy of PUVA for Vitiligo

Phototherapy is often used to treat vitiligo after failure of topical therapies and also in cases of extensive vitiligo where topical treatment is tedious and impractical. PUVA therapy has been the mainstay of vitiligo treatment for many years, and there are several studies which have confirmed its efficacy in treating vitiligo.

In a 10-year retrospective study of 97 patients with vitiligo undergoing PUVA treatment, 8 patients had complete repigmentation, 59 had moderate to extensive response and 30 had poor

or no response. Patients who retained their pigmentation for 2 years were less likely to relapse [5]. The younger the age of starting the treatment, the better the pigmentation retained compared to those starting at an older age.

Tallab et al. showed in his retrospective study of 32 patients undergoing PUVA treatment that 59% of patients had good improvement with PUVA. The face, trunk, arms and legs showed good response, but peri-orificial and acral areas had the poorest response [6].

In a comparative prospective study of oral PUVA versus oral PUVASol for the treatment of generalized vitiligo, 35 patients were recruited, 18 in the oral PUVA group and 17 in oral PUVASol group. At the end of 36 weeks, the mean percentage improvement in vitiligo in the oral PUVA group was 46.4% vs 26.1% in the oral PUVASol group. However, more phototoxic side effects were noted in the oral PUVA group [7].

Acral sites are known to respond poorly to photochemotherapy. It has been postulated that acral areas have lower hair follicle densities, lower melanocyte densities and stem cell reservoirs and therefore decreased repigmentation rates [8].

El Mofty et al. had carried out a prospective, randomized controlled study comparing BB UVA alone (without psoralen) with oral PUVA treatment in the treatment of vitiligo [9]. While the PUVA patients had faster improvement, at the end of study (5 months, 60 treatments), the BB UVA group treated at a dose of 15 mJ/cm^2 had similar efficacy compared with the PUVA group, suggesting that UVA alone may be effective in cases where oral psoralens are contraindicated.

Overall, oral PUVA is effective for vitiligo with the face, trunk and limbs showing the best response.

PUVASol

PUVASol is the treatment with psoralen and UVA obtained from natural sunlight. This can be used in areas where phototherapy facilities are not available or when there is difficulty in getting to the phototherapy facility. The main difficulty in using PUVASol is the variability of the UVA intensity in natural sunlight as it can be affected by the time of the day, atmospheric conditions, seasonal variation and latitude. There is little published data on the efficacy of PUVASol treatment.

In a randomized right-left comparison study of PUVASol vs PUVASol with topical calcipotriol in the treatment of vitiligo, treatment with PUVASol alone achieved marked or complete improvement in the vitiligo in 35% of the patients compared with 70% in the PUVASol- and calcipotriol-treated group, showing the increased efficacy with the combination therapy [10].

In a retrospective analysis of the efficacy of different modalities of vitiligo treatment, Handa et al. reported that with PUVASol treatment, 48 (84%) out of 57 patients had moderate to excellent repigmentation [11].

PUVASol, while an effective treatment, is difficult to deliver consistently due to variability in ambient light intensity. Therefore, in places where phototherapy facilities are readily available, PUVASol should not be encouraged.

Topical PUVA

Topical PUVA is a form of localized phototherapy where the psoralen is applied topically to the affected area with subsequent irradiation with UVA (Fig. 16.1). As it is a targeted form of phototherapy, it limits the side effects to the treated areas only, and it is therefore safer than systemic PUVA where the side effects are more generalized. However, the risk of phototoxicity with topical PUVA is higher, and therefore care should be taken when delivering the treatment.

The psoralen is available as a cream or lotion. It is applied to the affected area and left on for about 20 min before the irradiation [12]. The concentration of the psoralen applied is usually between 0.01% and 0.1%. The treatment is given one to three times a week. Topical khellin and topical TMP have also been used [13]. There may be significant hyperpigmentation on the margins

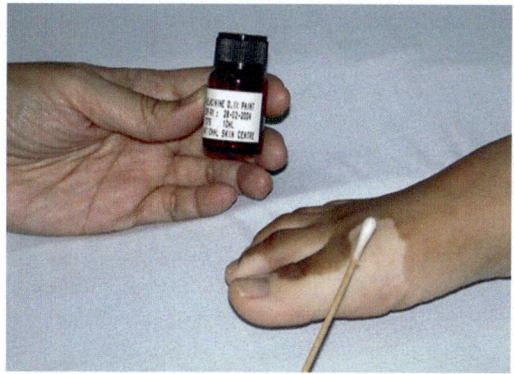

Fig. 16.1 Topical PUVA for vitiligo (Source: National Skin Centre, Singapore)

of the treated lesions which may make it difficult to continue with the treatment although this can resolved with time upon discontinuation of treatment.

Khellin + UVA (KUVA)

Oral khellin has been reported to be effective in the treatment of vitiligo. Khellin is a furanochromone and a photosensitizer. In a small study of 28 patients, 25 were treated with oral KUVA 3 times a week, and 3 patients were treated with topical khellin, with treatment given 3 times a week [14]. More than 70% repigmentation was achieved in 41% of patients who had received between 100 and 200 treatments. Mild elevation of liver enzymes was noted in seven patients, and the treatment was discontinued. Skin phototoxicity was not observed. However, there have been reports of marked elevation of transaminases with KUVA treatment [15]. The hepatotoxic effects of khellin may limit its use systemically. Topical khellin has also been shown to be effective in vitiligo [13]. In a study by Vlakova et al. comparing topical KUVA to systemic PUVA treatment, topical KUVA needed a longer duration and higher doses of UVA to achieve a comparable degree of repigmentation as systemic PUVA [13].

Side Effects of PUVA Treatment

PUVA treatment is associated with a number of side effects, both short term and long term. Nausea associated with oral psoralens, the need for sun avoidance on the day of treatment, cataract formation and increased risk of skin cancer are the main limiting factors in the use of PUVA compared to the newer NBUVB phototherapy. The side effects of PUVA treatment include:

Short-term side effects:

1. Nausea and vomiting
2. Sunburn reaction – erythema and blistering
3. Skin tanning
4. Herpes simplex virus reactivation
5. Photo-onycholysis [16] and melanonychia [17]
6. Central nervous system side effects – dizziness, headaches, depression and hyperactivity [18]

Long-term side effects:

1. Photoageing
2. Cataract formation
3. Skin malignancies, the risk of non-melanoma skin cancers (NMSC) is associated with high cumulative exposure of PUVA, especially squamous cell carcinoma. The risk of skin cancers persists even after discontinuation of the treatment [19, 20]. The risk of non-melanoma skin cancer with PUVA was also found to be increased in the PUVA cohort study by Stern et al. [21]

Photocarcinogenicity remains the main concern with long-term PUVA therapy, limiting its use particularly in patients with lighter skin types. The risk is much higher in skin type I–III individuals, and a lifetime limit of 200–250 treatments is generally advised.

Narrowband Ultraviolet B

Narrowband ultraviolet B (NB-UVB) represents a specific narrow segment of the ultraviolet light spectrum with a wavelength of 311 ± 2 nm. Prior to the introduction of NB-UVB, broadband ultraviolet B (BB-UVB) which has a wavelength range of 280–320 nm has been used as early as the 1920s for the treatment of psoriasis, notably in combination with crude coal tar as part of the Goeckerman regimen [22].

The therapeutic use of NB-UVB phototherapy first came to prominence in 1977 when Fischer discovered that ultraviolet light at a wavelength of 313 nm achieved effective clearance of plaque psoriasis and had the advantage of being less erythemogenic at higher doses compared to BB-UVB [23]. This heralded the development of the TL-01 fluorescent lamp (Philips, Eindhoven, the Netherlands) which is today a widely used light source for NB-UVB (Fig. 16.2). Over the years, NB-UVB phototherapy has established itself as a relatively safe and cost-effective therapeutic modality for a wide range of UVB-responsive dermatoses [24]. In the field of pigmentary disorders, NB-UVB phototherapy occupies an important position in the therapeutic armamentarium of vitiligo (Fig. 16.3).

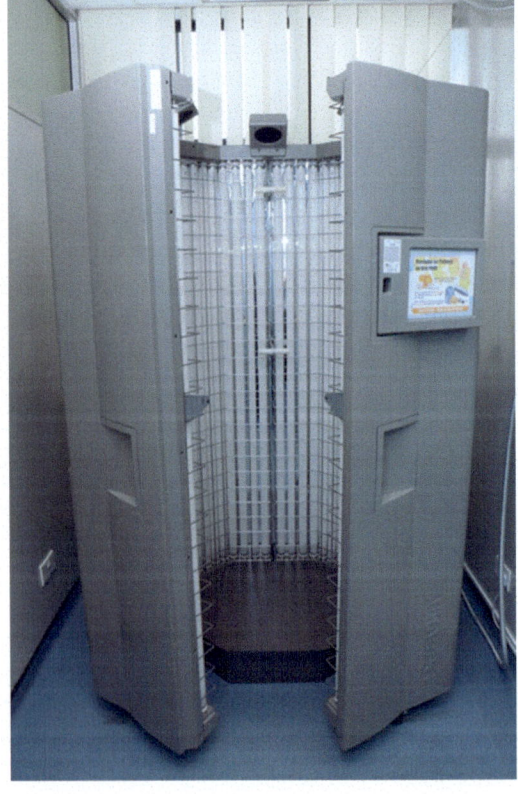

Fig. 16.2 Narrowband UVB cabin (Daavlin, USA)

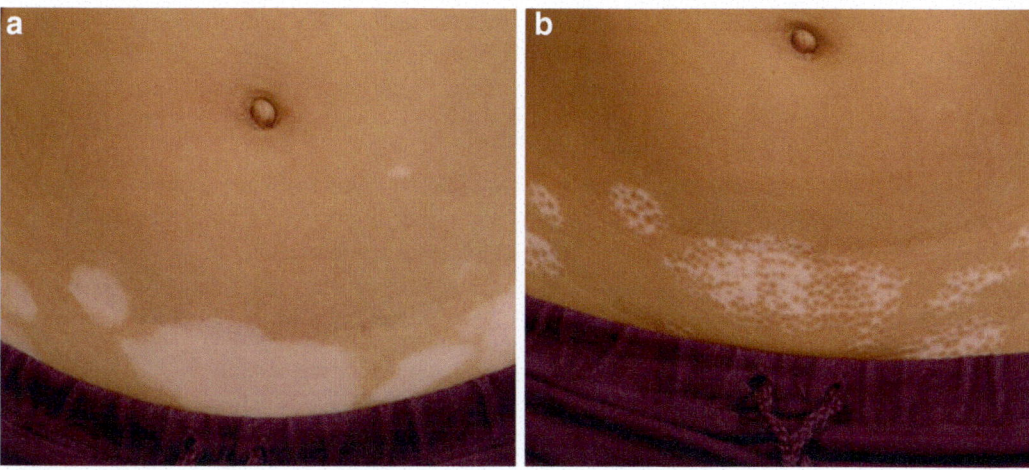

Fig. 16.3 (**a**) Baseline vitiligo on lower abdomen. (**b**) Follicular repigmentation after 24 sessions of NBUVB twice a week (Source: National Skin Centre, Singapore)

Mechanism of Action

The depth of penetration of ultraviolet light into the skin is influenced by factors such as its wavelength and the extent of reflection or absorption in the skin. NB-UVB traverses through the epidermis to the depth of the stratum basale, where it is absorbed by epidermal chromophores such as nucleic acids, urocanic acid, keratin and melanin [25].

NB-UVB phototherapy induces repigmentation in vitiligo via three main mechanisms. Firstly, it exerts immunosuppressive effects by depleting the number of Langerhans cells in the epidermis and impairing their antigen presentation and migration to draining lymph nodes [26]. Depletion of epidermal Langerhans cells has been observed in repigmentation of vitiligo, and this may be explained by their possible inhibitory effect on epidermal melanocyte proliferation [27]. Another immunosuppressive effect of NB-UVB can be seen in the inhibition of autoreactive CD4 and CD8 T-lymphocytes that are implicated in autoimmune melanocyte destruction, via induction of T-cell apoptosis and upregulation of interleukin-10 in the epidermis to induce regulatory T-cells [26].

Secondly, it has been demonstrated that ultraviolet radiation stimulates the cellular division, proliferation and migration of inactive melano-cytes from the outer root sheaths of hair follicles to the surrounding epidermis, to form clinically visible repigmenting islands [28, 29].

Thirdly, NB-UVB upregulates the expression of tyrosinase, the rate-limiting enzyme required for melanin synthesis [30].

NB-UVB for Vitiligo

Adult Vitiligo

The initial use of NB-UVB phototherapy for vitiligo was reported by Westerhof and Nieuweboer-Krobotova in 1997, who demonstrated that NB-UVB was superior to topical psoralen with ultraviolet A (PUVA) in achieving repigmentation [31]. Since then, several studies have established the therapeutic efficacy of NB-UVB in vitiligo. A retrospective review showed that five of seven vitiligo patients treated with NB-UVB thrice weekly achieved over 75% repigmentation fairly rapidly, with a mean of 19 treatments [32]. In 2004, a prospective randomized controlled left-right comparison trial evaluated 22 patients with symmetrically distributed vitiligo treated with NB-UVB thrice weekly to one-half of the body for either 60 treatments or 6 months, while their untreated contralateral half served as a control. The treated side achieved 43% repigmentation, markedly greater than the 3% repigmentation observed at the untreated side [33]. In another retrospective analysis of 60 Asian patients with predominantly generalized vitiligo recalcitrant to either topical corticosteroids or topical PUVA, who were then treated with NB-UVB twice weekly till maximal repigmentation, 42% of the cohort achieved over 50% repigmentation [34].

Paediatric Vitiligo

NB-UVB phototherapy is also effective and safe in paediatric vitiligo. In an open-label study of 51 children with generalized vitiligo who underwent twice weekly NB-UVB phototherapy for up to 1 year, over 75% overall repigmentation was achieved in approximately half the subjects, while stabilization of vitiligo was seen in 80%. There was significant improvement in quality of life which correlated with repigmentation, and adverse effects were minor and transient [35]. Another study evaluated 26 children with generalized vitiligo treated with NB-UVB phototherapy thrice weekly up to a maximum period of 1 year. The excellent efficacy of NB-UVB was evidenced by 75% of subjects achieving marked to complete repigmentation, and another 20% attaining mild to moderate repigmentation. A mean of 34 treatment sessions was required to achieve 50% repigmentation. No major adverse effects were reported [36]. While NB-UVB is useful for childhood vitiligo, its main limitation here is that it can only be used in children from a certain age who are mature enough to cooperate with the requirement of standing still in the phototherapy cabin for a few minutes.

NB-UVB Versus PUVA

In comparative studies, it has been shown that NB-UVB phototherapy had similar efficacy with fewer adverse effects compared to topical PUVA in the treatment of generalized vitiligo [31]. A randomized double-blind trial of 56 patients with non-segmental vitiligo found NB-UVB superior to oral PUVA, with two-thirds of patients achieving over 50% repigmentation in the NB-UVB group compared to one-third of patients in the PUVA group. Furthermore, there was excellent colour match of repigmented skin in all patients in the NB-UVB group, compared to 44% of

patients in the PUVA group [37]. Similarly, in childhood vitiligo, NB-UVB has demonstrated better overall repigmentation rates and safety profile than either topical or oral PUVA [38].

NB-UVB Versus Excimer Light

While the superiority of NB-UVB to PUVA in the treatment of vitiligo is clear, comparison studies between NB-UVB and 308-nm excimer light for vitiligo are mixed. A multicentre left-right intra-individual study of 21 patients showed that NB-UVB phototherapy may be less effective than excimer light in terms of the efficacy and onset of repigmentation [39]. These findings contrast with that of another intra-individual randomized controlled study of 11 patients which showed that localized 311-nm NB-UVB achieved a greater degree of repigmentation compared to 308-nm monochromatic excimer light [40]. More recently, a systematic review and meta-analysis of six studies found no significant differences between NB-UVB and excimer light in repigmentation efficacy in vitiligo [41]. In clinical practice, the choice between starting NB-UVB versus excimer light phototherapy for a patient with vitiligo is influenced by various considerations, such as the extent of vitiligo, cost and duration of treatment as well as resource constraints.

NB-UVB Combined with Topical Calcineurin Inhibitors

Apart from topical corticosteroids, topical calcineurin inhibitors such as tacrolimus and pimecrolimus are effective treatments for vitiligo and are frequently used in conjunction with phototherapy to enhance repigmentation [42]. A prospective single-blind left-right comparison study evaluated 74 patients with symmetrically distributed vitiligo who applied tacrolimus 0.1% ointment twice daily to only the left-sided lesions and underwent whole-body NB-UVB phototherapy thrice weekly. The authors observed a greater extent and faster onset of repigmentation for the side treated with both NB-UVB and tacrolimus ointment, compared to the corresponding NB-UVB-only side [43]. In a double-blind randomized trial comparing NB-UVB with pimecrolimus 1% cream versus NB-UVB with placebo for 3 months, there was significantly greater repigmentation for vitiliginous patches on the face in the NB-UVB with pimecrolimus group, but no significant differences between both groups for the other body sites [44]. On current evidence, topical calcineurin inhibitors appear to be a useful adjunctive treatment to NB-UVB phototherapy and may benefit patients by reducing the cumulative NB-UVB dose required to attain satisfactory repigmentation, thereby reducing cutaneous carcinogenic risk.

NB-UVB Combined with Topical Vitamin D Analogues

Unlike topical calcineurin inhibitors, the efficacy of topical vitamin D analogues in combination with NB-UVB phototherapy remains equivocal. In a prospective study of 24 patients with generalized vitiligo, NB-UVB phototherapy was administered thrice weekly over 6 months, and calcipotriol cream was applied on only the right side of the body. There was a faster onset and greater degree of repigmentation seen on the side with NB-UVB and calcipotriol [45]. A similar left-right study on 30 patients with symmetrical vitiligo showed that NB-UVB with topical tacalcitol ointment was superior in repigmentation efficacy and onset compared to NB-UVB alone [46].

However, these results contrast with that of several other studies showing that the addition of topical vitamin D analogues did not confer additional benefit in vitiligo. A prospective single-blinded right-left comparison study of 20 patients with symmetrical vitiligo showed that NB-UVB itself was effective for repigmentation, and addition of topical calcipotriol did not improve treatment outcome [47]. In a randomized study of 40 patients with generalized vitiligo split into two groups comparing NB-UVB with topical calcipotriol ointment versus NB-UVB alone, there was no statistically significant difference in repigmentation rates between both groups after a mean of 30 treatment sessions [48]. More recently, another right-left comparison study of 27 vitiligo patients treated over 6 months supported prior observations that the addition of topical calcipotriol did not enhance the time to onset and efficacy of repigmentation in patients treated with NB-UVB phototherapy [49]. In view that the existing studies on this issue have all been carried out on relatively small cohorts, larger randomized controlled trials are necessary to assess if there is any true benefit of add topical vitamin D analogues to NB-UVB phototherapy in the treatment of vitiligo.

NB-UVB Combined with Antioxidants

The aetiology of vitiligo is multifactorial, part of which includes increased oxidative stress characterized by higher levels of reactive oxygen species and hydrogen peroxide in the epidermis which impairs tyrosinase activity [50]. As such, there have been studies looking at the potential synergistic role of antioxidants in conjunction with NB-UVB phototherapy in vitiligo.

Polypodium leucotomos, a herbal extract originating from a tropical fern, has been shown in several studies to exert a range of antioxidant, photoprotective and immunomodulatory effects, which are potentially beneficial for a number of skin disorders [51]. In a randomized controlled trial, 50 patients with vitiligo vulgaris were assigned to either NB-UVB twice weekly plus oral *Polypodium leucotomos* 250 mg thrice daily or NB-UVB plus placebo over approximately 6 months. In the treatment group, there was a clear trend towards a greater extent of repigmentation in the head and neck area, particularly in patients of lighter skin types II and III [52]. *Polypodium leucotomos* is generally well tolerated across various doses ranging from 120 to 1080 mg daily, and it possesses an excellent safety profile with minimal risk of adverse effects [53]. Overall, oral *Polypodium leucomotos* appears to be a promising adjunctive treatment in combination with NB-UVB phototherapy for vitiligo, though its accessibility may be limited by cost.

Other oral antioxidants have been studied for their potential benefit in enhancing the efficacy of NB-UVB phototherapy in vitiligo. In a prospective study, 24 vitiligo patients were randomized to either NB-UVB plus oral vitamin E or NB-UVB phototherapy alone. In the vitamin E group, there was a higher proportion of patients achieving marked to excellent repigmentation (73% versus 56%), as well as a significant reduction in plasma malondialdehyde, a byproduct of polyunsaturated fatty acid peroxidation. These results suggest that the addition of oral vitamin E may play a role in increasing the repigmentation efficacy of NB-UVB phototherapy by inhibiting lipid peroxidation in the cell membranes of melanocytes [54].

Dell'Anna and colleagues evaluated 28 patients undergoing NB-UVB phototherapy for non-segmental vitiligo in a randomized, double-blind, placebo-controlled multicentre trial. In addition to phototherapy, patients in the treatment group took an oral antioxidant supplement comprising alpha-lipoic acid, vitamins C and E and polyunsaturated fatty acids beginning 2 months prior and throughout the 6 months of phototherapy. Significantly higher repigmentation of greater than 75% was observed in the treatment group compared to the placebo group (47% vs 18%). In addition, the treatment group recorded a significant increase in the activity of catalase (an enzyme that breaks down hydrogen peroxide) and reduction in the level of reactive oxygen species in peripheral blood mononuclear cells [55]. By counteracting vitiligo-associated oxidative stress, oral antioxidants may be a beneficial adjuvant treatment when combined with NB-UVB phototherapy for vitiligo.

NB-UVB Combined with Afamelanotide

Alpha-melanocyte-stimulating hormone (α-MSH) plays an important role in stimulating melanogenesis and melanocyte proliferation, and it is known that patients with vitiligo have lower levels of α-MSH in their plasma and lesional vitiliginous skin [56]. Afamelanotide is a potent synthetic analogue of α-MSH that exerts a longer duration of action compared to native α-MSH, and is administered via subcutaneous injection [57].

In a recent randomized multicentre trial, Lim and colleagues studied 28 patients with non-segmental vitiligo who received either combination therapy comprising afamelanotide and NB-UVB phototherapy or NB-UVB monotherapy. In the combination therapy group, afamela-

notide 16 mg was administered subcutaneously monthly for 4 months, beginning after 1 month of NB-UVB phototherapy. A statistically significant superior and faster repigmentation response was observed for the face and upper limbs in the combination therapy group. The improvement was more pronounced in patients with skin types IV to VI, which is encouraging because patients with darker skin types are likely to have more visually conspicuous vitiligo [58]. Large-scale dose-ranging studies are necessary to determine the optimal treatment regime for afamelanotide in combination with NB-UVB phototherapy.

Predictors of Response

Factors influencing clinical response of vitiligo to NB-UVB phototherapy may vary between populations. In a study of 70 patients with vitiligo treated twice weekly with NB-UVB phototherapy in Greece, factors associated with greater repigmentation included facial vitiligo, darker skin phototypes (types III to V) and early response to treatment within the first 1 month [59]. An Italian study of 60 vitiligo patients demonstrated that predictive factors of greater response to NB-UVB were the anatomical sites of vitiligo (the face, neck and trunk repigmented more than the limbs), younger age of under 20 years and recent onset [60]. Early commencement of NB-UVB phototherapy for generalized vitiligo has been associated with a significantly higher response rate [61].

It is well known that non-segmental vitiligo is more treatment-responsive than segmental vitiligo. Generally, the anatomical sites which respond well to phototherapy are the face, neck, trunk and proximal extremities, while the distal acral sites such as the hands, feet and genitalia tend to respond poorly (Fig. 16.4). It is well known that hair-bearing areas are more responsive to phototherapy, which may be explained by the reservoir of melanocyte stem cells in the outer root sheaths of hair follicles that are activated by ultraviolet irradiation.

Relapse Rate

As in many other UVB-responsive chronic dermatoses, vitiligo may relapse after a successful

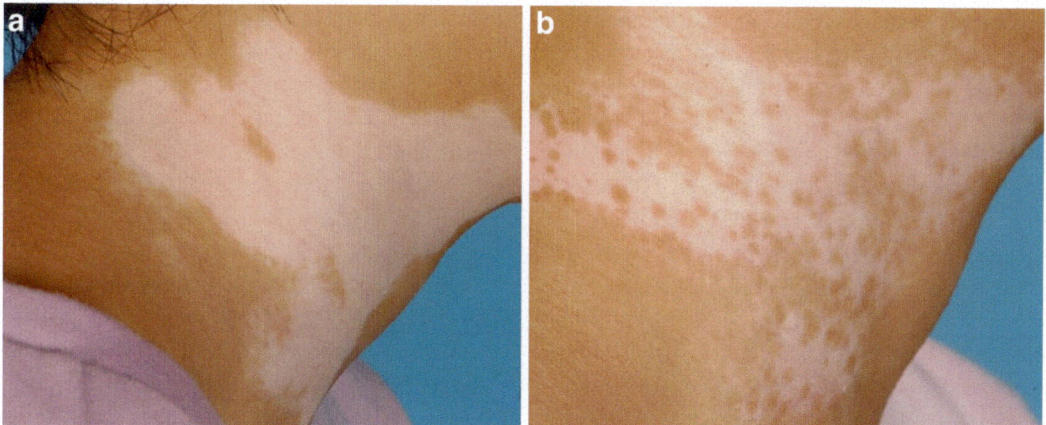

Fig. 16.4 (**a**) Baseline vitiligo on the neck. (**b**) Follicular repigmentation after 24 sessions of NBUVB twice a week (Source: National Skin Centre, Singapore)

course of NB-UVB phototherapy. There is, however, a paucity of published data on the durability of repigmentation following cessation of phototherapy. In a follow-up trial, Sitek and colleagues monitored 11 patients with generalized vitiligo who achieved over 75% repigmentation after a course of NB-UVB thrice weekly for up to 12 months and followed them up for the subsequent 2 years. Approximately half the patients experienced relapse of vitiligo (majority within 6 months post-treatment cessation), while the other half continued to maintain stable repigmentation at 24 months post-treatment [62].

NB-UVB for Progressive Macular Hypomelanosis

Progressive macular hypomelanosis (PMH) is an acquired hypopigmentary disorder characterized by the gradual development of asymptomatic non-scaly hypopigmented macules predominantly on the trunk and upper limbs, in the absence of preceding skin inflammation [63]. Though its exact pathogenesis remains a mystery, the currently accepted view is that PMH may be caused by a hypothetical depigmenting agent secreted by *Propionibacterium acnes* bacteria overgrowing in the pilosebaceous units of hair follicles in the lesional skin [64].

At present, there is no established first-line treatment for PMH. In view of the postulation that *Propionibacterium acnes* may be a causative agent, topical antimicrobial therapies such as clindamycin lotion and benzoyl peroxide have been used for PMH, with variable success [65, 66].

NB-UVB phototherapy has bacteriostatic properties and appears to be an effective treatment for PMH, though relapse may occur following cessation of treatment. A randomized left-right comparison study evaluated ten patients with PMH who received NB-UVB combined with an antimicrobial gel on one side of the trunk and NB-UVB monotherapy on the contralateral side for 8 weeks. Significant repigmentation was observed in all patients, without any significant difference between both sides [67]. Kim and colleagues conducted a prospective open study on 16 patients with PMH treated with NB-UVB phototherapy once to twice weekly. The majority (81%) achieved at least 50% repigmentation with an excellent colour match. Approximately half of the cohort had over 90% repigmentation. Recurrence was observed in 31% of the patients within 1–2 years [68]. A retrospective review of 32 PMH cases in Singapore treated with NB-UVB phototherapy twice to thrice weekly demonstrated an excellent response of greater than 80% repigmentation in 90% of the cohort. Repigmentation was noticeable within 4–8 sessions of phototherapy, reaching a peak response at approximately 22 sessions. The relapse rate was 6%, occurring on average within 7 months of discontinuing treatment [66].

In a retrospective analysis in Brazil, 84 cases of PMH were treated with either NB-UVB phototherapy (57 cases) or oral PUVA photochemotherapy (27 cases). The majority (81%) of patients achieved a good repigmentation response of greater than 50%, and there was no significant difference between NB-UVB and oral PUVA in repigmentation efficacy [69]. The authors proposed that NB-UVB is preferred to PUVA for treating PMH because of the former's better safety profile.

On current evidence, a combination of antimicrobial therapy and NB-UVB phototherapy is likely to offer the greatest benefit for PMH.

Contraindications

Prior to starting a patient on NB-UVB phototherapy, it is important to first exclude contraindications to this treatment modality [70]. Absolute contraindications to NB-UVB include severe medical illness or haemodynamic instability that precludes independent standing in the phototherapy cabin, photosensitive dermatoses such as connective tissue disorders (lupus erythematosus, dermatomyositis) and genophotodermatoses (such as xeroderma pigmentosum), photosensitivity and a personal history of melanoma.

Relative contraindications to NB-UVB include a personal history of non-melanoma skin cancer or atypical nevus syndrome, presence of premalignant skin lesions (such as actinic keratoses), a family history of skin cancer, poorly controlled epilepsy, intake of photosensitizing drugs, previous exposure to arsenic or ionizing radiation and treatment with immunosuppressive drugs such as ciclosporin that significantly increase the risk of cutaneous carcinogenesis.

Dosimetry

Based on published guidelines by Zanolli and Feldman, NB-UVB phototherapy is usually started at a frequency of two or three times a week [71]. The initial dose of NB-UVB (in units of mJ/cm^2) can be determined by either assessing the minimal erythema dose (MED) or by Fitzpatrick skin phototype.

In our phototherapy centre, after determining the patient's MED, NB-UVB is then started at a dose equivalent to 70% of the MED. As for the skin phototype method, the patient with vitiligo is assumed to have skin phototype I, and NB-UVB is started at a dose of 300 mJ/cm^2. It should be noted that there is a wide variation between different institutions with regard to the starting dose of NB-UVB for vitiligo, which can range from 100 to 740 mJ/cm^2 [72]. As the MED-based regime is individually tailored, it is considered to be a safer starting dosimetry compared to the skin phototype regime [73]. In clinical practice, the skin phototype regime is more convenient and preferred in some busy phototherapy centres with heavy patient loads, as it may not be feasible to conduct MED testing for all patients.

At each visit, the patient is assessed for the degree of erythema and side effects, if any, in order to decide on the appropriate dose adjustment. It has been shown that two-thirds of patients with vitiligo may develop photoadaptation with repeated phototherapy sessions [74]. Therefore, the dose of NB-UVB can be increased at each session, in increments of either 50 or 100 mJ/cm^2 (equivalent to approximately 10–20% of the previous dose), to counteract the epidermal hyperplasia and tanning effect of phototherapy. To optimize therapeutic response, the practitioner should aim to deliver a suberythemogenic dose of NB-UVB so as to maintain a mild perceptible erythema throughout the treatment course [75].

Safety

NB-UVB phototherapy is widely considered to be a relatively safe therapeutic modality. Patients should nevertheless be counselled on potential risks and written informed consent be obtained prior to commencing treatment. Acute and short-term risks include phototherapy burn, skin blistering, tanning, xerosis, pruritus and, rarely, reactivation of herpes simplex virus [76].

Long-term risks of NB-UVB phototherapy include photoageing and, more crucially, photocarcinogenesis. It has been shown that absorption of UVB radiation by DNA nucleotides induces formation of DNA photoproducts such as cyclobutane pyrimidine dimers and 6–4 photoproducts. When unrepaired, these mutagenic photoproducts trigger UVB signature mutations (C-T or CC-TT) in the p53 tumour suppressor gene, leading to proliferation of tumour cells [77]. In addition, UVB-induced DNA damage promotes the growth of tumour cells by activating transcription factors such as nuclear factor-κB and activator protein-1 that are key to the regulation of cellular proliferation, differentiation and survival [78].

Interestingly, genetic studies have suggested that vitiligo may confer a lower susceptibility to developing melanoma. As polymorphisms in the tyrosinase gene have been detected in both vitiligo and melanoma, it has been postulated that the strong autoimmune anti-tyrosinase expression in vitiligo may confer protection against melanoma [79, 80]. These findings have been supported by observations in large-scale epidemiological studies. A retrospective cohort analysis of 1307 vitiligo patients in Holland revealed that patients with vitiligo had a threefold lower probability of developing melanoma and non-melanoma skin cancers compared to non-vitiligo controls. Subgroup analyses of patients treated with NB-UVB and PUVA did not show any dose-related increases in age-adjusted lifetime prevalence of melanoma or non-melanoma skin cancers [81]. Similarly, Paradisi and colleagues demonstrated in their large Italian cohort of 10,040 patients that patients with vitiligo had a fourfold lower relative risk of melanoma and a fivefold lower relative risk of non-melanoma skin cancers, when compared to non-dermatology patients seen in the vascular surgery clinics. However, subgroup analyses of patients within the vitiligo cohort showed that those who underwent phototherapy had a significantly higher risk of developing melanoma (6% versus 0.8%) and non-melanoma skin cancers (14.1% versus 3.2%) compared to vitiligo patients who did not undergo phototherapy [82]. Nevertheless, these findings

should be interpreted with caution, as the study did not distinguish between NB-UVB and PUVA in the phototherapy group.

Overall, while NB-UVB phototherapy appears to be fairly safe in the short to medium term, the true long-term risk of photocarcinogenesis remains to be fully elucidated. As such, there is currently no internationally agreed consensus as to the maximum number of phototherapy sessions an individual can receive in one's lifetime. Individual risk stratification is recommended, and risk factors such as a family history of skin cancer and concomitant systemic immunosuppressive therapy should be taken into account in the planning of an individualized phototherapy regimen.

Home Phototherapy Treatment

Home-based phototherapy is an attractive option as it offers convenience to the patients as attendance for institutional phototherapy can be time-consuming and can lead to inconsistent treatment. The efficacy of home-based therapy has been shown in a few recent studies.

Ninety-three vitiligo patients were recruited in a home phototherapy study by Shan et al. [83]. Patients were prescribed with a hand-held NB-UVB home phototherapy. Patients were examined at baseline and every 3 months for a year. At the end of a year, 17% of patients achieved between 51% and 75% repigmentation and 38% >75% repigmentation. The treatments were well tolerated with burning, pruritus and mild dryness reported in 11 patients.

In a randomized parallel group trial comparing home-based phototherapy with institution-based 308-nm excimer lamp for the treatment of focal vitiligo, 44 vitiligo patient were randomized into 2 groups – 1 group using home-based phototherapy (Daavlin DermaPal® system) 3 times a week and the other group undergoing institution-based therapy twice a week with the excimer lamp [84]. At the end of 6 months, 72% and 50% of patients achieved good and excellent repigmentation in the home-based phototherapy group compared with 54%

and 36% in the excimer group. This may be explained by the better adherence in the home-based phototherapy group with 92% adhering to the prescribed treatment compared with 72% in the institutional excimer group.

Excimer Laser and Lamp

The excimer xenon chloride laser system delivers ultraviolet light at 308 nm wavelength. The light is delivered as a monochromatic and coherent beam, through a hand-held piece, and is used for targeted phototherapy. The advantage is that the light can be delivered at higher fluence to a targeted area. It received FDA approval in 2000. More recently, the 308-nm excimer lamps have been introduced (Fig. 16.5). Smaller hand-held excimer lamp units are also now available in the market. The excimer laser requires frequent gas exchanges and has higher maintenance cost compared to the excimer lamps.

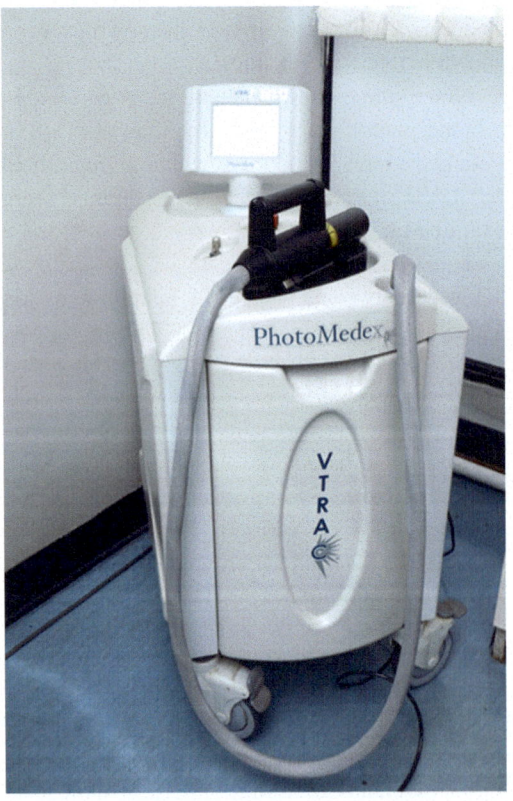

Fig. 16.5 VTRAC™ excimer lamp (PhotoMedex, USA)

Treatment Protocol for Excimer Laser

The excimer laser is delivered two to three times a week. Some protocols require the minimal erythema to be determined, while others have starting doses dependent on the site. The usual starting dose is in the range of 100–200 mJ/cm².

After each treatment, it is important to look for erythema, and a hint of erythema is the ideal endpoint. In the absence of erythema, the dose can be increased by 50 mJ/cm². If the erythema is persistent beyond a day, the dose should be reduced by 50 mJ/cm². If blistering occurs, the dose is dropped to the penultimate dose [85].

Efficacy of Excimer Laser for Vitiligo

The efficacy was first reported by Baltas in a case series of six patients [85]. Patients were treated twice a week for 24 weeks, and repigmentation was noted after 8 weeks.

Hadi et al. had reported the results of a retrospective review of 32 patients with 55 vitiligo spots [86]. The best improvement was seen in vitiligo on the face compared with acral areas. Overall, 71.5% of facial spots achieved over 75% repigmentation. This was in contrast to acral lesions with only 20% showing 50% or more improvement in the lesions. In a further retrospective review of 97 patients with 221 vitiligo patches, Hadi et al. again demonstrated that 50% of the treated lesions showed over 75% repigmentation, with the face showing the best improvement [87].

Zhang et al. reported the efficacy of excimer laser after 30 treatments in 36 patients with 44 vitiligo patches. Overall 61.4% (27/44) of the patches had achieved over 75% repigmentation. The percentages of the face, trunk and extremity lesions showing over 50% repigmentation were 74%, 100% and 25%, respectively [88]. Pigmentation was noticed as early as after four treatments in Asian skin.

In a small prospective study of 13 patients, Hofer et al. showed that the improvement in vitiligo correlated with the treatment number and not the treatment frequency. Improvement was seen faster in three times a week-treated group vs two times a week-treated group, but the ultimate repigmentation depended on the number of treatments and not the frequency [89]. The repigmentation was stable in most patients on a 12-month follow-up.

A controlled prospective study involving 34 Asian patients similarly showed the face with the best repigmentation, followed by the trunk with the hands and feet the least responsive. The response was also better seen in patients with higher skin phototype. The average number of treatments to repigmentation was 11 [90].

In a large prospective study of 979 Chinese patients with vitiligo treated with the excimer laser, 34% of patients showed over 76% repigmentation, 6% showed 51–75% repigmentation, 16% showed 26–50% repigmentation and 44% showed less than 25% repigmentation [91]. The face showed the best response, while the acral area showed the poorest response. The degree of repigmentation correlated negatively with duration. In the presence of poliosis, the vitiligo was more resistant to treatment.

Efficacy of Excimer Lamp

The excimer lamp is increasingly used in place of the excimer laser as it is more cost-effective and much easier to maintain. There are fewer published data on the efficacy of the excimer lamp, although most of the data shows similar efficacy to the excimer laser (Fig. 16.6).

In a randomized comparative study between the excimer laser and excimer lamp, Le Duff treated 20 patients with 104 vitiligo lesions, one side with the excimer lamp and the other side with excimer laser [92]. The results showed similar efficacy for repigmentation of at least 50%, but there was increased erythema with the excimer lamp.

Another small randomized bilateral comparison study comparing the 308-nm excimer laser with the 308-nm excimer lamp in the treatment showed similar repigmentation rates between the two groups [93].

In a meta-analysis of the efficacy of excimer lamp vs excimer laser and NB-UVB, there was no significant difference in the efficacy between excimer laser and lamp in outcome measure of >50% and 75% repigmentation [94]. There was also no significant difference in the efficacy between excimer lamp and NB-UVB.

Combination Therapy

Excimer Laser with Topical Calcineurin Inhibitors

Topical calcineurin inhibitors like tacrolimus and pimecrolimus are used as monotherapy in the treatment of vitiligo with good effect. There are now several studies demonstrating the improved efficacy of combination therapy with these topical calcineurin inhibitors and the excimer laser.

A pilot study by Kawalek et al. compared the efficacy of excimer laser alone vs excimer laser

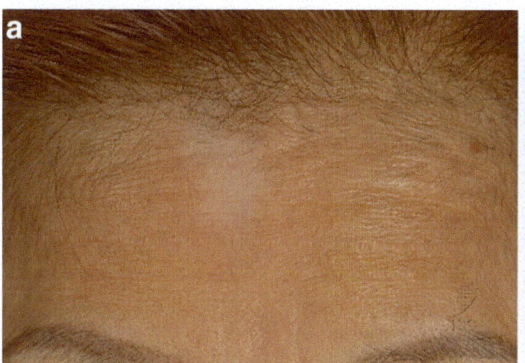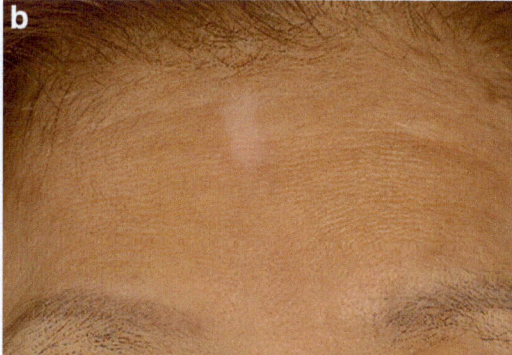

Fig. 16.6 (**a**) Baseline vitiligo on the forehead. (**b**) 50% marginal repigmentation after 35 sessions of excimer light phototherapy twice weekly (Source: National Skin Centre, Singapore)

with topical tacrolimus 0.1% in the treatment of vitiligo. After 24 treatments or 10 weeks of treatment at 3 times a week, the excimer laser alone led to a greater than 75% repigmentation in 20% of patches compared to 50% when combined with topical tacrolimus [95].

In another intra-individual randomized prospective study, greater than 75% repigmentation was achieved in 70% (16/23) of the vitiligo patches treated with excimer laser and topical tacrolimus vs 20% (4/20) in those treated with excimer laser alone. The improvement was especially good for traditional UV-resistant sites [96]. Adverse events were minimal and well tolerated.

The efficacy of combination therapy of excimer laser and topical tacrolimus was further corroborated by findings of a randomized controlled study by Nistico el al [97]. In this study, there were 53 vitiligo patients treated for 12 weeks with either excimer laser twice a week with oral vitamin E, excimer laser twice a week with topical tacrolimus once a day and oral vitamin E or with vitamin E alone. The best response was seen in the group with topical tacrolimus with good repigmentation in 40% of patients and excellent repigmentation in 30%. A retrospective study from Matin and colleagues also showed a better response of vitiligo in combination with tacrolimus [98].

Of interest is a study by Park et al. which showed that the improvement of vitiligo treated with combination therapy of excimer laser with tacrolimus was useful during induction for up to 6 months and that the benefit was not seen beyond 6 months, suggesting that continued therapy beyond 6 months may not have a better outcome than monotherapy [99].

In a single-blinded study examining the combination of topical pimecrolimus and excimer laser versus excimer laser alone in childhood vitiligo, 71% of patients in the combination group achieved grade 3 or 4 repigmentation compared with 50% in the comparator group. Treatment was also well tolerated [100].

A recent meta-analysis examined the efficacy of the 308-nm excimer laser/light and topical agent combination therapy versus excimer laser/light monotherapy. Combination therapy with

calcineurin inhibitors was superior to monotherapy, but there was insufficient evidence to support the combination of topical vitamin D3 analogues and corticosteroids [101].

Safety of Excimer Laser/Lamp

The excimer laser is generally well tolerated. Most of the side effects are localized and mild, and no systemic complication are seen. From the published studies, the main side effects are transient erythema which is mild and a burning sensation that is mild. Blistering or a localized sunburn reaction can occur. In general, the treatment is very well tolerated with high patient satisfaction.

With a low side effect profile, early repigmentation and good efficacy, the excimer laser is an ideal treatment option for localized vitiligo sites. For generalized vitiligo, the treatment is too time-consuming and not practical to be used.

Conclusion

Phototherapy remains one of the main treatments for vitiligo. Traditional PUVA therapy is still an effective treatment, but NB-UVB and excimer are effective and safer options which are now more commonly employed. Phototherapy can be used in combination with other treatments like topical calcineurin inhibitors for greater efficacy. The face, trunk and limbs are the more likely sites to respond to treatment, and the acral areas are much more treatment-resistant.

References

1. Ceoviae R, Pasiae A, Lipozenciase J, Jakiae-Razumoviae J, Szirovicza L, Kostoviae K. Antiproliferative, antiangiogenic, and apoptotic effect of photochemotherapy (PUVA) in psoriasis. Coll Anthropol. 2007;31:551–6.
2. Falabella R, Barona MI. Update on skin repigmentation therapies in vitiligo. Pigment Cell Melanoma Res. 2008;22:42–65.
3. Wu CS, Lan CC, Wang LF, Chen GS, Wu CS, Yu HS. Effects of psoralen plus ultraviolet A irradiation

on cultured epidermal cells in and patients with psoriasis in vivo. Br J Dermatol. 2007;156:122–9.

4. Ibbotson SH, Farr PM. The time-course of psoralen ultraviolet A (PUVA) erythema. J Invest Dermatol. 1999;113:346–50.

5. Kwok YK, Anstey AV, Hawk JL. Psoralen photochemotherapy (PUVA) is only moderately effective in widespread vitiligo: a 10-year retrospective study. Clin Exp Dermatol. 2002;27(2):104–10.

6. Tallab T, Joharji H, Bahamdan K, Karkashan E, Mourad M, Ibrahim K. Response of vitiligo to PUVA therapy in Saudi patients. Int J Dermatol. 2005;44(7):556–8.

7. Singh S, Khandpur S, Sharma VK, et al. Comparison of efficacy and side-effect profile of oral PUVA vs. oral PUVA sol in the treatment of vitiligo: a 36 week prospective study. J Eur Acad Dermatol Venereol. 2013;27(11):1344–51.

8. Esmat SM, El-Tawdy AM, Hafez GA, et al. Acral lesions of vitiligo: why are they resistant to photochemotherapy. J Eur Acad Dermatol. 2012;26(9):1097–104.

9. El Mofty M, Bosseila M, Mashaly HM, Gawdat H, Makaly H. Broadband ultraviolet A vs psoralen in the treatment of vitiligo: a randomized controlled trial. Clin Exp Dermatol. 2013;38(8):830–5.

10. Parsad D, Saini R, Verma N. Combination of PUVAsol and topical calcipotriol in vitiligo. Dermatology. 1998;197(2):167–70.

11. Handa S, Pandhi R, Kaur I. Vitiligo: a retrospective comparative analysis of treatment modalities in 500 patients. J Dermatol. 2001;28:461–6.

12. Halpern SM, Anstey AV, Dawe RS, et al. Guidelines for topical PUVA: a report of a workshop of the British Photodermatology group. Br J Dermatol. 2000;142:22–31.

13. Valkova S, Trashlieva M, Christova P. Treatment of vitiligo with local khellin and UVA: comparison with systemic PUVA. Clin Exp Dermatol. 2004;29(2):180–4.

14. Ortel B, Tanew A, Honigsmann H. Treatment of vitiligo with khellin and ultraviolet A. J Am Acad Dermatol. 1998;90(5):720–4.

15. Duschet P, Schwartz T, Pusch M, Gschnait F. Marked increase of liver transaminases after Khellin and UVA therapy. J Am Acad Dermatol. 1989;21(3 Pt 1):592–4.

16. Morison WL, Marwaha S, Beck L. PUVA-induced phototoxicity: incidence and causes. J Am Acad Dermatol. 1997;36:183–5.

17. Ledbetter LS, Hsu S. Melanonychia associated with PUVA therapy. J Am Acad Dermatol. 2003;4:S31–2.

18. Pathak MA, Mosher DB, Fitzpatrick TB. Safety and therapeutic effectiveness of 8 methoxypsoralen4,5′,8-trimethlypsoralen, and psoralen in vitiligo. Natl Cancer Inst Monogr. 1984;66:165–73.

19. Stern RS, Laird N, Melski J, Parrish JA, Fitzpatrik TB, Bleich NL. Cutaneous squamous cell carcinoma in patients treated with oral methoxsalen photochemotherapy for psoriasis. N Engl J Med. 1984;310:1156–61.

20. Nijsten TE, Stern RS. The increase risk of skin cancer is persistent after discontinuation of psoralen + ultraviolet A: a cohort study. J Invest Dermatol. 2003;121:252–8.

21. Stern RS, Nichols KT, Vakeva LH. Malignant melanoma in patients treated for psoriasis with methoxalen (psoralen) and ultraviolet A radiation (PUVA): the PUVA follow-up study. N England J Med. 1997;336:1041–5.

22. Goekerman WH. The treatment of psoriasis. Northwest Med. 1925;24:229–31.

23. Fischer T. Comparative treatment of psoriasis with UV-light, trioxsalen plus UV-light, and coal tar plus UV-light. Acta Derm Venereol. 1977;57:345–50.

24. Bandow GD, Koo JY. Narrow-band ultraviolet B radiation: a review of the current literature. Int J Dermatol. 2004;43:555–61.

25. Anderson RR, Parrish JA. The optics of human skin. J Invest Dermatol. 1981;77:13–9.

26. el-Ghorr AA, Norval M. Biological effects of narrow-band (311 nm TL01) UVB irradiation: a review. J Photochem Photobiol B. 1997;38:99–106.

27. Kao CH, Yu HS. Depletion and repopulation of Langerhans cells in nonsegmental type vitiligo. J Dermatol. 1990;17:287–96.

28. Staricco RG, Miller-Milinska A. Activation of the amelanotic melanocytes in the outer root sheath of the hair follicle following ultra violet rays exposure. J Invest Dermatol. 1962;39:163–4.

29. Cui J, Shen LY, Wang GC. Role of hair follicles in the repigmentation of vitiligo. J Invest Dermatol. 1991;97:410–6.

30. Wu CS, Lan CC, Yu HS. Narrow-band UVB irradiation stimulates the migration and functional development of vitiligo-IgG antibodies-treated pigment cells. J Eur Acad Dermatol Venereol. 2012;26:456–64.

31. Westerhof W, Nieuweboer-Krobotova L. Treatment of vitiligo with UV-B radiation vs topical psoralen plus UV-A. Arch Dermatol. 1997;133:1525–8.

32. Scherschun L, Kim JJ, Lim HW. Narrow-band ultraviolet B is a useful and well-tolerated treatment for vitiligo. J Am Acad Dermatol. 2001;44:999–1003.

33. Hamzavi I, Jain H, McLean D, et al. Parametric modeling of narrowband UV-B phototherapy for vitiligo using a novel quantitative tool: the Vitiligo Area Scoring Index. Arch Dermatol. 2004;140:677–83.

34. Natta R, Somsak T, Wisuttida T, et al. Narrowband ultraviolet B radiation therapy for recalcitrant vitiligo in Asians. J Am Acad Dermatol. 2003;49:473–6.

35. Njoo MD, Bos JD, Westerhof W. Treatment of generalized vitiligo in children with narrow-band (TL-01) UVB radiation therapy. J Am Acad Dermatol. 2000;42:245–53.

36. Kanwar AJ, Dogra S. Narrow-band UVB for the treatment of generalized vitiligo in children. Clin Exp Dermatol. 2005;30:332–6.

37. Yones SS, Palmer RA, Garibaldinos TM, et al. Randomized double-blind trial of treatment of vitiligo: efficacy of psoralen-UV-A therapy vs narrowband-UV-B therapy. Arch Dermatol. 2007;143:578–84.

38. Jekler J, Larkö O. Vitiligo treatment in childhood: a state of the art review. Pediatr Dermatol. 2010;27:437–45.

39. Casacci M, Thomas P, Pacifico A, et al. Comparison between 308-nm monochromatic excimer light and narrowband UVB phototherapy (311-313 nm) in the treatment of vitiligo – a multicentre controlled study. J Eur Acad Dermatol Venereol. 2007;21:956–63.

40. Verhaeghe E, Lodewick E, van Geel N, et al. Intrapatient comparison of 308-nm monochromatic excimer light and localized narrow-band UVB phototherapy in the treatment of vitiligo: a randomized controlled trial. Dermatology. 2011;223:343–8.

41. Lopes C, Trevisani VF, Melnik T. Efficacy and safety of 308-nm monochromatic excimer lamp versus other phototherapy devices for vitiligo: a systematic review with meta-analysis. Am J Clin Dermatol. 2016;17:23–32.

42. Wong R, Lin AN. Efficacy of topical calcineurin inhibitors in vitiligo. Int J Dermatol. 2013;52:491–6.

43. Majid I. Does topical tacrolimus ointment enhance the efficacy of narrowband ultraviolet B therapy in vitiligo? A left-right comparison study. Photodermatol Photoimmunol Photomed. 2010;26:230–4.

44. Esfandiarpour I, Ekhlasi A, Farajzadeh S, et al. The efficacy of pimecrolimus 1% cream plus narrow-band ultraviolet B in the treatment of vitiligo: a double-blind, placebo-controlled clinical trial. J Dermatolog Treat. 2009;20:14–8.

45. Goktas EO, Aydin F, Senturk N, et al. Combination of narrow band UVB and topical calcipotriol for the treatment of vitiligo. J Eur Acad Dermatol Venereol. 2006;20:553–7.

46. Leone G, Pacifico A, Iacovelli P, et al. Tacalcitol and narrow-band phototherapy in patients with vitiligo. Clin Exp Dermatol. 2006;31:200–5.

47. Ada S, Sahin S, Boztepe G, et al. No additional effect of topical calcipotriol on narrow-band UVB phototherapy in patients with generalized vitiligo. Photodermatol Photoimmunol Photomed. 2005;21:79–83.

48. Arca E, Taştan HB, Erbil AH, et al. Narrow-band ultraviolet B as monotherapy and in combination with topical calcipotriol in the treatment of vitiligo. J Dermatol. 2006;33:338–43.

49. Khullar G, Kanwar AJ, Singh S, et al. Comparison of efficacy and safety profile of topical calcipotriol ointment in combination with NB-UVB vs. NB-UVB alone in the treatment of vitiligo: a 24-week prospective right-left comparative clinical trial. J Eur Acad Dermatol Venereol. 2015;29:925–32.

50. Westerhof W, d'Ischia M. Vitiligo puzzle: the pieces fall in place. Pigment Cell Res. 2007;20:345–59.

51. Choudhry SZ, Bhatia N, Ceilley R, et al. Role of oral Polypodium leucotomos extract in dermatologic diseases: a review of the literature. J Drugs Dermatol. 2014;13:148–53.

52. Middelkamp-Hup MA, Bos JD, Rius-Diaz F, et al. Treatment of vitiligo vulgaris with narrow-band UVB and oral Polypodium leucotomos extract: a randomized double-blind placebo-controlled study. J Eur Acad Dermatol Venereol. 2007;21:942–50.

53. Winkelmann RR, Del Rosso J, Rigel DS. Polypodium leucotomos extract: a status report on clinical efficacy and safety. J Drugs Dermatol. 2015;14:254–61.

54. Elgoweini M, Nour El Din N. Response of vitiligo to narrowband ultraviolet B and oral antioxidants. J Clin Pharmacol. 2009;49:852–5.

55. Dell'Anna ML, Mastrofrancesco A, Sala R, et al. Antioxidants and narrow band-UVB in the treatment of vitiligo: a double-blind placebo controlled trial. Clin Exp Dermatol. 2007;32:631–6.

56. Thody AJ. Alpha-MSH and the regulation of melanocyte function. Ann N Y Acad Sci. 1999;885:217–29.

57. Fabrikant J, Touloei K, Brown SM. A review and update on melanocyte stimulating hormone therapy: afamelanotide. J Drugs Dermatol. 2013;12:775–9.

58. Lim HW, Grimes PE, Agbai O, et al. Afamelanotide and narrowband UV-B phototherapy for the treatment of vitiligo: a randomized multicenter trial. JAMA Dermatol. 2015;151:42–50.

59. Nicolaidou E, Antoniou C, Stratigos AJ, et al. Efficacy, predictors of response, and long-term follow-up in patients with vitiligo treated with narrowband UVB phototherapy. J Am Acad Dermatol. 2007;56:274–8.

60. Brazzelli V, Antoninetti M, Palazzini S, et al. Critical evaluation of the variants influencing the clinical response of vitiligo: study of 60 cases treated with ultraviolet B narrow-band phototherapy. J Eur Acad Dermatol Venereol. 2007;21:1369–74.

61. Hallaji Z, Ghiasi M, Eisazadeh A, et al. Evaluation of the effect of disease duration in generalized vitiligo on its clinical response to narrowband ultraviolet B phototherapy. Photodermatol Photoimmunol Photomed. 2012;28:115–9.

62. Sitek JC, Loeb M, Ronnevig JR. Narrowband UVB therapy for vitiligo: does the repigmentation last? J Eur Acad Dermatol Venereol. 2007;21:891–6.

63. Guillet G, Helenon R, Gauthier Y, et al. Progressive macular hypomelanosis of the trunk: primary acquired hypopigmentation. J Cutan Pathol. 1988;15:286–9.

64. Relyveld GN, Menke HE, Westerhof W. Progressive macular hypomelanosis: an overview. Am J Clin Dermatol. 2007;8:13–9.

65. Santos JB, Almeida OL, Silva LM, et al. Efficacy of topical combination of benzoyl peroxide 5% and clindamycin 1% for the treatment of progressive macular hypomelanosis: a randomized, double-blind, placebo-controlled trial. An Bras Dermatol. 2011;86:50–4.

66. Thng ST, Long VS, Chuah SY, et al. Efficacy and relapse rates of different treatment modalities for progressive macular hypomelanosis. Indian J Dermatol Venereol Leprol. 2016;82:673–6.

67. Sim JH, Lee DJ, Lee JS, et al. Comparison of the clinical efficacy of NBUVB and NBUVB with

benzoyl peroxide/clindamycin in progressive macular hypomelanosis. J Eur Acad Dermatol Venereol. 2011;25:1318–23.

68. Kim MB, Kim GW, Cho HH, et al. Narrowband UVB treatment of progressive macular hypomelanosis. J Am Acad Dermatol. 2012;66:598–605.

69. Duarte I, Nina BI, Gordiano MC, et al. Progressive macular hypomelanosis: an epidemiological study and therapeutic response to phototherapy. An Bras Dermatol. 2010;85:621–4.

70. Bilsland D, Dawe RS. Ultraviolet phototherapy and photochemotherapy of skin disease. In: Ferguson J, Dover JS, editors. Photodermatology. London: Manson Publishing Ltd; 1996. p. 113–24.

71. Zanolli MD, Feldman SR. Phototherapy treatment protocols for psoriasis and other phototherapy-responsive dermatoses. New York: Taylor & Francis Group; 2004.

72. Madigan LM, Al-Jamal M, Hamzavi I. Exploring the gaps in the evidence-based application of narrowband UVB for the treatment of vitiligo. Photodermatol Photoimmunol Photomed. 2016;32:66–80.

73. Kist JM, Van Voorhees AS. Narrowband ultraviolet B therapy for psoriasis and other skin disorders. Adv Dermatol. 2005;21:235–50.

74. Hexsel CL, Mahmoud BH, Mitchell D, et al. A clinical trial and molecular study of photoadaptation in vitiligo. Br J Dermatol. 2009;160:534–9.

75. Schneider LA, Hinrichs R, Scharffetter-Kochanek K. Phototherapy and photochemotherapy. Clin Dermatol. 2008;26:464–76.

76. Ibbotson SH, Bilsland D, Cox NH, et al. An update and guidance on narrowband ultraviolet B phototherapy: a British Photodermatology Group Workshop Report. Br J Dermatol. 2004;151:283–97.

77. de Gruijl FR, Rebel H. Early events in UV carcinogenesis – DNA damage, target cells and mutant p53 foci. Photochem Photobiol. 2008;84:382–7.

78. Cooper SJ, Bowden GT. Ultraviolet B regulation of transcription factor families: roles of nuclear factor-kappa B (NF-kappaB) and activator protein-1 (AP-1) in UVB-induced skin carcinogenesis. Curr Cancer Drug Targets. 2007;7:325–34.

79. Bishop DT, Demenais F, Iles MM, et al. Genome-wide association study identifies three loci associated with melanoma risk. Nat Genet. 2009;41:920–5.

80. Jin Y, Birlea SA, Fain PR, et al. Variant of TYR and autoimmunity susceptibility loci in generalized vitiligo. N Engl J Med. 2010;362:1686–97.

81. Teulings HE, Overkamp M, Ceylan E, et al. Decreased risk of melanoma and nonmelanoma skin cancer in patients with vitiligo: a survey among 1307 patients and their partners. Br J Dermatol. 2013;168:162–71.

82. Paradisi A, Tabolli S, Didona B, et al. Markedly reduced incidence of melanoma and nonmelanoma skin cancer in a nonconcurrent cohort of 10,040 patients with vitiligo. J Am Acad Dermatol. 2014;71:1110–6.

83. Shan X, Wang C, Tian H, Yang B, Zhang F. Narrowband ultraviolet B home phototherapy for vitiligo. Indian J Dermatol Venereol Lepro. 2014;80(4):336–8.

84. Tien Guan ST, Theng C, Chang A. Randomized, parallel group trial comparing home-based phototherapy with institution-based 308 excimer lamp for the treatment of focal vitiligo vulgaris. J Am Acad Dermatol. 2015;72(4):733–73.

85. Baltas E, Csoma Z, Ignacz F, et al. Treatment of vitiligo with the 308-nm xenon chloride excimer laser. Arch Dermatol. 2002;138:1619–20.

86. Hadi SM, Spencer JM, Lebwohl M. Treatment of vitiligo using the 308-nm excimer laser for the treatment of vitiligo. Dermatol Surg. 2004;30(7):983–6.

87. Hadi S, Tinio P, Al-Ghaithi K, Al-Quari H, Al-Helalat M, Lebwohl M, Spencer J. Treatment of vitiligo using the 308nm excimer laser. Photomed Laser Surg. 2006;24:354–7.

88. Zhang XY, He LY, Dong J, et al. Clinical efficacy of the 308-nm excimer laser in the treatment of vitiligo. Photodermatol Photoimmunol Photomed. 2010;26:138–42.

89. Hofer A, Hassan AS, Legat FJ, et al. The efficacy of excimer laser (308 nm) for vitiligo at different body sites. J Eur Acad Dermatol Venereol. 2006;20:558–64.

90. Al-Otaibi SR, Zadeh VB, Al-Abdulrazzaq AH, et al. Using a 308-nm excimer laser to treat vitiligo in Asians. Acta Dermatovenereol Alp Panonica Adriat. 2009;18(1):13–9.

91. Fa Y, Lin Y, Chi WH, et al. Treatment of vitiligo with 308-nm excimer laser: our experience from a 2 year follow-up of 979 Chinese patients. J Eur Acad Dermatol Venereol. 2017;31(2):337–40.

92. Le Duff F, Fontas E, Giacchero D, et al. 308 excimer lamp vs 308-nm excimer laser for treating vitiligo: a randomized study. Br J Dermatol. 2010;163:188–92.

93. Shi Q, Li K, Fu J, Wang Y, Ma C, Li Q, Li C, Gao T. Comparison of the 308-nm ecimer laser with the 308-nm excimer lamp in the treatment of vitiligo – a randomized bilateral comparison study. Photodermatol Photoimmunol Photomed. 2013;29(1):27–33.

94. Lopes C, Trevisanni VF, Melnik T. Efficacy and safety of 308-nm monochromatic Excimer lamp versus other phototherapy devices for vitiligo: a systemic review and meta-analysis. Am J Dermatol. 2016;17(1):23–32.

95. Kawalek AZ, Spencer JM, Phelps RG. Combined excimer laser and topical tacrolimus for the treatment of vitiligo: a pilot study. Dermatol Surg. 2004;30(2Pt1):130–5.

96. Passeron T, Ostovari N, Zakaria W, Fontas E, Larrouy JC, Lacour JP, Ortonne JP. Topical tacrolimus and the 308-nm excimer laser: a synergistic combination for the treatment of vitiligo. Arch Dermatol. 2004;140(9):1065–9.

97. Nistico S, Chiricozzi A, Saraceno R, Schipani C, Chimenti S. Vitiligo treatment with monochromatic excimer light and tacrolimus: results of an open

randomized controlled study. Photomed Laser Surg. 2012;30(1):26–30.

98. Matin M, Latifi S, Zoufan N, Koushki D, Mirhafari Daryasari SA, Rahdari F. The effectiveness of excimer laser on vitiligo treatment in comparison with a combination therapy of Excimer laser and tacrolimus in an Iranian population. J Cosmet Laser Ther. 2014;16(5):241–5.

99. Park OJ, Park GH, Choi JR, Jung HJ, ES O, Choi JH, Lee MW, Chang SE. A combination of excimer laser treatment and topical tacrolimus is more effective in treating vitiligo than either therapy alone for the initial 6 months, but not thereafter. Clin Exp Dermatol. 2016;41(3):236–41.

100. Hui-Lan Y, Xiao-Yan H, Jian-Yong F, Zong-Rong L. Combination of 308-nm excimer laser with topical pimecrolimus for the treatment of childhood vitiligo. Paediatr Dermatol. 2009;26(3):354–6.

101. Bae JM, Hong BY, Lee JH, Lee JH, Kim GM. The efficacy of 308-nm excimer laser/light (EL) and topical agent combination therapy versus EL monotherapy for vitiligo: a systematic review and meta-analysis of randomized controlled trials (RCTs). J Am Acad Dermatol. 2016;74(5):907–15.

Chemical Peels in Pigmentary Disorders

17

Rashmi Sarkar and Shivani Bansal

Chemical peeling is the application of a chemical agent to the skin, which causes the controlled destruction of a part or of the entire epidermis, with or without the dermis, leading to exfoliation and removal of superficial lesions, followed by the regeneration of new epidermal and dermal tissues. They act by thinning the stratum corneum, promoting epidermolysis, dispersing basal layer melanin and increasing collagen genes expression. Although melasma is the most prominent condition, chemical peels are used for various other pigmentary disorders like post-inflammatory hyperpigmentation, facial melanoses, freckles and lentigines and other skin conditions (Table 17.1). Chemical peeling has become an increasingly popular treatment modality for melasma, particularly as it eliminates pigment through exfoliation. It is an economical and relatively safe office procedure requiring minimal technical expertise [1].

The use of chemical peels for beautifying the skin dates back to ancient Egypt when sour milk (lactic acid) was used by Cleopatra to produce a more cosmetically elegant appearance of the skin

[2]. Dermatologists pioneered skin peeling for therapeutic purposes. In 1882, Unna described the use of salicylic acid, resorcinol, phenol and trichloroacetic acid (TCA) as skin peels, and in 1903, Mackee first started using phenol peels in acne scarring [3]. Stegman's work in the early 1980s on both animal and human models compared the histological changes of wound injury after chemical peeling, paving the way for chemical peeling in a controlled and scientific way on the human skin [4]. With Richard Glogau sensible photoaging classification and depth knowledge of wounding techniques, peeling can be accomplished by more technical accuracy than at any point in the history [5].

Many agents are available for chemical peeling today depending upon the depth of peeling (Table 17.2). New agents are being researched, and older agents are being used in different combinations and formulations to create new ways of peeling. The choice becomes relatively limited in treating a patient with a Fitzpatrick skin type IV or above [6]. This is because there is risk of prolonged hyperpigmentation in dark-skinned patients by deep chemical peels.

R. Sarkar (✉)
Department of Dermatology, Maulana Azad Medical College, New Delhi, India

S. Bansal
Kaya Skin Clinic, Preet Vihar, India

Alpha Hydroxy Peels

This family of naturally occurring acids includes glycolic acid, which is present in sugarcane; lactic acid, which is present in sour milk; malic acid,

© Springer International Publishing AG, part of Springer Nature 2018
P. Kumarasinghe (ed.), *Pigmentary Skin Disorders*, Updates in Clinical Dermatology,
https://doi.org/10.1007/978-3-319-70419-7_17

Table 17.1 Indications of chemical peel

1. *Pigmentary disorders* – melasma, freckles, lentigines, post-inflammatory hyperpigmentation, facial melanoses

2. *Acne* – acne vulgaris, comedonal acne, post-acne pigmentation, superficial scars

3. *Aesthetic* – photoaging, dilated pores, fine superficial wrinkles

4. *Epidermal growth* – wart, milia, seborrhoeic keratosis, actinic keratosis, dermatoses papulosa nigra

Table 17.2 Chemical peeling agents used in dark skin (Mark Rubin classification) [7]

Superficial peeling agents (epidermis to upper papillary dermis)
Trichloroacetic acid 10–35%
Glycolic acid solution 30–50% or glycolic gel 70%
Salicylic acid 20–30% in ethanol
Jessner's solution (Combes' formula)
Medium-depth peeling agents (epidermis to upper reticular dermis)
Trichloroacetic acid 50%
Glycolic acid solution 70%
Trichloroacetic acid 25% + glycolic gel 70%
Jessner's solution and trichloroacetic acid

which is present in apples; citric acid, which is present in oranges and other fruits; and tartaric acid, which is present in grapes. Of all the alpha hydroxy acids used as chemical peels for treatment of melasma, glycolic acid is considered the safest and most versatile peeling agent because it has the smallest molecule and penetrates the epidermis the best. It is used in solutions at concentrations varying between 25% and 70% and at a pH between 1 and 3; tolerance is generally good. The higher the concentration and the lower the pH, the more intense the peeling will be, but it remains superficial. Glycolic acid is always used over several sessions (generally six) several weeks apart (Fig. 17.1). As sessions progress, the concentration of the solution used and application time are progressively increased depending on tolerance [4]. It is less favourable as a peeling agent for melasma and post-inflammatory hyperpigmentation (PIH) because it may induce PIH in skin types V and VI. There have been ample

studies using GA for melasma in the ethnic skin. In most of these studies, there was a moderate improvement achieved in almost one-half of the patients [8–11]. As expected, the epidermal form showed the best response, followed by the mixed type, whereas the dermal variant was almost resistant to the effect of chemical peels. It is the only peel that is time dependent, can be neutralized easily, and has been found to be efficacious in dark-skinned patients such as Indians.

Lactic acid, also an alpha hydroxy acid having action similar to GA, has surprisingly not been used extensively as a peeling agent in the treatment of melasma, although it is a cheap and readily available agent. Sharquie et al. [12] did first pilot study on lactic acid and found it to be a safe and effective peeling agent for melasma in skin type IV. In their study of 20 patients, 92% pure lactic acid was applied for a maximum of six sessions, and a significant fall in MASI (56%) was observed in all the 12 patients who completed the study.

Alpha Keto Peels

Alpha keto acid is less hydrophilic than alpha hydroxyl acids; hence they are well suited for greasy surface. One member of this group which has gained significant attention in recent years is pyruvic acid. It has keratolytic, comedolytic, antimicrobial and sebostatic properties, and at dermal level it stimulates the formation of new collagen and elastic fibres. Apart from being effective for acne, photodamage and superficial scarring, the agent has also shown benefit in an epidermal and mixed melasma in light-skinned patients [13].

Beta Hydroxy Peels

Salicylic acid is the beta hydroxy acid family member which is a naturally occurring substance found in the bark of the willow tree. It functions as a keratolytic and comedolytic agent. It is one of the older peeling agents with first documented use by Unna, a German dermatologist. Salicylic acid due to its properties is used for acne but also

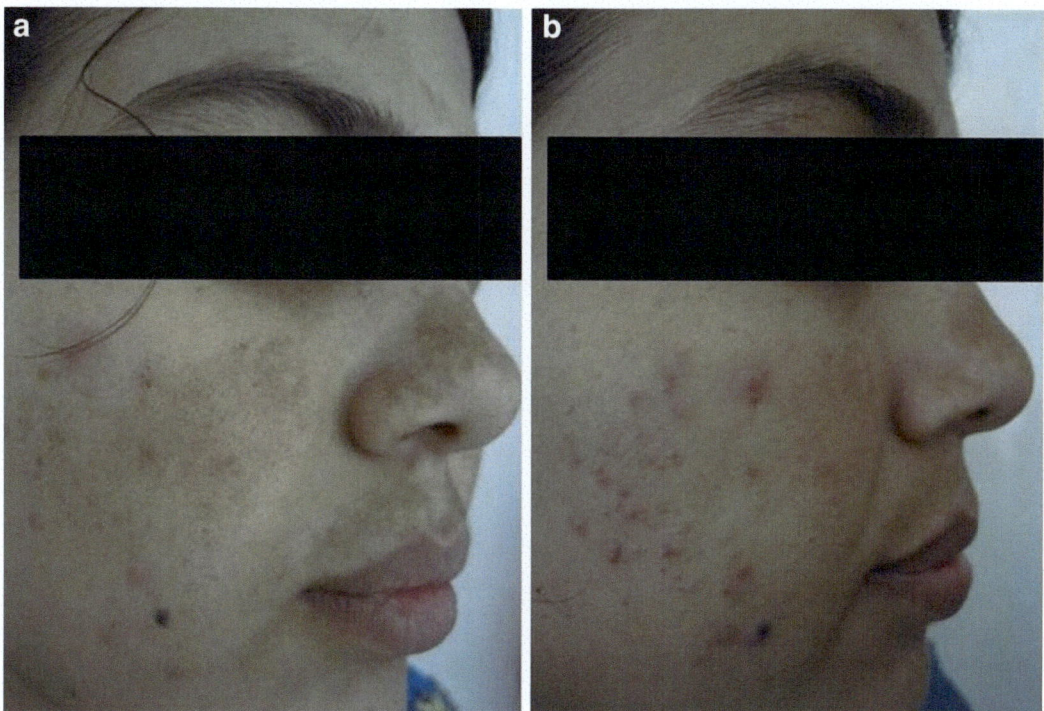

Fig. 17.1 Patient's photographs at baseline (**a**) and at 12 weeks (**b**) of treatment with glycolic acid peel

has been tried in pigmentary disorders like melasma. In fact, ethanol solutions of salicylic acid are excellent peeling agents for numerous conditions in dark-skinned individuals including acne, melasma and PIH. It has a diffuse whitening effect on the skin as shown in one study [14]. In a pilot study by Grimes et al. on dark-skinned individuals, 20–30% salicylic acid peel was used to treat acne, PIH and melasma, and it was observed that almost two-thirds of the patients with melasma showed a moderate improvement. Only mild side effects were noted in 16% patients which were transient and resolved in 1–2 weeks [15].

Salicylic-Mandelic Acid Peels

Salicylic-mandelic (SM) acid peel is a combination of an alpha hydroxy acid with a beta hydroxy acid. Mandelic acid (MA), because of its large molecular weight (MW), tends to remain on the skin surface longer and penetrates stratum corneum slowly thus producing a uniform epidermal

effect. Salicylic acid penetrates the skin quickly and provides an additional benefit of decreasing the PIH. Thus, the combination of these two agents would serve as an effective peeling agent especially for the ethnic skin. In our own experience, the combination does really well for various skin conditions like acne, post-acne scarring and pigment dyschromias including melasma. Decreasing MASI score was well-tolerated and better received by the patient (Fig. 17.2). In one recent study, SM peels had better sustained efficacy and fewer side effects than GA, presumably due to greater lipophilicity of SA and larger molecular size of MA. Mild, transient burning sensation was noted [16].

Trichloroacetic Acid Peels

Trichloroacetic acid (TCA) was first described by Roberts in 1926. It is usually prepared by a weight-to-volume aqueous solution. One hundred percent TCA is available in crystalform, which is colourless and ready to be diluted

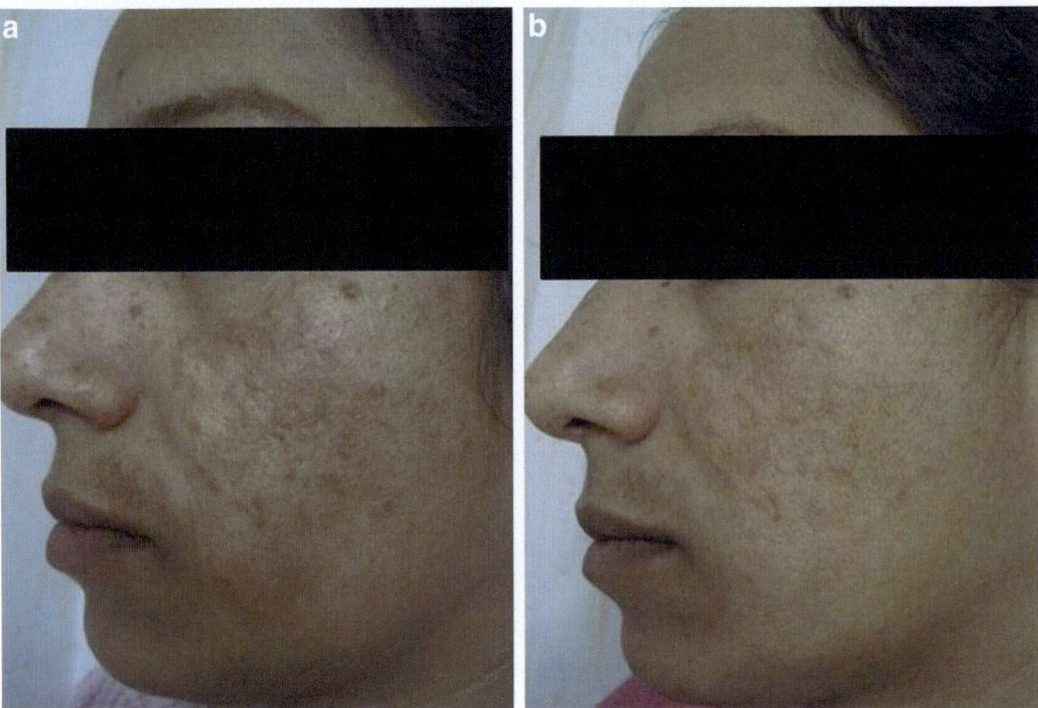

Fig. 17.2 Patient's photographs at baseline (**a**) and at 12 weeks (**b**) of treatment with salicylic-mandelic peel

withwater. To prepare a 30% concentration, 30 g of TCA crystals are added to distilled water to get a total volume of 100 mL. Similarly, various other concentrations can be prepared. The solution must be prepared fresh every 6 months. As the crystals are hygroscopic, they have to be stored in tightly capped, acid-resistant plastic or glass. Application of 10–25% TCA to the skin causes precipitation of proteins and coagulative necrosis. It causes necrosis of collagen in the papillary and reticular dermis in higher concentrations. It may be used alone or in combination with other agents such as glycolic acid or salicylic acid. Trichloroacetic acid is self-neutralizing and does not require water or bicarbonate to terminate the peeling action. The typical endpoint of a TCA peel is a white frost. In lighter complexions, this is sometimes a desirable effect; however, in skin types IV–VI, a frost is not desired and may carry risks of post peel dyschromia and scarring.

When used, only a low concentration of TCA (10–35%) is preferred which reaches up to the upper papillary dermis, and hence TCA peels are not appropriate for treating dermal and mixed forms of melasma [17]. In a comparative study on 40 Indian women by Kumari et al. [18], the decrease fall in MASI after six TCA (10–20%) peels proved to be an equally effective treatment modality as compared to similar number of 10–35% GA peels. But GA group has less side effects as compared to TCA group. To conclude, though, TCA peels may be as effective as GA peels for the treatment of pigment dyschromias.

Jessner's Solution

Formulated by Dr. Max Jessner, Jessner's solution is as follows: 14 g of resorcinol, 14 g of salicylic acid, 14 mL of lactic acid (85%), and add sufficient quantity to 100 mL ethyl alcohol(95%). The advantages of this formulation are that there is a synergistic effect caused by three keratolytic agents, as well as the additional of a phenolic skin-lightening agent (resorcinol) as one of the components [19]. Some authors combine Jessner's solutionwith a 35% TCA peel in the same session to obtain a medium-depth peel [19, 20]. The limitation of Jessner's solution is the storage requirement of a dark bottle to prevent photo-oxidation.

Tretinoin Peels

Retinol peels are having strong keratolytic, sebostatic and pigment elimination properties. Pigment elimination, textural improvements and photodamage correction are marked with this peel. In spite of the extensive use of topical tretinoin cream both alone and as a part of Kligman's formula for treating melasma, there is still a paucity of literature on the peel formulation of the agent which has shown favourable results in a few of the recent studies. RA is useful as a slow release peel as it can be used sequentially after SA or TCA peels.

The first successful use of tretinoin peel for melasma was done by Cuce et al. [21] in fair-skinned patients. Following this, a pilot study was carried out in dark-skinned patients by Khunger et al. [22], who compared 1% tretinoin peel with a standard 70% GA peel. Ten female patients of melasma were taken up for an open left-right comparison study of 12 weeks. One percent tretinoin peel was applied on one-half of the face, whereas 70% GA was applied on the other at weekly intervals. The fall in MASI at 6 and 12 weeks with tretinoin peel was similar to that achieved with the standard glycolic solution, with only minimal side effects.

Newer Peels

A number of newer peeling agents are being explored for various pigmentary dyschromias including melasma. An important drawback associated with the application of alpha hydroxyl peels on the skin is the need for neutralization and defining the exact time of neutralization. If the peel is neutralized too quickly, it fails to produce the desired effects; whereas, if the neutralization is delayed, it might lead to unwanted side effects. Easy phytic solution (50%) is a slow

release commercial proprietary product that is composed of phytic acid, in addition to a mixture of glycolic acid, lactic acid and phenyl glycolic (mandelic) acid and requires no external neutralization; hence the danger of overpeeling is avoided [23]. The peel allows progressive and sequential actuation of its acid in a nonaggressive manner. Phytic acid (2–4%) has proven to be efficient in the treatment of epidermal melasma, especially when associated with glycolic acid or retinoic acid. The typical burning sensation seen with the glycolic peel is not observed with the phytic acid peels. There was a statistically significant reduction in MASI in phytic group at the end of 12 weeks although the results were less gratifying than glycolic and SM peels [16].

Another agent is the Obagi blue peel. It is composed of a fixed concentration of TCA with the blue peel base (containing glycerine, saponins and a nonionic blue colour base). A reduction in the surface tension of TCA, water and glycerine occurs which ensures a slow and more uniform penetration of TCA [24]. In a split-face study of 18 Korean women, the Obagi blue peel was compared with a single sitting of 1550 nm erbium fibre laser. There was no difference between laser treatment and TCA peeling with respect to any outcome measure [25].

Another new peeling agent is acidified amino acid peels, which are carboxylated acidic amino acids, created by dissolution and acidification of natural amino acids due to their potent antioxidants, tyrosinase inhibitory and exfoliant action and are, therefore, effective against melasma [26]. As they have an alkaline pH (close to physiological pH), they are well-tolerated, especially in patients with dry and sensitive skin. They also offer hydration benefits by virtue of their amino acid group and are well-tolerated by patients. In a single-blind, randomized study, 31 patients with melasma were treated with 12 serial GA and amino fruit peels every 2 weeks for 6 months. There was significant decrease in MASI scoring ($P < 0.05$) at 3 and 6 months on both sides. Amino acid peels were less irritating [27].

In a recent study of 42 patients of melasma, efficacy and safety of (20% azelaic acid +10% resorcinol +6% phytic acid) were compared with

50% glycolic acid in split-face design. The efficacy of combination formula (azelaic acid, resorcinol and phytic acid) was similar to glycolic acid but with fewer complications [28].

Contraindications

Pregnant or nursing women, patients with hypersensitivity to the formulations, patients on any concurrent therapy, systemic illness and history of herpes labialis, keloidal tendencies, unrealistic expectations and women on oral contraceptives were few contraindications for chemical peeling.

Post Peel Instructions

To minimize complications and ensure early recovery, patients are advised to use broad-spectrum sunscreens and only bland moisturizers until peeling is complete. This is most important in dark-skinned patients in whom pigmentary alterations are common. Mild soap or a non-soap cleanser may be used.

Role of Priming Agents

The biggest drawback with the use of chemical peels for melasma in the ethnic skin is PIH which can either occur between the treatment sessions or after stopping treatment. This can be decreased by priming or preparing the skin. They help toachieve a more uniform penetration of peeling agents and accelerate healing and have a lightening effect by enhancing dispersion of melanin granules. In another study by Nanda et al., 2% hydroquinone was superior as a priming agent as compared to 0.025% tretinoin when used as an adjunct with 10–30% TCA peels [29]. In a study by Garg et al., 60 Indian patients with melasma were randomly allocated into three groups, receiving only glycolic peel, GA primed with 0.025% tretinoin and 2% hydroquinone, respectively [29]. The fall in MASI was the highest in the group receiving 2% hydroquinone as a priming agent with minimum relapse and PIH. In

another study by Nanda et al., 2% hydroquinone was superior as a priming agent as compared to 0.025% tretinoin when used as an adjunct with 10–30% TCA peels [30].

Summary

Treatment of melasma still remains challenging due to the prolonged duration of therapy. The substantial relapse rate, mainly attributed to inevitable persistence of the exacerbating factors (sun exposure), is still an obstacle. Chemical peels are used in various pigmentary disorders. It produces consistent reproducible results in people with dark complexions. There are many agents available for chemical peeling. The traditional glycolic peels prove to be the best both in terms of safety and efficacy. Lactic acid peels being relatively inexpensive and having shown equally good results in a few studies definitely need further experimentation. Easy phytic solution, a commonly used agent in our setup, might as well replace the conventional alpha hydroxy acids because of its unique properties, whereas the TCA peels still need to be used with caution in dark skin owing to the risk of pigment dyschromias. Patient selection is critical to outcome. With attention to skin type, peeling agent, peel concentration and duration of peel, you can achieve a high degree of satisfaction in patients of skin of colour.

References

1. Grimes PE. Melasma. Etiologic and therapeutic considerations. Arch Dermatol. 1995;131(12):1453–7.
2. Brody HJ, Monheit GD, Resnick SS, et al. A history of chemical peeling. Dermatol Surg. 2000;26:405–9.
3. Mackee GM, Karp FL. The treatment of post acne scars with phenol. Br J Dermatol. 1952;64:456–9.
4. Stegman SJ. A comparative histologic study of the effects of three peeling agents and dermabrasion on normal and sun damaged skin. Aesthet Plast Surg. 1982;6:123–35.
5. Glogou RG. Chemical peeling and aging skin. J Geriatr Dermatol. 1994;2:30–5.
6. Roberts WE. Chemical peeling in ethnic/dark skin. Dermatol Ther. 2004;17:196–205.

7. Rubin ME. Superficial and medium depth, Manual of chemical peels. Philadelphia: Lippincott; 1995. p. 17–25.
8. Lim JT, Tham SN. Glycolic acid peels in the treatment of melasma among Asian women. Dermatol Surg. 1997;23:177–9.
9. Javaheri SM, Handa S, Kaur I, Kumar B. Safety and efficacy of glycolic acid facial peel in Indian women with melasma. Int J Dermatol. 2001;40:354.
10. Grover C, Reddu BS. The therapeutic value of glycolic acid peels in dermatology. Indian J Dermatol Venereol Leprol. 2003;69:148–50.
11. Godse KV, Sakhia J. Triple combination and glycolic acid peels in melasma in Indian patients. J Cosmet Dermatol. 2011;10:68–9.
12. Sharquie KE, Al-Tikreety MM, Al-Mashhadani SA. Lactic acid as a new therapeutic peeling agent in melasma. Dermatol Surg. 2005;31:149–54.
13. Griffin TD, Van Scott EJ, Maddin S. The use of pyruvic acid as a chemical peeling agent. J Dermatol Surg Oncol. 1989;15:13.
14. Ahn HH, Kim IH. Whitening effect of salicylic acid peels in Asian patients. Dermatol Surg. 2006;32:372–5.
15. Grimes PE. The safety and efficacy of salicylic acid chemical peels in darker racial-ethnic groups. Dermatol Surg. 1999;25(1):18–22.
16. Sarkar R, Garg V, Bansal S, Sethi S, Gupta C. Comparative evaluation of efficacy and tolerability of glycolic acid, salicylic mandelic acid, and phytic acid combination peels in melasma. Dermatol Surg. 2016;42(3):384–91.
17. Zakopoulou N, Kontochristopoulos G. Superficial chemical peels. J Cosmet Dermatol. 2006;5:246–53.
18. Kumari R, Thappa DM. Comparative study of trichloroacetic acid versus glycolic acid chemical peels in the treatment of melasma. Indian J Dermatol Venereol Leprol. 2010;76:447.
19. Lawrence N, Cox SE, Brody HJ. Treatment of melasma withJessner's solution versus glycolic acid: a comparison ofclinical efficacy and evaluation of the predictive ability ofWood's light examination. J Am Acad Dermatol. 1997;36:589–93.
20. Monheit GD. The Jessner's trichloroacetic acid peel. Anenhanced medium-depth chemical peel. Dermatol Clin. 1995;13:277–83.
21. Cuce LC, Bertino MC, Scattone L, Birkenhauer MC. Tretinoin peeling. Dermatol Surg. 2001;25:12–4.
22. Khunger N, Sarkar R, Jain RK. Tretinoin peels versus glycolic acid peels in the treatment of Melasma in dark-skinned patients. Dermatol Surg. 2004;30:756–60.
23. Deprez P. Easy phytic solution: a new alpha hydroxy acid peel with slow release and without neutralization. Int J Cosmet Surg Aesth Dermatol. 2003;5:45–51.
24. Obagi ZE, Obagi S, Alaiti S, Stevens MB. TCA-based blue peel: a standardized procedure with depth control. Dermatol Surg. 1999;25:773–80.
25. Hong SP, Han SS, Choi SJ, Kim MS, Won CH, Lee MW, et al. Split-face comparative study of 1550 nm fractional photothermolysis and trichloroacetic acid 15% chemical peeling for facial melasma in Asian skin. J Cosmet Laser Ther. 2012;14:81–6.
26. Klein M. Amino fruit acids: the new cosmeceutical. Cosmet Dermatol. 2000;13:25–8.
27. Ilknur T, Bicak MU, Demirtaroglu M, Ozkan S. Glycolic acid peels versus amino fruit acid peels in the treatment of melasma. Dermatol Surg. 2010;36:490–5.
28. Faghihi G, Taheri A, Shahmoradi Z, Nilforoushzadeh MA. Solution of azelaic acid (20%), resorcinol (10%) and phytic acid (6%) versus glycolic acid (50%) peeling agent in the treatment of female patients with facial melasma. Adv Biomed Res. 2017;6:9.
29. Garg VK, Sarkar R, Agarwal R. Comparative evaluation of beneficiary effects of priming agents (2% hydroquinone and 0.025% retinoic acid) in the treatment of melasma with glycolic acid peels. Dermatol Surg. 2008;34:1032–40.
30. Nanda S, Grover C, Reddy BS. Efficacy of hydroquinone (2%) versus tretinoin (0.025%) as adjunct topical agents for chemical peeling in patients of melasma. Dermatol Surg. 2004;30:385–8.

Depigmenting Agents

18

Priyadarshani Galappatthy
and Deepani Rathnayake

Introduction

Depigmenting agents are widely used in the treatment of melasma and other disorders of hyperpigmentation. Some agents are used widely in cosmetic skin lightening products. Depigmenting agents are sometimes misused in ethnicities with pigmented skin. Although a large number of products are available as depigmenting agents, most agents have only limited evidence of their efficacy and long-term safety [1]. Most of the agents used as depigmenting agents target melanin found in pigment-producing cells, the melanocytes, which are responsible for skin pigmentation. The depigmenting agents act by inhibiting melanogenesis, interrupting melanosome transfer, accelerating epidermal desquamation and melanin turnover, antioxidant effects and by other methods [2].

Melanogenesis

Production of melanin in melanocytes is a key step which is targeted by several depigmenting agents as increased melanogenesis is responsible for pigmentation in most hyperpigmentory disorders. UV radiation activates tyrosinase, the key enzyme of melanogenesis [2]. Tyrosinase is a glycoprotein located in the membrane of the melanosome, where melanogenesis takes place. Tyrosinase catalyses the first two steps of melanin production (Fig. 18.1), the hydroxylation of L-tyrosine to L-dihydroxyphenylalanine (L-DOPA) and, the next step, oxidation of L-DOPA to L-dopaquinone which is subsequently converted to melanin [3, 4]. Oestrogens have shown to stimulate melanogenesis through the synthesis of melanogenic enzymes such as tyrosinase, tyrosinase-related proteins 1 and 2 (TRP-1, TRP-2). As tyrosinase catalyses main steps in melanin production, tyrosinase inhibitors are a main class of depigmenting agents.

Agents That Act by Tyrosinase Inhibition or Inhibiting Melanogenesis

Hydroquinone

Hydroquinone (HQ) is a hydroxyphenolic compound, and its depigmenting properties were discovered about 50 years ago [5]. HQ has been the gold standard for treating hyperpigmentation ever since. HQ acts by inhibiting tyrosinase, the rate-limiting enzyme in melanogenesis [6]. It inhibits

P. Galappatthy (✉)
Department of Pharmacology, Faculty of Medicine, University of Colombo, Colombo, Sri Lanka
e-mail: p.galappatthy@pharm.cmb.ac.lk

D. Rathnayake
Sinclair Dermatology,
East Melbourne, Victoria, Australia

© Springer International Publishing AG, part of Springer Nature 2018
P. Kumarasinghe (ed.), *Pigmentary Skin Disorders*, Updates in Clinical Dermatology,
https://doi.org/10.1007/978-3-319-70419-7_18

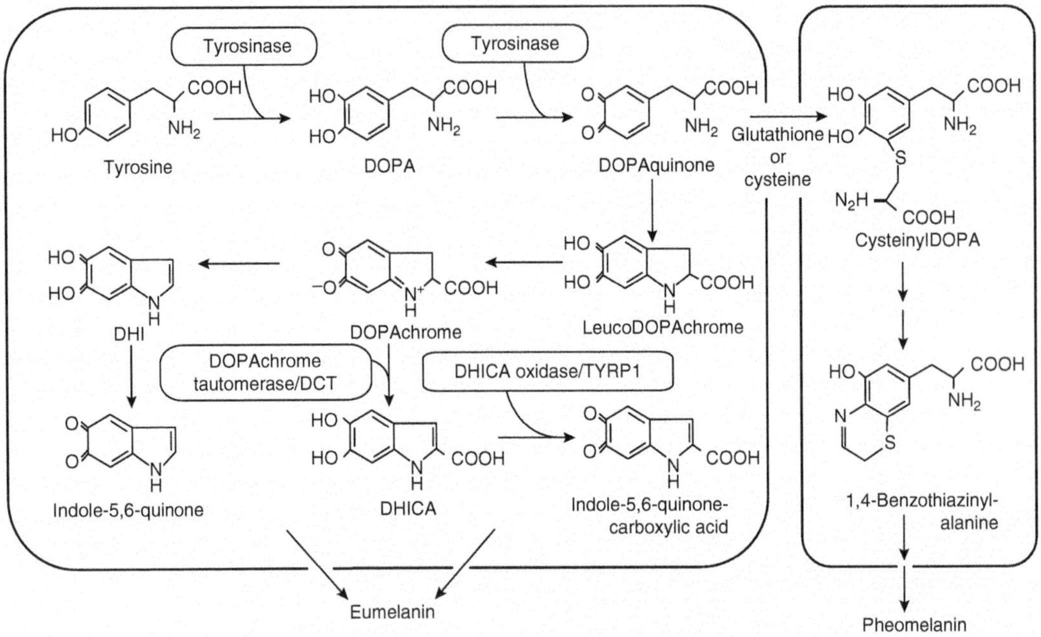

Fig. 18.1 Schematic of the melanin biosynthetic pathway. *DHI* - 5,6-dihydroxyindole, *DHICA* - 5,6-dihydroxyindole-2-carboxylic acid, *TRP* - tyrosinase-related protein, *DOPA* - 3,4-dihydroxyphenylalanine (Reproduced with permission from John Wiley and Sons and Copyright Clearance Center (License number 3982371163774, dated 5th Nov 2016) [146])

the conversion of l-3,4-dihydroxyphenylalanine to melanin by the competitive inhibition of tyrosinase. HQ also induces degradation of melanosomes and destruction of melanocytes by inhibiting DNA and RNA synthesis. HQ's oxidative products also cause oxidative damage to membrane lipids and proteins. HQ is a ubiquitous chemical found in many foods such as red wine, coffee, tea, wheat and fruits and herbal medications [5].

When applied to the skin, 45% of total dose of hydroquinone is absorbed quickly, and 30% reach the bloodstream in 1 h [7]. HQ is excreted slowly via urine, 35% getting excreted after 24 h [8]. The major part of HQ is metabolised and detoxified via the glucuronide and sulphate route which is excreted via the kidney. In humans, a small amount of HQ is not metabolised in the liver, and another small amount is converted into p-benzoquinone. The non-metabolised HQ and the p-benzoquinone are further conjugated with glutathione. These glutathione conjugates of HQ, which impair mitochondrial function, are known

to be nephrotoxins [7]. With normal use, the cream is applied every 24 h, and as excretion takes approximately every 72 h, it is likely that accumulation of HQ could occur.

HQ concentrations of 2–4% are commonly used to treat hyperpigmentation, but higher concentrations up to 10% can be compounded and used in refractory cases [9, 10]. HQ is widely prescribed by medical practitioners for the treatment of hyperpigmentation, and preparations with lower concentrations can be obtained over the counter in many parts of the world. HQ is also misused as skin whitening agents especially in dark-skinned populations.

Clinical Efficacy

A double-blind comparative placebo-controlled study comparing efficacy and tolerability of 4% HQ versus sunscreens used as placebo in melasma showed 40% of the patients having complete improvement compared to 10% in placebo group after 12 weeks of the treatment [11]. All patients given HQ showed some improvement, while 20% of the patients on placebo did not have any improvement. No serious adverse events were reported. Studies comparing HQ 4% cream versus 3% and 6% formulations did not show a significant difference in efficacy. However higher concentration showed more skin irritation [11]. It usually takes 5–7 weeks before the effect is apparent, and the treatment needs to be continued for 3–12 months [12]. HQ is also effective in the treatment of postinflammatory hyperpigmentation (PIH) [13, 14], which is seen more in darker-skinned patients [15].

HQ can be combined with other depigmenting agents to enhance efficacy. HQ 4% in combination with fluocinolone acetonide 0.01% and tretinoin 0.05% (triple-combination cream, TCC) is widely used in the treatment of melasma. Exfoliating effects of retinoid enhance penetration of HQ and steroids reduce skin irritation. TCC is approved by the US FDA for the treatment of facial melasma. Complete clearance of melasma was seen in 26% of patients after 8 weeks of TCC in one study [16]. Extended daily use of TCC for 12 months showed clearance of lesions in over 90% of patients. Although over 50% of participants experienced some form of side effects, these were transient and minimal and were confined to the application site. Only 1% withdrew from the study due to side effects [17]. A multicentre, randomised, controlled, blinded, parallel comparison study comparing TCC therapy with 4% hydroquinone in Asian patients for melasma showed TC therapy to be more effective [18]. Current evidence suggests that TCC treatment is an effective and safe treatment in melasma.

HQ 4% is also used in combinations with 10% buffered glycolic acid, vitamin C, vitamin E and sunscreen with good results [19]. Skin irritation was more common compared to control group which used sunscreen alone but could be managed with moisturisers [19]. Sequential treatment with TCC alternating with glycolic acid peels in patients with moderate to severe melasma showed excellent improvement of objectively assessed parameters of efficacy in over 90% of the participants, and treatments were well tolerated [20].

Most of the patients who were treated with TCC were able to achieve a good improvement of their melasma after 12 weeks of treatment. About half of treated patients were able to commence twice-weekly maintenance therapy after 12 weeks. However, majority of patients relapse during maintenance therapy [21]. In a multicentre study done in Brazil and Mexico, about 78% of patients were able to commence maintenance therapy after 8 weeks of daily treatment with TCC [22]. Twice-weekly maintenance therapy showed to be more effective in postponing relapses compared to tapering regimen (thrice weekly for 1 month, twice weekly for 1 month, weekly for 1 month). Therefore maintenance treatment is an important aspect in management of melasma [22]. However TCC should not be used beyond 6 months because of the possibility of steroid-induced atrophy and it cannot be used as maintenance therapy for melasma.

Tolerability and Safety

Even though HQ is an effective treatment for hyperpigmentation, controversies exist regarding its safety [23]. The side effects of HQ are dose and duration dependent. Skin irritation, erythema and transient hypopigmentation are common but do not need stopping medication. Small dots of depigmentation within the macules of melasma have been reported in some patients.

Paradoxical postinflammatory hyperpigmentation also can occur. Nail discoloration has been reported in some cases which is self-limiting on discontinuation of treatment [24, 25]. Exogenous ochronosis is an often feared side effect that can occur after prolonged use of high-concentration HQ [26]. It occurs due to accumulation of homogentisic acid causing degeneration of collagen and elastic fibres, leading to deposition of ochre-coloured fibres. This is usually a rare side effect seen mostly in dark-skinned people and clinically manifests as grey-brown hyperpigmentation and pinpoints hyperchromic papules. As exogenous ochronosis is difficult to treat, differentiating it from melasma and stopping of HQ is necessary. Dermoscopy is an important tool in diagnosing exogenous ochronosis [27] which shows densely pigmented structures obliterating some follicular openings. This typical appearance helps in early diagnosis and spares the need for a biopsy. Maintenance therapy with HQ has shown that daily treatment for 8 weeks is safe and able to maintain the effects achieved [28].

Nephrotoxicity, hepatic and renal adenomas and leukaemia have been reported in animal models following systemic absorption of HQ [7]. Because of the concerns of these side effects in humans, US FDA and many other regulatory authorities have banned HQ in over-the-counter skin lightening products. However some dermatologists are not in agreement with the ban as cancers are not reported in humans, and exogenous ochronosis is a very rare side effect with only 22 cases reported in the USA over the last 50 years [29]. The ban on hydroquinone in cosmetic products has led to research on many HQ-free skin lightening products which have shown promising results [30–32].

Monobenzyl Ether of Hydroquinone

Monobenzyl ether of hydroquinone (MBEH) destroys melanocytes causing permanent depigmentation [33]. It is approved by the US Food and Drug Administration (USFDA) in treatment of extensive vitiligo to permanently depigment the remaining normal skin. Confetti-like depigmentation occurs in parts other than where it is used when MBEH is wrongly used in melasma. It should never be used in melasma as it almost always causes permanent depigmentation.

Arbutin and Deoxyarbutin

Arbutin (hydroquinone-O-β-D-glucopyranoside), a derivative of hydroquinone, is a botanically derived compound found in cranberries, blueberries, wheat and pears. Deoxyarbutin is a synthetic form of arbutin. Arbutin acts as a depigmenting agent by inhibiting tyrosinase and thereby production of melanin [34]. Arbutin inhibit tyrosinase activity without affecting its mRNA expression. However arbutin and deoxyarbutin have less cytotoxicity on melanocytes than

HQ. Deoxyarbutin is as effective as HQ in treating hyperpigmentation and considered safe and less cytotoxic than HQ [35, 36]. Therefore arbutin and derivatives were considered to have the potential to become an important agent in cosmetic skin lightning creams [37].

The mild effect of arbutin is attributed to the controlled release of hydroquinone as a result of in vivo cleavage of the glycosidic bond. Concentrations up to 3% are used as skin whitening agents [38]. Higher concentrations of arbutin are more efficacious than lower concentrations but may cause paradoxical hyperpigmentation [39]. Arbutin derivatives may release hydroquinone under high temperature due to in vivo cleavage of the glycosidic bond, or they can be hydrolysed to HQ by skin bacteria during use [40].

Tolerability and Safety

The Scientific Committee on Consumer Safety (SCCS) recently reviewed the evidence on safety of deoxyarbutin for use in cosmetic products. As significant amounts of HQ can be formed when using 3% deoxyarbutin in face creams, the committee concluded that cosmetic products containing up to 3% deoxyarbutin are not safe to use [41].

Kojic Acid

Kojic acid (5-hydroxy-2-[hydroxymethyl]-4H-pyran-4-one) is derived from naturally occurring fungi like *Acetobacter* and *Aspergillus*. It reduces pigmentation by inhibiting production of free tyrosinase through chelation of copper in tyrosinase and inhibiting NF-κB in keratinocytes [42]. Kojic acid (KA) is used as a skin lightening agent in several cosmetic products [43]. KA originated in Japan and is also used as a food additive for preventing enzymatic browning of foods. KA is often produced during the fermentation of normal dietary food items. KA is used in concentrations ranging from 1% to 4% in topical preparations, and percutaneous absorption is 17% [44]. It is metabolised probably similar to dietary hexoses. Toxicity resulting from oral administration has not been reported [45].

Clinical Efficacy

KA 2% combined with HQ 2% was shown to be superior to glycolic acid (GA) 10% and HQ 2% in one double-blind study [46]. GA 5% with either 4% HQ or 4% KA for 3 months has shown equal efficacy in another study [47]. Concentrations over 2% have shown similar efficacy with other commonly used depigmenting agents, and adding KA has further improved melasma. One Indian study has shown that combination of KA and HQ has better synergistic effects in treating melasma than HQ and betamethasone valerate [48]. Concentrations lower than 1% are not as effective as 2% [49].

Tolerability and Safety

Allergic contact dermatitis is a concern when using KA concentrations higher than 1% in cosmetic skin lightening products [50, 51]. In vitro and in vivo mammalian studies have not shown mutagenicity or genotoxicity [44]. KA reversibly inhibits iodine uptake by the thyroid gland, leading to decreased thyroid hormone production and increased TSH, promoting thyroid hyperplasia and carcinogenesis (adenomas) in animal studies. However risk of affecting iodine metabolism and inducing thyroid adenomas in humans appears to be extremely low. Evaluation of toxicity of consuming KA at levels normally found in food and in topical applications has concluded that it does not present a concern for safety [44, 45]. Cosmetic Ingredient Review (CIR) expert panel concluded that KA concentrations up to 1% are safe to use in cosmetic products [52].

Azelaic Acid

Azelaic acid (AzA) is a naturally occurring compound originally derived from *Pityrosporum ovale*. It was discovered after investigation of hypopigmentation observed in pityriasis versicolor infections. AzA was initially developed as a topical treatment for acne. It is also used as a treatment for hyperpigmentation like melasma and PIH. Mechanisms of action include tyrosinase inhibition, inhibition of DNA synthesis and inhibiting mitochondrial enzymes in abnormal and hyperactive melanocytes inducing direct cytotoxic effects [53, 54]. Topical AzA has no depigmentation effect on normally pigmented skin as AzA has selective effects on abnormal melanocytes [55]. Free radicals are believed to contribute to hyperpigmentation following acne, and AzA also act by reducing free radical production [56]. AzA also has antibacterial properties on several dermal microflora including *Staphylococcus aureus*, *Staphylococcus epidermidis* and *Propionibacterium acnes* making it useful in treatment of acne. Percutaneous absorption is 3% from application of 20% AzA, but increased absorption up to 8% was noted with different vehicles used. Parenterally administered AzA is rapidly distributed and extensively eliminated via urinary excretion [57]. Animal studies have shown that AzA is non-toxic, non-mutagenic and non-teratogenic [54].

Clinical Efficacy

Topical AzA 20% cream is used as an off-label treatment in melasma. However it is available by prescription and should be applied twice daily, and treatment should be given for at least 2–3 months. AzA 20% is available to treat acne as well as for treatment of postinflammatory hyperpigmentation in acne. A 16-week controlled study of 15% AzA in mild to moderate acne in patients with dark skin showed improvement of both acne and the hyperpigmentation [58]. A 24-week multicentre, randomised, double-blind, parallel-group study of assessing the efficacy, safety and tolerability of AzA 20% cream, compared with its vehicle for the treatment of facial hyperpigmentation, showed that the AzA group had significant improvement of the pigmentation [56]. AzA 20% cream has also shown to be as effective as 4% HQ in the treatment of melasma [59]. An open-label study of 20% AzA twice-daily application found that it is more effective than 4% HQ cream daily for melasma [60]. Combination of AzA 20% with glycolic acid 15% showed comparable efficacy when compared to 4% HQ in treating facial pigmentation with more irritation in Aza and GA group. This study did not show any benefit of adding GA to AzA, but patients had more irritant side effects [61]. Combining AzA and retinoic acid is especially helpful in PIH in acne [62].

Tolerability and Safety

Side effects of AzA are mostly mild and transient and do not need stopping the medication. Pruritus, burning, stinging, tingling, erythema and skin peeling had been reported in less than 5% of patients. Skin peeling and dermatitis are rarer side effects. After 4 weeks of use, significantly more burning and stinging were seen in patients compared to vehicle [56].

4-n-Butylresorcinol

Anti-melanogenic compound, 4-n-butylresorcinol, has been shown to inhibit the activities of tyrosinase and tyrosinase-related protein-1 (TRP-1) in vitro [63]. A randomised, double-blind split-face study of liposome-encapsulated 4-n-butylresorcinol showed a significant improvement in the treated side of the face compared with the control side without any adverse events [64].

Antioxidants

Antioxidants are thought to cause skin lightening effects primarily by preventing melanogenesis induced by ultraviolet radiation. Oxidative effects and production of reactive oxygen species (ROS) by UV radiation induce melanogenesis by activating tyrosinase. Antioxidants can also reduce direct photo-oxidation of pre-existing melanin. Ascorbic acid and alpha tocopherol are two main antioxidants used in skin lightening products.

Ascorbic Acid

Ascorbic acid (AsA) or vitamin C is a water-soluble vitamin and is the most abundant antioxidant in the human skin. AsA interferes with melanin synthesis by inhibiting tyrosinase through chelation of copper ions at the active site of tyrosinase. AsA also acts by scavenging ROS by neutralising free radicals [65]. Vitamin C and

its several derivatives are available as creams, serum and dermal patches in the market. Magnesium ascorbyl phosphate (MAP) is the most stable derivative. MAP is a lipophilic molecule and theoretically easily absorbed in to the skin. Active form of vitamin C, L-ascorbic acid, is colourless and unstable and on exposure to light is converted to dehydroascorbic acid giving it a yellow colour [66]. The stability of vitamin C is maintained at pH less than 3, at which it is non-ionised and penetrates well through the stratum corneum [67].

Optimum percutaneous absorption is seen at maximum concentration of 20%. Daily application for 3 days saturates dermal concentration and takes 4 days to disappear from the skin. As UV light reduces vitamin C levels, it is better to apply after exposure to UV light. Other derivatives of vitamin C such as MAP, ascorbyl-6-parmitate and dehydroascorbic acid were shown to be poorly absorbed through the skin [67]. Recommended oral dose of ascorbic acid is 60 mg daily. When vitamin C is taken more than 60 mg daily orally, tissue stores get saturated and urinary elimination occurs. However in some healthy volunteers, urinary excretion does not occur until 100 mg is taken and absorption and bioavailability declines after 500 mg [68]. 1000–3000 mg daily dose is recommended for skin lightening effects, and lower than 400 mg daily probably has no clinical value. Even though toxicity of vitamin C is rare, doses over 1000 mg daily can cause gastrointestinal discomfort. Therefore, topical application of vitamin C can achieve higher concentration in the skin than oral vitamin C and more beneficial as a skin whitening agent.

Clinical Efficacy

A double-blind study comparing 5% AsA and 4% HQ in melasma found 62.5% and 93% improvement in the two groups, respectively [69]. Side effects were present in 68.7% with HQ versus 6.2% with AsA. The study concluded that even though HQ showed better efficacy, AsA may play a role in melasma and as a skin whitening product as it is almost devoid of any side effects [69]. In another study, 25% l-ascorbic acid and a chemical penetration enhancer showed significant improvement of pigmentation in melasma patients after 16 weeks [70].

MAP is part of many cosmetic products. Although one in vitro study has shown poor absorption of MAP [67], another clinical study has shown 10% MAP to have significant skin lightening effects in melasma and senile freckles [71]. More patient satisfaction and improvement had been seen in melasma patients treated with Q-switched Nd:YAG combining with ultrasonic application of vitamin C in a split-face study [72].

Human studies of oral vitamin C in melasma have been mostly done in combination with other oral agents. A randomised, double-blind, placebo-controlled trial was done comparing an oral product containing procyanidin with vitamins A, C and E for melasma among 60 Filipino women [73]. This trial which used 60 mg of vitamin C evaluated changes in pigmentation using a mexameter. The study showed significant improvement in the Melasma Area and Severity Index (MASI) and concluded that oral procyanidin given with vitamins A, C and E was safe and effective for epidermal melasma when given orally for a period of 8 weeks.

Tolerability and Safety

Topical vitamin C has high safety profile. It can be used on a daily basis for a long duration. AsA can safely be combined with other depigmenting and anti-ageing products like retinoic acid, glycolic acid and sunscreens. Oxidative changes of topical vitamin C on the skin can cause yellowish discoloration of the skin and can stain cloths. Stinging and erythema are rare side effects [74].

Vitamin E

Vitamin E is a lipophilic antioxidant in the body. Increasing intracellular glutathione, interference with lipid peroxidation of melanocyte membranes and inhibiting tyrosinase bring about its depigmenting effects. Vitamin E consists of eight naturally occurring compounds having vitamin E activity, four tocopherols and four tocotrienols [75]. In humans, alpha tocopherol is the most abundant vitamin E derivative, followed by gamma tocopherol. Alpha tocopherol is the most commonly used compound [76]. There is limited data on the efficacy of vitamin E in treating hyperpigmentation or as a skin lightening agent. It is however commonly used in combination with other products.

Alpha tocopherol is the predominant vitamin E in the human skin, and gamma tocopherol is also found in epidermis, dermis and stratum corneum [77]. After exposure to UV light, the amount of alpha tocopherol decreases by about 50%. Depletion of alpha tocopherol in the skin is an early and sensitive indicator of photo-oxidative damage to the skin. Alpha tocopherol is regenerated from photo-oxidised alpha tocopherol in the presence of other antioxidants such as ascorbate which gets regenerated by glutathione. Vitamin E is shown to be the predominant antioxidant barrier in the human skin [78]. Nonnucleated stratum corneum lacks antioxidants compared to the nucleated epidermal and dermal layers. Therefore application of these antioxidants, vitamin E and vitamin C, prior to UV exposure reduces acute sun damage as well as chronic photoaging and also improves pigmentation [79]. Most vitamin E products are available as esters for stability which act as prodrugs and have to be hydrolysed to active vitamin E after dermal absorption. Bioconversion of vitamin E esters to vitamin E is much less in stratum corneum than in dermal layers [80]. Different skincare products contain variable amounts of vitamin E esters ranging from 2% to 36%, and there is a lack of data on dose-response relationship of effects of different vitamin E preparations.

Clinical Efficacy

A double-blind study showed a significant improvement of melasma and pigmented contact dermatitis lesions using topical vitamins E and C [81]. Combination of vitamins has been more effective than either agent as monotherapy. Another randomised double-blind trial using a facial lotion containing 4% niacinamide, 0.5% panthenol and 0.5% tocopheryl acetate daily in Indian women showed skin lightening effects and improvement of pigmentation [82]. An animal study investigating the

effects of oral and topical preparations of vitamin E in mice has shown that supplementation
with topical α-tocopherol or topical tocopheryl
succinate or oral α-tocopheryl acetate can
reduce the incidence of acute and chronic damage to the skin induced by UVR such as sunburn, pigmentation and skin cancer [83].
Another study in mice showed oral vitamin E
alone or combined with L-selenomethionine
was effective in protection against UV-induced
blistering, pigmentation and skin cancer [84].
The study which showed efficacy of an oral
product containing procyanidin with vitamins
A, C and E for melasma had 15IU of D-alpha-
tocopherol acetate [73].

Tolerability and Safety

Topical application of vitamin E is well tolerated
except for mild transient burning sensation.
However long-term use of oral vitamin E supplements above daily requirement could be harmful
and has potential haemorrhagic risks.

Glutathione

Glutathione is a ubiquitous compound found in
our body containing SH groups which interact
with biological systems. It exists in cells in
reduced form (GSH) and gets oxidised into oxidised glutathione (GSSG) which gets converted
back to GSH catalysed by glutathione reductase
[85]. Glutathione has depigmenting effects due to
inhibition of tyrosinase by binding to copper containing active site of the enzyme and antioxidant
effects due to the presence of SH groups and
shifting melanogenesis from eumelanin to pheomelanin synthesis.

Glutathione is available as topical preparations (creams and face washes), oral preparations
(capsules and sublingual tablets) and intravenous
injections. Oral glutathione is marketed as a
dietary supplement or a nutraceutical either alone
or in combination with vitamin C and other antioxidants. It is absorbed by upper jejunum and
excreted via the kidneys. After absorption, it is
broken down to the amino acids and reformed
intracellularly [79].

Clinical Studies

Topical GSSG 2% lotion twice-daily application
was found to significantly improve melanin
index, moisture content of the stratum corneum,
skin smoothness, skin elasticity and wrinkle formation over placebo after 10 weeks [86]. GSSG
was preferred as GSH is unstable in aqueous
solutions. There are only two studies published
up to now on efficacy and safety of oral glutathione. One randomised, double-blind, placebo-
controlled study conducted among 60 Thai
medical students demonstrated skin lightening
with oral glutathione 250 mg twice daily taken
for 1 month compared to placebo [87]. A second
recent open-label study also demonstrated similar skin lightening effects in 30 subjects who
received a lozenge formulation containing
reduced L-glutathione with selenium, vitamin C,
vitamin D3, vitamin E and grapeseed extract
[88]. There is one published clinical trial to date
evaluating efficacy and safety of parenteral glutathione for skin lightening. Sixteen healthy
Pakistani women aged 25–47 years were given iv
glutathione with vitamin C twice weekly for
6 weeks compared to placebo group who were
given iv normal saline. There was improvement
of skin tone in 37%, but the improvement was
gradually lost after stopping treatment in all participants but one. There were significant side
effects with the treatment [89].

However this route is now increasingly used
without much evidence of its efficacy and with
serious risks of side effects particularly when
used by unqualified practitioners.

Tolerability and Safety

Postulated and observed adverse effects of glutathione include lightening of hair colour, hypopigmented patches and depletion of natural hepatic
stores of glutathione with long-term supplementation, which could have potentially dangerous consequences. Systemic glutathione could
also increase the susceptibility to melanoma as
long-term administration switches eumelanin to
pheomelanin [79]. As there is insufficient data
on efficacy and safety of glutathione products,
no regulatory authority has granted approval
for its use as a skin whitening agent. US FDA

in 2015 issued a warning to consumers on the dangers associated with the use of injectable skin lightening agents, such as glutathione [90]. Philippine FDA also has issued a similar warning where use of glutathione is common. Other recent publications have also warned about the dangers and unethical use of glutathione for skin whitening [91–93]. The other adverse effects reported with the use of intravenous glutathione include toxicity to the kidneys, liver and nervous system and serious cutaneous eruptions such as Stevens–Johnson syndrome and toxic epidermal necrolysis.

Methimazole

Methimazole is an oral antithyroid agent which has been used for that purpose over 50 years. It causes depigmentation of the skin when used topically due to inhibition of melanin synthesis [94]. Methimazole causes inhibition of peroxidase both in thyroid cells and melanocytes interfering with different steps in the biosynthesis of eumelanin and pheomelanin pigments. It is also an inhibitor of tyrosinase. Topical methimazole had been tested as a hydroquinone free skin depigmenting agent over the recent years after concerns of cytotoxic and mutagenic side effects of HQ. After a single topical application of 5% methimazole, it was undetectable in the serum from 15 min up to 24 h, but after oral administration, methimazole was detected in serum in 15 min and remained detectable in serum up to 24 h [95]. Long-term topical methimazole applications in melasma patients did not induce any significant changes in thyroid functions.

Clinical Efficacy
Depigmenting effects of topical methimazole in the human skin was first reported in 2005 by Kasraee et al. in a single case report [94]. Topical application of 5% methimazole daily showed improvement of PIH following acid burns in a 27-year-old male after 6 weeks. Two patients with melasma who were resistant to topical HQ reported significant improvement after 8 weeks of topical 5% methimazole [96]. Current data on

the efficacy of methimazole as a depigmenting agents are limited to a few case studies. There is a need for randomised controlled trials using a large number of patients to further determine its efficacy.

Tolerability and Safety
Topical methimazole is very well tolerated and not melanocytotoxic. Long-term topical use of 5% methimazole in 20 melasma patients did not show significant changes in serum TSH, free thyroxine and free triiodothyronine levels [95]. There were no reported cutaneous side effects. However topical methimazole is not recommended as a skin bleaching cream on a large skin area in normal individuals.

Agents Interrupting Melanosome Transfer

Niacinamide

Niacinamide is a biologically active form of niacin (vitamin B3) and is an important precursor of cellular coenzymes, NADH (nicotinamide adenine dinucleotide) and NADPH (nicotinamide adenine dinucleotide phosphate). The effect of niacinamide on hyperpigmentation is believed to occur through inhibition of melanosome transfer from melanocytes to keratinocytes. Niacinamide has shown to inhibit 35–68% of melanosome transfer [97].

Topical niacin and niacinamide in concentrations up to 5% are used as hypopigmenting agents [98]. Both are readily absorbed from the skin, blood and the intestines and are widely distributed throughout the body. Excretion is primarily through the urinary tract. Both are relatively nontoxic [99]. They have shown efficacy when used alone or in combination with other agents such as HQ [100], N-acetyl glucosamine [101], vitamin C [102], sunscreens and N-undecyl-10-enoyl-L-phenylalanine [103]. Although oral niacinamide is used as a pharmacological agent for a variety of other conditions [104], there were no studies showing efficacy of oral niacinamide in skin whitening.

Clinical Efficacy

A double-blind, randomised clinical trial of nia-cinamide 4% versus HQ 4% in a split-face study in 27 patients with melasma showed improve-ment in MASI score in 44% of patients in nico-tinamide group compared to 55% in HQ group [100]. The effects were evident in 4 weeks in HQ group and in 8 weeks in nicotinamide group. Topical nicotinamide had significantly less side effects. The study concluded that nicotinamide is safe and effective for treatment of melasma and safe to use over long term. Daily use of niacina-mide and sunscreens showed better skin lighten-ing effects compared to sunscreens alone [90].

Five percent topical niacinamide had shown improvement of pigmentation in another 12-week double-blind placebo-controlled split-face study, compared to the control [105]. The study also showed improvement of features of skin ageing such as fine wrinkles, texture, blotchiness and yellowing.

Topical nicotinamide works well in combina-tion with other depigmenting agents. Topical for-mulation containing niacinamide and N-acetyl glucosamine was significantly more effective than vehicle control in one study [101]. Combination of topical vitamin C and niacina-mide was an effective treatment for pigmentation and addition of ultrasound radiation-enhanced epidermal delivery of the agents [102].

Tolerability and Safety

Side effects of topical niacinamide are rare and minor and improve with continuous use. Mild skin burning, pruritus and erythema had been reported [100]. Both niacin and niacinamide are accepted for use in cosmetics in Japan and the European Union. The cosmetics ingredient review panel considered niacin and niacinamide at its current low concentrations used in cosmet-ics as safe [99].

Lectins

Lectins improve hyperpigmentation by revers-ibly inhibiting melanosome transfer from mela-nocytes to keratinocytes. Lectins and niacinamide combination has enhanced depigmenting effects [98]. Lectins have shown 15–44% inhibition of melanosome transfer under experimental condi-tions [2].

Agents Accelerating Epidermal Desquamation and Melanin Turnover

Retinoids

Depigmenting effects of retinoids are brought about by interfering with pigment transfer, accel-erating epidermal desquamation, enhancing cell turnover and, therefore, pigment loss. Tretinoin, or retinoic acid (RA), also inhibits transcription of the key melanin synthesis enzyme tyrosinase. Retinoids are used in combination with HQ and enhance its penetration and efficacy [53, 106, 107]. Topical retinoids, tretinoin and adapalene are used in gel, cream and liquid forms in con-centrations ranging from 0.01% to 0.1%. Adapalene is a synthetic retinoid having greater selectivity than tretinoin for certain retinoic acid receptors. When used in combination with HQ and steroids, retinoids enhance the depigmenting effect of HQ and minimise skin atrophy caused by steroids.

Clinical Efficacy

Topical retinoids are commonly used in treat-ment of acne and photoaging. It is a useful ther-apy in PIH following acne. It is not approved as monotherapy in the treatment of melasma. However retinoid, HQ and steroid triple therapy is FDA approved to treat melasma.

Several studies showed improvement of melasma and PIH with topical retinoids given as monotherapy. Griffiths et al. showed 68% clini-cal improvement of melasma in Caucasian women after treatment with 0.1% tretinoin, while worsening of pigmentation was noted in control group [108]. Another double-blind, randomised controlled study in 30 African-American patients showed improvement of melasma with 0.1% tret-inoin compared to vehicle group at 40 weeks [109]. Tretinoin 0.1% cream showed 40% improvement of PIH on the face and arms after 40 weeks of treatment in patients with black skin

[110]. Topical tretinoin 0.1% cream showed 90% improvement of pigmentation associated with photoaging, after 40 weeks in Chinese and Japanese patients [111].

Adapalene 0.1% was found to have comparable efficacy to tretinoin 0.05% cream in melasma with fewer side effects [112]. Even though available clinical studies show good clinical efficacy of topical retinoids as monotherapy in treating melasma and PIH, better results are obtained in combination with other depigmenting agents. Moreover retinoids as monotherapy needs to be used for a longer periods to obtain the results. Topical tretinoin 0.1% has been effective in treating PIH in combination with GA peels and hydroquinone in dark-skinned individuals [113].

Tolerability and Safety

Retinoid dermatitis is the most common side effects of topical retinoids and usually seen in the first few weeks of starting treatment. Burning sensation, itching, erythema, scaling and dry skin are commonly seen. These side effects are reversible on discontinuation of therapy. Mild skin irritation settle after a few weeks of usage. PIH or hypopigmentation is more common in dark skin and can persist for few months after discontinuation of treatment. In the study done by Griffith et al., the cutaneous reactions were reported in 88% of patients compared to 29% on vehicle group [108]. Photosensitivity has been reported with topical retinoids. Therefore retinoid creams should be used at night, and sunscreens are needed during daytime. Topical retinoids should not be used in pregnant women due to potential teratogenic effects.

Hydroxy Acids and Other Acids

Hydroxy acids are a group of natural compounds found in sugar cane, citrus fruits and milk. Alpha hydroxy acid has the smallest molecule size of the group and has the advantage of better penetration of the epidermis. Alpha hydroxy acid accelerates the epidermal desquamation and improves skin pigmentation [114]. Concentrations up to 10% are commonly available in skincare products like creams, cleansers and soaps. Alpha hydroxy acids are more commonly used in chemical peels for melasma, acne and in products used for treatment of skin wrinkling. Higher concentrations are used in chemical peels. Skin irritation, erythema and itching are some commonly reported side effects of alpha hydroxy acids, and concomitant use of sunscreens are recommended to minimise skin irritation.

Salicylic acid and linoleic acid improve hyperpigmentation by accelerating turnover of stratum corneum. Salicylic acid is also used as a peeling agent to treat hyperpigmentation.

Other Agents

Tranexamic Acid

Tranexamic acid (TXA) is a synthetic derivative of lysine, indicated in preventing abnormal fibrinolysis to reduce blood loss. It reversibly blocks the lysine-binding sites on plasminogen molecules, inhibiting the plasminogen activator from converting plasminogen to plasmin. Plasminogen also exists in human epidermal keratinocytes. Ultraviolet light induces plasmin activity which can activate precursors of the melanogenesis like membrane phospholipids, arachidonic acid and prostaglandins [115]. TXA inhibits plasminogen activation, binding of plasminogen to the keratinocytes resulting in reduction in formation of prostaglandins and arachidonic acid, which are inflammatory mediators involved in melanogenesis. TXA is probably the only treatment that can prevent the activation of melanocyte by various stimuli such as sunlight, hormones and injured keratinocytes through the inhibition of the plasminogen activation. It can also reduce the likelihood of recurrence of pigmentation after other treatments that damage the melanocytes (peels, lasers), which activate melanogenesis. TXA also inhibits the melanin synthesis via decreasing the α-melanocyte-stimulating hormone (α-MSH). TXA has also been reported to suppress neovascularization induced by basic fibroblast growth factor.

Topical, oral, intradermal, intravenous and other methods of delivery of TXA have been used as hypopigmenting agents with varying results [115]. Topical TXA up to 5% are used as monotherapy or in combination with HQ and steroids for treatment of melasma. A liposomal formulation of topical TXA is available [116]. Iontophoresis of TA using chemical enhancer and constant electric current is also possible [117]. Oral doses of 250 mg twice a day for 6 months [118] and 750 mg three times a day for 2 months have been used in treating melasma [119]. Usual effective dose of TXA for depigmentation is 250 mg 2–3 times daily, much lower than the doses used to reduce excessive bleeding. Clinical response is seen in about 1 month [120]. Intravenous TXA is also used at a dose of 500 mg every 2–4 weeks, as a bolus intravenous injection or as an infusion with normal saline together with ascorbic acid. Absorption of TXA is not affected by food, and peak plasma concentrations are reached within 3 h, and 90% of the drug is eliminated in 1 day. TA can cross the blood–brain barrier and the placenta. TXA seems to have a very safe profile in recent studies involving over 20,000 patients given TXA following trauma, and the theoretical thrombotic risk is shown to be very low [120].

Clinical Studies

Topical TXA 2% showed improvement in the pigmentation in 80% of subjects when given for 5–18 weeks with no significant side effects [121]. A study using 5% TXA in Asian patients in a split-face study showed no effect after 3 months of application compared to the vehicle, with more skin irritation seen with TXA [122]. In another study comparing the safety and efficacy of 3% topical TXA with 3% hydroquinone and 0.01% dexamethasone showed that the TXA is as effective as the cumulative effect of hydroquinone and dexamethasone, with lesser side effects [123]. Another split-face study comparing 5% liposomal TXA with 4% HQ showed equal results after 12 weeks [121, 122]. Skin irritation was noticed in HQ group without any irritation noted with TXA. In 100 women with melasma, intradermal microinjection of TXA for 12 weeks resulted in 76.5% improvement of MASI score with no significant side effects [124].

A number of studies reported in literature have evaluated varying doses of oral TXA either alone or in combination with other agents for treatment of melasma. In one of the first studies, Hajime et al. in 1985 showed reduction of melasma severity in 33 out of 40 patients following 10 weeks of oral TA 1–1.5 g daily [115]. Over 90% of 74 patients showed improvement of melasma with oral TA 250 mg twice daily taken for 6 months in another study [125]. A prospective, randomised controlled trial with TA at a dose of 250 mg twice a day for 3 months compared to usual topical therapy in 260 patients with melasma showed significant decrease in the mean MASI score at 8 and 12 weeks [126]. Addition of oral tranexamic acid to fluocinolone-based TCC was shown to produce faster and sustained improvement of melasma. Oral TXA has also shown efficacy when given in combination with light or laser therapy in patients with melasma without serious adverse effects [127, 128]. Oral TXA 250 mg twice daily in 25 patients with refractory melasma showed 70% improvement of MASI score after 3–4 months of use in another study [129]. A recent retrospective study done by Lee HC et al. in 561 Asian patients with melasma showed 89% of patients showing improvement in pigmentation with oral TXA [1]. There was one case of DVT reported who was later found to have familial protein S deficiency. The authors suggested screening for coagulation disorders before commencing oral TXA for melasma. According to available clinical studies, the usual effective dose of TXA in treating pigmentary disorders is 250–500 mg daily, much lower than the doses used to treat bleeding. The duration of treatment and repeated courses of treatments appear to be more effective than increasing dose.

Tolerability and Safety

The commonly reported side effects of TXA are nausea, diarrhoea and orthostatic hypotension. No mutagenic activity or harmful foetal effects have been reported. Adverse events that have been reported include anaphylactic shock, skin reaction and acute renal cortical necrosis. TXA has no effect on coagulation parameters. TXA seems to have a very safe profile, and the theoretical thrombotic risk is very low. However proper history should be taken, and a clinical examination should be done to exclude any potential risk of thromboembolism. Coagulation screening needs to be done when relevant. Skin irritation could occur with topical TXA.

Steroids

The exact mechanisms of skin lightening effects of topical steroids are not completely known, but possible mechanisms include vasoconstriction, reduction of activity and number of melanocytes and reducing MSH activity. Steroids might also alter melanocyte function by inhibition of prostaglandin or production of melanogenic cytokines such as endothelin-1 and granulocyte macrophage colony-stimulating factor [131]. Steroids can inhibit these cytokine mediated UV-induced melanogenesis by various cells of the epidermis.

It is used in treatment of hyperpigmentation as part of triple-combination treatment under regular medical supervision [18, 21, 22, 32]. When used in TCC, steroids reduce skin irritation caused by retinoids. Topical hydrocortisone, mometasone, and fluocinolone acetonide are used in combination with other depigmenting agents to treat melasma [132]. The use of stronger topical steroids in skin lightening creams in large body areas had been reported in some African countries. The misuse of potent topical steroids for long term causes significant side effects such as steroid-induced acne, skin infections, striae, telangiectasia and even systemic effects such as diabetes mellitus and Cushing's disease [132]. Therefore steroid-containing preparations should not be used for more than 6 months for maintenance therapy in hyperpigmented conditions.

Natural and Other Agents

Many natural plant extracts have been identified to have potentially active compounds which inhibit melanin synthesis and having skin lightening properties [133, 134]. Most of these agents which act by different methods have been tested in combination with other agents for their hypopigmenting effects. N-acetylglucosamine,

tested alone or with niacinamide, inhibits enzymatic glycosylation in converting inactive protyrosinase to active tyrosinase, inhibiting melanin production [101]. Anti-inflammatory and antioxidant properties are also proposed for glucosamine compounds. N-undecyl-10-enoyl-L-phenylalanine acts by antagonising alpha melanocyte-stimulating hormone (MSH) receptor, reducing melanin production [101]. Resveratrol, a natural extract derived from the roots of the Japanese Knotweed, is shown to be effective in the treatment of melasma. It has proven antioxidant activity by a 14-fold increase in the action of superoxide dismutase 2 in cells treated with resveratrol 0.05% [135].

Other topical applications that have resulted in hypopigmentation of the skin in animal studies after UV irradiation include linolenic acid, linoleic acid, oleic acid and phospholipase D2 [136]. The effect is via the stimulation of tyrosinase ubiquitination and proteasomal degradation. Other compounds that modify tyrosinase structures at glycosylation sites to induce hypopigmentation in vitro include glucosamine and tunicamycin [137]. Calcium D-pantetheine-S-sulfonate also has shown hypopigmenting effects by modifying glycosylation of tyrosinase and TRP1, which are key enzymes for melanogenesis [138].

Grapeseed Extracts

Grapeseed extracts (GSE) containing proanthocyanidin have shown strong antioxidant properties and reduce melanin biosynthesis as well as UV-induced hyperpigmentation [139]. Oral intake of GSE for 6 months was shown to improve melasma in 10 out of 12 women studied [140].

Pomegranate Extract

A pomegranate extract (PE) containing 90% ellagic acid has skin whitening effects due to inhibition of the tyrosinase in melanocytes and also by inhibiting proliferation of melanocytes [141]. The magnitude of inhibition is comparable to arbutin [142]. In a clinical study involving 13 young women, oral intake of 100 and 200 mg of ellagic acid containing PE was shown to be effective in reducing UVR-induced skin pigmentation [143].

Licorice

Licorice extracts are derived from licorice root. There are number of active ingredients. Glabridin, the main ingredient in hydrophobic fraction of licorice extracts, improves hyperpigmentation mainly by inhibiting tyrosinase [144]. The other main ingredient of licorice extracts, liquiritin, acts by dispersing melanin.

Other Natural Agents

Several other agents such as mequinol, gentisic acid, flavonoids, aloesin and soybeans and a variety of other plant extracts such as mulberry, orchid and green tea are used as depigmenting agents [133, 134]. A skin whitening formula containing ferulic acid, *Ginkgo biloba*, lipohydroxy acid, niacinamide and thermal spring water was safe and improved melasma compared to placebo after administration for 3 months [145]. Topical plant extracts are increasingly used in skin lightening cosmeceuticals as they have probably less side effects. These products could be considered for combined use with standard depigmenting agents. Further properly conducted clinical trials are needed to assess their efficacy and safety.

A large number of studies had been done in search of newer effective depigmenting agents having a better safety profile. Most of these studies have been done for short periods and have involved a small number of subjects. There is a need for properly designed large-scale studies to evaluate the efficacy and safety of these newer agents (Table 18.1).

Table 18.1 Depigmenting agents

Depigmenting agents classified according to mode of action	Topical agents	Oral agents	Others (intradermal, mesotherapy, intravenous use)
1. Inhibitors of melanogenesis (tyrosinase inhibitors)	Hydroquinone [5–8, 11, 16, 17, 28–30] and monobenzyl ether of hydroquinone [33], arbutin [34, 38, 40], deoxyarbutin [35–37, 41], kojic acid [42–46, 48–50, 52], azelaic acid [53–62], ascorbic acid [65–71], magnesium ascorbyl phosphate [67, 71], 4-n-butylresorcinol [63], alpha tocopherol [75–85], glutathione [79, 85–93], methimazole [94–96], mequinol, gentisic acid, flavonoids, aloesin [133, 134], licorice extracts containing glabridin [144], pomegranate extracts containing ellagic acid [141–143], resveratrol [135]	Ascorbic acid [73], vitamin E [73], procyanidin [73], glutathione [87–89], grapeseed extracts	Q-switched Nd:YAG with ultrasonic application of vitamin C [72], ultrasonic application of vitamin C and niacinamide, intravenous glutathione [79, 90–92]
2. Interrupting melanosome transfer	Niacinamide [89, 97–105], soybeans [133, 134], lectins and neoglycoproteins [2, 97]		
3. Accelerating epidermal desquamation and melanin turnover	Retinoids [53, 106–111], adapalene [112], hydroxy acids [114], glycolic acids [114], salicylic acids, linoleic acids		
4. Agents acting by other methods and other natural agents	Tranexamic acid [115–124], steroids (18, 21, 22, 32) [131, 132], other plant extracts [133, 134], grapeseed extracts containing proanthocyanidin [139, 140], gentisic acid, flavonoids, soybeans, lectins, ferulic acid, *Ginkgo biloba*, lipohydroxy acid [145], thermal spring water [145], N-undecyl-10-enoyl-L-phenylalanine, N-acetyl glucosamine [101], linolenic acid, linoleic acid, oleic acid, and phospholipase D2 [136], glucosamine, tunicamycin [137] and calcium D-pantetheine-S-sulfonate [138]	Tranexamic acid [115, 125–130]	Intradermal [124], intravenous [121] and iontophoresis of tranexamic acid [119]

Conclusion

Disorders of hyperpigmentation are a common encounter in dermatology practice and often challenging to treat. There is no universal effective treatment. Hyperpigmentation especially in melasma tends to recur. Most of the currently used depigmenting agents act by inhibiting tyrosinase, the rate limiting enzyme in melanin synthesis. Topical modalities still remain the first choice. Hydroquinone is the gold standard for therapy though there are concerns of its safety, especially for long-term use. Combinations of topical therapies are preferred as the agents with different mechanisms of action have synergistic effects, and some agents reduce side effects and skin irritation induced by the other. Triple-combination cream containing hydroquinone, retinoic acid and a topical steroid is the most widely used treatment. Topical tranexamic acid, niacinamide, kojic acid and azelaic acid are the other important topical agents used. Oral tranexamic acid has gained popularity as a safe and effective adjuvant treatment in treating refractory melasma, and it has the benefit of inhibiting pigmentation induced by UV light and postinflammatory pigmentation induced by treatments themselves. Maintenance treatment is an important aspect of managing hyperpigmentation in sustaining clinical improvement. Concomitant use of broad spectrum sunscreens needs to be encouraged to achieve an effective depigmenting effect with any form of treatment. Multiple natural agents like grapeseed extracts, licorice, flavonoids, mequinol and mulberry extracts have evaluated for their skin lightening properties. Most natural agents are not as effective as hydroquinone and other commonly used depigmenting agents.

References

1. Jutley GS, Rajaratnam R, Halpern J, Salim A, Emmett C. Systematic review of randomized controlled trials on interventions for melasma: an abridged Cochrane review. J Am Acad Dermatol. 2014;70(2):369–73.
2. Gillbro JM, Olsson MJ. The melanogenesis and mechanisms of skin-lightening agents–existing and new approaches. Int J Cosmet Sci. 2011;33(3):210–21.
3. Hearing V. Unraveling the melanocyte. Am J Hum Genet. 1993;52(1):1.
4. Ito S, Fujita K, Takahashi H, Jimbow K. Characterization of melanogenesis in mouse and guinea pig hair by chemical analysis of melanins and of free and bound dopa and 5-S-cysteinyldopa. J Investig Dermatol. 1984;83(1):12–4.
5. Nordlund JJ. Hyperpigmentation: its historical treatment and the development of hydroquinone. J Pigment Disord. 2015;2: 221. doi:10.4172/2376-0427.1000221
6. Palumbo A, d'Ischia M, Misuraca G, Prota G. Mechanism of inhibition of melanogenesis by hydroquinone. Biochim Biophys Acta. 1991; 1073(1):85–90.
7. Westerhof W, Kooyers T. Hydroquinone and its analogues in dermatology–a potential health risk. J Cosmet Dermatol. 2005;4(2):55–9.
8. Xiaoying RCWJM, Hongbo HRCSS, Maibach ZDQHI. Human in vivo and in vitro hydroquinone topical bioavailability, metabolism, and disposition. J Toxicol Environ Health A. 1998;54(4):301–17.
9. Katsambas AD, Stratigos AJ. Depigmenting and bleaching agents: coping with hyperpigmentation. Clin Dermatol. 2001;19(4):483–8.
10. Rendon M, Berneburg M, Arellano I, Picardo M. Treatment of melasma. J Am Acad Dermatol. 2006;54(5):S272–S81.
11. Ennes SBP, Paschoalick RC, Alchorne MMDA. A double-blind, comparative, placebo-controlled study of the efficacy and tolerability of 4% hydroquinone as a depigmenting agent in melasma. J Dermatol Treat. 2000;11(3):173–9.
12. Prignano F, Ortonne J-P, Buggiani G, Lotti T. Therapeutical approaches in melasma. Dermatol Clin. 2007;25(3):337–42.
13. Grimes PE. A microsponge formulation of hydroquinone 4% and retinol 0.15% in the treatment of melasma and postinflammatory hyperpigmentation. Cutis. 2004;74(6):362–8.
14. Davis EC, Callender VD. Postinflammatory hyperpigmentation: a review of the epidemiology, clinical features, and treatment options in skin of color. J Clin Aesthet Dermatol. 2010;3(7):20.
15. Hexsel D, Arellano I, Rendon M. Ethnic considerations in the treatment of Hispanic and Latin-American patients with hyperpigmentation. Br J Dermatol. 2006;156(s1):7–12.
16. Taylor SC, Torok H, Jones T, Lowe N, Rich P, Tschen E, et al. Efficacy and safety of a new triple-combination agent for the treatment of facial melasma. Cutis. 2003;72(1):67–72.
17. Torok HM, Jones T, Rich P, Smith S, Tschen E. Hydroquinone 4%, tretinoin 0.05%, fluocinolone acetonide 0.01%: a safe and efficacious 12-month treatment for melasma. Cutis. 2005;75(1):57–62.
18. Chan R, Park KC, Lee MH, Lee ES, Chang SE, Leow YH, et al. A randomized controlled trial of the efficacy and safety of a fixed triple combination (fluocinolone acetonide 0· 01%, hydroquinone

4%, tretinoin 0· 05%) compared with hydroquinone 4% cream in Asian patients with moderate to severe melasma. Br J Dermatol. 2008;159(3):697–703.

19. Guevara IL, Pandya AG. Safety and efficacy of 4% hydroquinone combined with 10% glycolic acid, antioxidants, and sunscreen in the treatment of melasma. Int J Dermatol. 2003;42(12):966–72.

20. Rendon M, Cardona LM, Bussear EW, Benitez AL, Colon LE, Johnson LA. Successful treatment of moderate to severe melasma with triple-combination cream and glycolic acid peels: a pilot study. Cutis. 2008;82(5):372–8.

21. Grimes PE, Bhawan J, Guevara IL, Colón LE, Johnson LA, Gottschalk RW, et al. Continuous therapy followed by a maintenance therapy regimen with a triple combination cream for melasma. J Am Acad Dermatol. 2010;62(6):962–7.

22. Arellano I, Cestari T, Ocampo-Candiani J, Azulay-Abulafia L, Bezerra Trindade Neto P, Hexsel D, et al. Preventing melasma recurrence: prescribing a maintenance regimen with an effective triple combination cream based on long-standing clinical severity. J Eur Acad Dermatol Venereol. 2012;26(5):611–8.

23. Draelos ZD. Skin lightening preparations and the hydroquinone controversy. Dermatol Ther. 2007;20(5):308–13.

24. Glazer A, Sofen BD, Gallo ES. Nail discoloration after use of hydroquinone. JAAD Case Rep. 2016;2(1):57.

25. Ozluer SM, Muir J. Nail staining from hydroquinone cream. Australas J Dermatol. 2000;41(4):255–6.

26. Charlín R, Barcaui CB, Kac BK, Soares DB, Rabello-Fonseca R, Azulay-Abulafia L. Hydroquinone-induced exogenous ochronosis: a report of four cases and usefulness of dermoscopy. Int J Dermatol. 2008;47(1):19–23.

27. Mishra SN, Dhurat RS, Deshpande DJ, Nayak CS. Diagnostic utility of dermatoscopy in hydroquinone-induced exogenous ochronosis. Int J Dermatol. 2013;52(4):413–7.

28. Tse TW. Hydroquinone for skin lightening: safety profile, duration of use and when should we stop? J Dermatol Treat. 2010;21(5):272–5.

29. Levitt J. The safety of hydroquinone: a dermatologist's response to the 2006 Federal Register. J Am Acad Dermatol. 2007;57(5):854–72.

30. Makino ET, Mehta RC, Garruto J, Gotz V, Sigler ML, Herndon JH. Clinical efficacy and safety of a multimodality skin brightener composition compared with 4% hydroquinone. J Drugs Dermatol. 2013;12(3):s21–6.

31. Herndon JH Jr, Makino ET, Stephens TJ, Mehta RC. Hydroquinone-free skin brightener system for the treatment of moderate-to-severe facial hyperpigmentation. J Clin Aesthet Dermatol. 2014;7(5):27.

32. Doris Hexsel MD, Bsca CS. Objective assessment of erythema and pigmentation of melasma lesions and surrounding areas in long-term management regimens with triple combination. J Drugs Dermatol. 2014;13(4):444–8.

33. Oakley AMM. Rapid repigmentation after depigmentation therapy: vitiligo treated with monobenzyl ether of hydroquinone. Australas J Dermatol. 1996;37(2):96–8.

34. Maeda K, Fukuda M. Arbutin: mechanism of its depigmenting action in human melanocyte culture. J Pharmacol Exp Ther. 1996;276(2):765–9.

35. Chawla S, DeLong MA, Visscher MO, Wickett RR, Manga P, Boissy RE. Mechanism of tyrosinase inhibition by deoxyArbutin and its second-generation derivatives. Br J Dermatol. 2008;159(6):1267–74.

36. Chawla S, Kvalnes K, de Long MA, Wickett R, Manga P, Boissy RE. DeoxyArbutin and its derivatives inhibit tyrosinase activity and melanin synthesis without inducing reactive oxygen species or apoptosis. J Drugs Dermatol. 2012;11(10):e28–34.

37. Mov REB. Comparative efficacy and safety of deoxyarbutin, a new tyrosinase-inhibiting agent. J Cosmet Sci. 2006;57:291–308.

38. Lim Y-J, Lee EH, Kang TH, Ha SK, MS O, Kim SM, et al. Inhibitory effects of arbutin on melanin biosynthesis of α-melanocyte stimulating hormone-induced hyperpigmentation in cultured brownish guinea pig skin tissues. Arch Pharm Res. 2009;32(3): 367–73.

39. Parvez S, Kang M, Chung HS, Cho C, Hong MC, Shin MK, et al. Survey and mechanism of skin depigmenting and lightening agents. Phytother Res. 2006;20(11):921–34.

40. Bang SH, Han SJ, Kim DH. Hydrolysis of arbutin to hydroquinone by human skin bacteria and its effect on antioxidant activity. J Cosmet Dermatol. 2008;7(3):189–93.

41. Degen GH. Opinion of the Scientific Committee on Consumer safety (SCCS)–opinion on the safety of the use of deoxyarbutin in cosmetic products. Regul Toxicol Pharmacol. 2016;74:77–8.

42. Kahn V. Effect of kojic acid on the oxidation of DL-DOPA, norepinephrine, and dopamine by mushroom tyrosinase. Pigment Cell Res. 1995;8(5):234–40.

43. Cabanes J, Chazarra S, Garcia-Carmona F. Kojic acid, a cosmetic skin whitening agent, is a slow-binding inhibitor of Catecholase activity of tyrosinase. J Pharm Pharmacol. 1994;46(12):982–5.

44. Nohynek GJ, Kirkland D, Marzin D, Toutain H, Leclerc-Ribaud C, Jinnai H. An assessment of the genotoxicity and human health risk of topical use of kojic acid [5-hydroxy-2-(hydroxymethyl)-4H-pyran-4-one]. Food Chem Toxicol. 2004;42(1):93–105.

45. Burdock GA, Soni MG, Carabin IG. Evaluation of health aspects of kojic acid in food. Regul Toxicol Pharmacol. 2001;33(1):80–101.

46. Lim JTE. Treatment of melasma using kojic acid in a gel containing hydroquinone and glycolic acid. Dermatol Surg. 1999;25(4):282–4.

47. Garcia A, Fulton JE. The combination of glycolic acid and hydroquinone or kojic acid for the treatment of melasma and related conditions. Dermatol Surg. 1996;22(5):443–7.

48. Deo KS, Dash KN, Sharma YK, Virmani NC, Oberai C. Kojic acid vis-a-vis its combinations with hydroquinone and betamethasone valerate in melasma: a randomized, single blind, comparative study of efficacy and safety. Indian J Dermatol. 2013;58(4):281.

49. Monteiro RC, Kishore BN, Bhat RM, Sukumar D, Martis J, Ganesh HK. A comparative study of the efficacy of 4% hydroquinone vs 0.75% kojic acid cream in the treatment of facial melasma. Indian J Dermatol. 2013;58(2):157.

50. Nakagawa M, Kawai K, Kawai K. Contact allergy to kojic acid in skin care products. Contact Dermatitis. 1995;32(1):9–13.

51. García-Gavín J, González-Vilas D, Fernández-Redondo V, Toribio J. Pigmented contact dermatitis due to kojic acid. A paradoxical side effect of a skin lightener. Contact Dermatitis. 2010;62(1):63–4.

52. Burnett CL, Bergfeld WF, Belsito DV, Hill RA, Klaassen CD, Liebler DC, et al. Final report of the safety assessment of kojic acid as used in cosmetics. Int J Toxicol. 2010;29(6 suppl):244S–73S.

53. Briganti S, Camera E, Picardo M. Chemical and instrumental approaches to treat hyperpigmentation. Pigment Cell Res. 2003;16(2):101–10.

54. Nguyen QH, Bui TP. Azelaic acid: pharmacokinetic and pharmacodynamic properties and its therapeutic role in hyperpigmentary disorders and acne. Int J Dermatol. 1995;34(2):75–84.

55. Halder RM, Richards GM. Topical agents used in the management of hyperpigmentation. Skin Therapy Lett. 2004;9(6):1–3.

56. Lowe NJ, Rizk D, Grimes P, Billips M, Pincus S. Azelaic acid 20% cream in the treatment of facial hyperpigmentation in darker-skinned patients. Clin Ther. 1998;20(5):945–59.

57. Bertuzzi A, Gandolfi A, Salinari S, Mingrone G, Arcieri-Mastromattei E, Finotti E, et al. Pharmacokinetic analysis of azelaic acid disodium salt. Clin Pharmacokinet. 1991;20(5):411–9.

58. Kircik LH. Efficacy and safety of azelaic acid (AzA) gel 15% in the treatment of post-inflammatory hyperpigmentation and acne: a 16-week, baseline-controlled study. J Drugs Dermatol. 2011;10(6):586–90.

59. Baliña LM, Graupe K. The treatment of melasma 20% azelaic acid versus 4% hydroquinone cream. Int J Dermatol. 1991;30(12):893–5.

60. Farshi S. Comparative study of therapeutic effects of 20% azelaic acid and hydroquinone 4% cream in the treatment of melasma. J Cosmet Dermatol. 2011;10(4):282–7.

61. Kakita LS, Lowe NJ. Azelaic acid and glycolic acid combination therapy for facial hyperpigmentation in darker-skinned patients: a clinical comparison with hydroquinone. Clin Ther. 1998;20(5):960–70.

62. Woolery-Lloyd HC, Keri J, Doig S. Retinoids and azelaic acid to treat acne and hyperpigmentation in skin of color. J Drugs Dermatol. 2013;12(4):434–7.

63. Kim D-S, Kim S-Y, Park S-H, Choi Y-G, Kwon S-B, Kim M-K, et al. Inhibitory effects of 4-n-butylresorcinol on tyrosinase activity and melanin synthesis. Biol Pharm Bull. 2005;28(12):2216–9.

64. Huh SY, Shin JW, Na JI, Huh CH, Youn SW, Park KC. Efficacy and safety of liposome-encapsulated 4-n-butylresorcinol 0.1% cream for the treatment of melasma: a randomized controlled split-face trial. J Dermatol. 2010;37(4):311–5.

65. Farris PK. Topical vitamin C: a useful agent for treating photoaging and other dermatologic conditions. Dermatol Surg. 2005;31(s1):814–8.

66. Telang PS. Vitamin C in dermatology. Indian Dermatol Online J. 2013;4(2):143.

67. Pinnell SR, Yang H, Omar M, Riviere NM, Debuys HV, Walker LC, et al. Topical L-ascorbic acid: percutaneous absorption studies. Dermatol Surg. 2001;27(2):137–42.

68. Levine M, Conry-Cantilena C, Wang Y, Welch RW, Washko PW, Dhariwal KR, et al. Vitamin C pharmacokinetics in healthy volunteers: evidence for a recommended dietary allowance. Proc Natl Acad Sci. 1996;93(8):3704–9.

69. Espinal-Perez LE, Moncada B, Castanedo-Cazares JP. A double-blind randomized trial of 5% ascorbic acid vs. 4% hydroquinone in melasma. Int J Dermatol. 2004;43(8):604–7.

70. Hwang S-W, Oh D-J, Lee D, Kim J-W, Park S-W. Clinical efficacy of 25% L-ascorbic acid (C'ensil) in the treatment of melasma. J Cutan Med Surg. 2009;13(2):74–81.

71. Kameyama K, Sakai C, Kondoh S, Yonemoto K, Nishiyama S, Tagawa M, et al. Inhibitory effect of magnesium L-ascorbyl-2-phosphate (VC-PMG) on melanogenesis in vitro and in vivo. J Am Acad Dermatol. 1996;34(1):29–33.

72. Lee M-C, Chang C-S, Huang Y-L, Chang S-L, Chang C-H, Lin Y-F, et al. Treatment of melasma with mixed parameters of 1,064-nm Q-switched Nd: YAG laser toning and an enhanced effect of ultrasonic application of vitamin C: a split-face study. Lasers Med Sci. 2015;30(1):159–63.

73. Handog EB, Galang DAVF, Leon-Godinez D, Azirrel M, Chan GP. A randomized, double-blind, placebo-controlled trial of oral procyanidin with vitamins A, C, E for melasma among Filipino women. Int J Dermatol. 2009;48(8):896–901.

74. Traikovich SS. Use of topical ascorbic acid and its effects on photodamaged skin topography. Arch Otolaryngol Head Neck Surg. 1999;125(10):1091–8.

75. Sarkar R, Arora P, Garg KV. Cosmeceuticals for hyperpigmentation: what is available? J Cutan Aesthet Surg. 2013;6(1):4.

76. Thiele JJ, Hsieh SN, Ekanayake-Mudiyanselage S. Vitamin E: critical review of its current use in cosmetic and clinical dermatology. Dermatol Surg. 2005;31(s1):805–13.

77. Thiele JJ, Ekanayake-Mudiyanselage S. Vitamin E in human skin: organ-specific physiology and considerations for its use in dermatology. Mol Asp Med. 2007;28(5):646–67.

78. Thiele J, Schroeter C, Hsieh S, Podda M, Packer L. The antioxidant network of the stratum corneum. In: Oxidants and antioxidants in cutaneous biology, vol. 29. New York: Karger Publishers; 2001. p. 26–42.

79. Ritter EF, Axelrod M, Minn KW, Eades E, Rudner AM, Serafin D, et al. Modulation of ultraviolet light-induced epidermal damage: beneficial effects of tocopherol. Plast Reconstr Surg. 1997;100(4):973–80.

80. Baschong W, Artmann C, Hueglin D, Roeding J. Direct evidence for bioconversion of vitamin E acetate into vitamin E: an ex vivo study in viable human skin. J Cosmet Sci. 2000;52(3):155–61.

81. Hayakawa R, Ueda H, Nozaki T, Izawa Y, Yokotake J, Yazaki K, et al. Effects of combination treatment with vitamins E and C on chloasma and pigmented contact dermatitis. A double blind controlled clinical trial. Acta Vitaminol Enzymol. 1980;3(1):31–8.

82. Jerajani HR, Mizoguchi H, Li J, Whittenbarger DJ, Marmor MJ. The effects of a daily facial lotion containing vitamins B3 and E and provitamin B5 on the facial skin of Indian women: a randomized, double-blind trial. Indian J Dermatol Venereol Leprol. 2010;76(1):20.

83. Burke KE, Clive J, Combs GF, Commisso J, Keen CL, Nakamura RM. Effects of topical and oral vitamin E on pigmentation and skin cancer induced by ultraviolet irradiation in Skh: 2 hairless mice. Nutr Cancer. 2000;38(1):87–97.

84. Burke KE, Clive J, Combs GF, Nakamura RM. Effects of topical L-selenomethionine with topical and oral vitamin E on pigmentation and skin cancer induced by ultraviolet irradiation in Skh: 2 hairless mice. J Am Acad Dermatol. 2003;49(3):458–72.

85. Sonthalia S, Daulatabad D, Sarkar R. Glutathione as a skin whitening agent: facts, myths, evidence and controversies. Indian J Dermatol Venereol Leprol. 2016;82(3):262.

86. Watanabe F, Hashizume E, Chan GP, Kamimura A. Skin-whitening and skin-condition-improving effects of topical oxidized glutathione: a double-blind and placebo-controlled clinical trial in healthy women. Clin Cosmet Investig Dermatol. 2014;7:267.

87. Arjinpathana N, Asawanonda P. Glutathione as an oral whitening agent: a randomized, double-blind, placebo-controlled study. J Dermatol Treat. 2012;23(2):97–102.

88. Handog EB, Datuin MSL, Singzon IA. An open-label, single-arm trial of the safety and efficacy of a novel preparation of glutathione as a skin-lightening agent in Filipino women. Int J Dermatol. 2016;55(2):153–7.

89. Zubair S, Hafeez S, Mujtaba G. Efficacy of intravenous glutathione vs. placebo for skin tone lightening. J Pakistan Assoc Dermatol. 2017;26(3):177–81.

90. FDA Consumer Health Information. Injectable skin lightening products: what you should know. Epub 2015.

91. Dadzie OE. Unethical skin bleaching with glutathione. BMJ. 2016;354:i4386.

92. Tate SA. Nadinola and glutathione: refining and advancing a dangerous practice. In: Skin bleaching in black atlantic zones: shade shifters: Springer; Palgrave Pivot, Macmillan UK. 2016. p. 87–114.

93. Davids LM, van Wyk JC, Khumalo NP. Intravenous glutathione for skin lightening: inadequate safety data. SAMJ S Afr Med J. 2016;106(8):782–6.

94. Kasraee B, Handjani F, Parhizgar A, Omrani GR, Fallahi MR, Amini M, et al. Topical methimazole as a new treatment for postinflammatory hyperpigmentation: report of the first case. Dermatology. 2005;211(4):360–2.

95. Kasraee B, Safaee Ardekani G, Parhizgar A, Handjani F, Omrani G, Samani M, et al. Safety of topical methimazole for the treatment of melasma. Skin Pharmacol Physiol. 2008;21(6):300–5.

96. Malek J, Chedraoui A, Nikolic D, Barouti N, Ghosn S, Abbas O. Successful treatment of hydroquinone-resistant melasma using topical methimazole. Dermatol Ther. 2013;26(1):69–72.

97. Hakozaki T, Minwalla L, Zhuang J, Chhoa M, Matsubara A, Miyamoto K, et al. The effect of niacinamide on reducing cutaneous pigmentation and suppression of melanosome transfer. Br J Dermatol. 2002;147(1):20–31.

98. Greatens A, Hakozaki T, Koshoffer A, Epstein H, Schwemberger S, Babcock G, et al. Effective inhibition of melanosome transfer to keratinocytes by lectins and niacinamide is reversible. Exp Dermatol. 2005;14(7):498–508.

99. Panel CIRE. Final report of the safety assessment of niacinamide and niacin. Int J Toxicol. 2005;24:1.

100. Navarrete-Solís J, Castanedo-Cázares JP, Torres-µlvarez B, Oros-Ovalle C, Fuentes-Ahumada C, González FJ, et al. A double-blind, randomized clinical trial of niacinamide 4% versus hydroquinone 4% in the treatment of melasma. Dermatol Res Pract. 2011;2011:379173.

101. Kimball AB, Kaczvinsky JR, Li J, Robinson LR, Matts PJ, Berge CA, et al. Reduction in the appearance of facial hyperpigmentation after use of moisturizers with a combination of topical niacinamide and N-acetyl glucosamine: results of a randomized, double-blind, vehicle-controlled trial. Br J Dermatol. 2010;162(2):435–41.

102. Hakozaki T, Takiwaki H, Miyamoto K, Sato Y, Arase S. Ultrasound enhanced skin-lightening effect of vitamin C and niacinamide. Skin Res Technol. 2006;12(2):105–13.

103. Bissett DL, Robinson LR, Raleigh PS, Miyamoto K, Hakozaki T, Li J, et al. Reduction in the appearance of facial hyperpigmentation by topical N-undecyl-10-enoyl-l-phenylalanine and its combination with niacinamide. J Cosmet Dermatol. 2009;8(4):260–6.

104. Prousky J, Millman CG, Kirkland JB. Pharmacologic use of niacin. J Evid Based Complementary Altern Med. 2011;16(2):91–101.

105. Bissett DL, Miyamoto K, Sun P, Li J, Berge CA. Topical niacinamide reduces yellowing, wrinkling, red blotchiness, and hyperpigmented spots in aging facial skin1. Int J Cosmet Sci. 2004;26(5):231–8.

106. Lee J, Jung E, Huh S, Boo YC, Hyun CG, Kim YS, et al. Mechanisms of melanogenesis inhibition by 2, 5-dimethyl-4-hydroxy-3 (2H)-furanone. Br J Dermatol. 2007;157(2):242–8.

107. Solano F, Briganti S, Picardo M, Ghanem G. Hypopigmenting agents: an updated review on biological, chemical and clinical aspects. Pigment Cell Res. 2006;19(6):550–71.

108. Griffiths CEM, Finkel LJ, Ditre CM, Hamilton TA, Ellis CN, Voorhees JJ. Topical tretinoin (retinoic acid) improves melasma. A vehicle-controlled, clinical trial. Br J Dermatol. 1993;129(4):415–21.

109. Kimbrough-Green CK, Griffiths CEM, Finkel LJ, Hamilton TA, Bulengo-Ransby SM, Ellis CN, et al. Topical retinoic acid (tretinoin) for melasma in black patients: a vehicle-controlled clinical trial. Arch Dermatol. 1994;130(6):727–33.

110. Bulengo-Ransby SM, Griffiths C, Kimbrough-Green CK, Finkel LJ, Hamilton TA, Ellis CN, et al. Topical tretinoin (retinoic acid) therapy for hyperpigmented lesions caused by inflammation of the skin in black patients. N Engl J Med. 1993;328(20):1438–43.

111. Griffiths CEM, Goldfarb MT, Finkel LJ, Roulia V, Bonawitz M, Hamilton TA, et al. Topical tretinoin (retinoic acid) treatment of hyperpigmented lesions associated with photoaging in Chinese and Japanese patients: a vehicle-controlled trial. J Am Acad Dermatol. 1994;30(1):76–84.

112. Dogra S, Kanwar AJ, Parsad D. Adapalene in the treatment of melasma: a preliminary report. J Dermatol. 2002;29(8):539–40.

113. Burns RL, Prevost-Blank PL, Lawry MA, Lawry TB, Faria DT, Ftvenson DP. Glycolic acid peels for postinflammatory hyperpigmentation in black patients. Dermatol Surg. 1997;23(3):171–5.

114. Yamamoto Y, Uede K, Yonei N, Kishioka A, Ohtani T, Furukawa F. Effects of alpha-hydroxy acids on the human skin of Japanese subjects: the rationale for chemical peeling. J Dermatol. 2006;33(1):16–22.

115. Tse TW, Hui E. Tranexamic acid: an important adjuvant in the treatment of melasma. J Cosmet Dermatol. 2013;12(1):57–66.

116. Manosroi A, Podjanasoonthon K, Manosroi J. Development of novel topical tranexamic acid liposome formulations. Int J Pharm. 2002;235(1):61–70.

117. Todo H, Sugibayashi K. Usefulness of transdermal delivery of tranexamic acid with a constant-voltage iontophoresis patch containing chemical enhancer. Arch Pharm Pract. 2012;3(1):2.

118. Wu S, Shi H, Wu H, Yan S, Guo J, Sun Y, et al. Treatment of melasma with oral administration of tranexamic acid. Aesthet Plast Surg. 2012;36(4):964–70.

119. Mafune E, Morimoto Y, Iizuka Y. Tranexamic acid and melasma. Farumashia. 2008;44:437–42.

120. Cap AP, Baer DG, Orman JA, Aden J, Ryan K, Blackbourne LH. Tranexamic acid for trauma patients: a critical review of the literature. J Trauma Acute Care Surg. 2011;71(1):S9–S14.

121. Banihashemi M, Zabolinejad N, Jaafari MR, Salehi M, Jabari A. Comparison of therapeutic effects of liposomal tranexamic acid and conventional hydroquinone on melasma. J Cosmet Dermatol. 2015;14(3):174–7.

122. Kanechorn Na Ayuthaya P, Niumphradit N, Manosroi A, Nakakes A. Topical 5% tranexamic acid for the treatment of melasma in Asians: a double-blind randomized controlled clinical trial. J Cosmet Laser Ther. 2012;14(3):150–4.

123. Ebrahimi B, Naeini FF. Topical tranexamic acid as a promising treatment for melasma. J Res Med Sci Off J Isfahan Univ Med Sci. 2014;19(8):753.

124. Lee JH, Park JG, Lim SH, Kim JY, Ahn KY, MY KIM, et al. Localized intradermal microinjection of tranexamic acid for treatment of melasma in Asian patients: a preliminary clinical trial. Dermatol Surg. 2006;32(5):626–31.

125. Higashi N. Treatment of melasma with oral tranexamic acid. Skin Res. 1988;30:676–80.

126. Karn D, Kc S, Amatya A, Razouria E, Timalsina M. Oral tranexamic acid for the treatment of melasma. Kathmandu Univ Med J. 2014;10(4):40–3.

127. Cho HH, Choi M, Cho S, Lee JH. Role of oral tranexamic acid in melasma patients treated with IPL and low fluence QS Nd: YAG laser. J Dermatol Treat. 2013;24(4):292–6.

128. Shin JU, Park J, Oh SH, Lee JH. Oral tranexamic acid enhances the efficacy of low-fluence 1064-nm quality-switched neodymium-doped yttrium aluminum garnet laser treatment for melasma in Koreans: a randomized, prospective trial. Dermatol Surg. 2013;39(3pt1):435–42.

129. Tan AW, Sen P, Chua SH, Goh BK. Oral tranexamic acid lightens refractory melasma. Australas J Dermatol. 2016;58(3).

130. Lee HC, Thng TG, Goh CL. Oral tranexamic acid (TA) in the treatment of melasma: a retrospective analysis. J Am Acad Dermatol. 2016;75(2):385–92.

131. Gupta AK, Gover MD, Nouri K, Taylor S. The treatment of melasma: a review of clinical trials. J Am Acad Dermatol. 2006;55(6):1048–65.

132. Nnoruka E, Okoye O. Topical steroid abuse: its use as a depigmenting agent. J Natl Med Assoc. 2006;98(6):934.

133. Fisk WA, Agbai O, Lev-Tov HA, Sivamani RK. The use of botanically derived agents for hyperpigmentation: a systematic review. J Am Acad Dermatol. 2014;70(2):352–65.

134. Zhu W, Gao J, editors. The use of botanical extracts as topical skin-lightening agents for the improvement of skin pigmentation disorders. J Invest Dermatol Symp Proc. 2008;13(1):20–4. Nature Publishing Group.

135. Robb EL, Page MM, Wiens BE, Stuart JA. Molecular mechanisms of oxidative stress resistance induced

by resveratrol: specific and progressive induction of MnSOD. Biochem Biophys Res Commun. 2008;367(2):406–12.

136. Ando H, Ryu A, Hashimoto A, Oka M, Ichihashi M. Linoleic acid and α-linolenic acid lightens ultraviolet-induced hyperpigmentation of the skin. Arch Dermatol Res. 1998;290(7):375–81.

137. Mishima Y, Imokawa G. Selective aberration and pigment loss in melanosomes of malignant melanoma cells in vitro by glycosylation inhibitors: premelanosomes as glycoprotein. J Investig Dermatol. 1983;81(2):106–14.

138. Franchi J, Coutadeur MC, Marteau C, Mersel M, Kupferberg A. Depigmenting effects of calcium d-pantetheine-s-sulfonate on human melanocytes. Pigment Cell Res. 2000;13(3):165–71.

139. Yamakoshi J, Otsuka F, Sano A, Tokutake S, Saito M, Kikuchi M, et al. Lightening effect on ultraviolet-induced pigmentation of Guinea pig skin by oral administration of a proanthocyanidin-rich extract from grape seeds. Pigment Cell Res. 2003;16(6):629–38.

140. Yamakoshi J, Sano A, Tokutake S, Saito M, Kikuchi M, Kubota Y, et al. Oral intake of proanthocyanidin-rich extract from grape seeds improves chloasma. Phytother Res. 2004;18(11):895–9.

141. Yoshimura M, Watanabe Y, Kasai K, Yamakoshi J, Koga T. Inhibitory effect of an ellagic acid-rich pomegranate extract on tyrosinase activity and ultraviolet-induced pigmentation. Biosci Biotechnol Biochem. 2005;69(12):2368–73.

142. Ismail T, Sestili P, Akhtar S. Pomegranate peel and fruit extracts: a review of potential anti-inflammatory and anti-infective effects. J Ethnopharmacol. 2012;143(2):397–405.

143. Kasai K, Yoshimura M, Koga T, Arii M, Kawasaki S. Effects of oral administration of ellagic acid-rich pomegranate extract on ultraviolet-induced pigmentation in the human skin. J Nutr Sci Vitaminol. 2006;52(5):383–8.

144. Yokota T, Nishio H, Kubota Y, Mizoguchi M. The inhibitory effect of glabridin from licorice extracts on melanogenesis and inflammation. Pigment Cell Res. 1998;11(6):355–61.

145. Wang X, Li ZX, Zhang D, Li L, Sophie S. A double-blind, placebo controlled clinical trial evaluating the efficacy and safety of a new skin whitening combination in patients with chloasma. J Cosmet Dermatol Sci. 2014;4:92–98. http://dx.doi.org/10.4236/jcdsa.2014.42014

146. Hearing VJ. The regulation of melanin formation. In: Nordlund JJ, Boissy RE, Hearing VJ, King RA, Oetting WS, Ortonne J-P, editors. The pigmentary system: physiology and pathophysiology, vol. 10. 2nd ed. Blackwell Publishing Ltd; 2006. p. 193.

Index

© Springer International Publishing AG, part of Springer Nature 2018
P. Kumarasinghe (ed.), *Pigmentary Skin Disorders*, Updates in Clinical Dermatology,
https://doi.org/10.1007/978-3-319-70419-7

The manufacturer's authorised representative in the EU is Springer
Nature Customer Service Centre GmbH, Europaplatz 3, 69115 Heidelberg,
Germany. If you have any concerns regarding our products, please
contact ProductSafety@springernature.com

Printed and bound by CPI Group (UK) Ltd, Croydon, CR0 4YY
29/04/2026
02099451-0018